Anesthesiology

Edited by
Fun-Sun F. Yao, M.D., F.A.C.A.
Assistant Professor of Clinical Anesthesiology,
Cornell University Medical College.
Associate Attending Anesthesiologist,
The New York Hospital

Joseph F. Artusio, Jr., M.D., F.A.C.A.
Professor and Chairman of Anesthesiology,
Cornell University Medical College.
Anesthesiologist-in-Chief,
The New York Hospital

With four contributors

Anesthesiology
Problem-Oriented
Patient Management

J.B. Lippincott Company
Philadelphia London Mexico City New York
St. Louis São Paulo Sydney

Sponsoring Editor:
  Sanford Robinson
Manuscript Editor:
  Rachel Bedard
Indexer:
  Julie Schwager
Art Director:
  Maria Karkucinski

Designer:
  Ronald Dorfman
Production Supervisor:
  N. Carol Kerr
Production Coordinator:
  Charles Field
Compositor:
  Ruttle, Shaw & Wetherill, Inc.
Printer/Binder:
  Halliday Lithograph

The authors and publisher have exerted every effort to ensure that drug selection and dosage set forth in this text are in accord with current recommendations and practice at the time of publication. However, in view of ongoing research, changes in government regulations, and the constant flow of information relating to drug therapy and drug reactions, the reader is urged to check the package insert for each drug for any change in indications and dosage and for added warnings and precautions. This is particularly important when the recommended agent is a new or infrequently employed drug.

Copyright © 1983, by J. B. Lippincott Company. All rights reserved. No part of this book may be used or reproduced in any manner whatsoever without written permission except for brief quotations embodied in critical articles and reviews. Printed in the United States of America. For information write J. B. Lippincott Company, East Washington Square, Philadelphia, Pennsylvania 19105.

1   3   5   6   4   2

Library of Congress Cataloging in Publication Data
  Main entry under title:

  Anesthesiology.

    Includes bibliographies and index.
    1. Anesthesiology. I. Yao, Fun-Sun F., Date II. Artusio, Joseph Francis, Date. [DNLM: 1. Anesthesia. WO 200 C641]
RD81.A55   1983   617'.96   82-17281
ISBN 0-397-50509-4

To the former, present, and future
residents in anesthesiology
of The New York Hospital–
Cornell Medical Center

Contributors

Joseph F. Artusio, Jr., M.D., F.A.C.A.
Professor and Chairman of Anesthesiology
Cornell University Medical College;
Anesthesiologist-in-Chief
The New York Hospital
New York, New York

Vinod Malhotra, M.D., F.A.C.A.
Assistant Professor of Clinical Anesthesiology
Cornell University Medical College;
Assistant Attending Anesthesiologist
The New York Hospital
New York, New York

Michael Tjeuw, M.D., F.A.C.A.
Assistant Professor of Clinical Anesthesiology
Cornell University Medical College;
Associate Attending Anesthesiologist
The New York Hospital
New York, New York

Marjorie Topkins, M.D., F.A.C.A.
Professor of Clinical Anesthesiology
Cornell University Medical College;
Attending Anesthesiologist
The New York Hospital
New York, New York

Alan Van Poznak, M.D., F.A.C.A.
Professor of Anesthesiology
Cornell University Medical College;
Attending Anesthesiologist
The New York Hospital
New York, New York

Fun-Sun F. Yao, M.D., F.A.C.A.
Assistant Professor of Clinical Anesthesiology
Cornell University Medical College;
Associate Attending Anesthesiologist
The New York Hospital
New York, New York

Preface

ANESTHESIOLOGY: PROBLEM-ORIENTED PATIENT MANAGEMENT was written to present a group of important clinical entities covering the most critical anesthetic problems. It is intended to provide logical and scientific fundamentals for individualized patient management.

We have organized *Anesthesiology* by organ systems into eight sections, consisting of 37 chapters. Each chapter begins with a brief case presentation followed by essential problems of each disease entity, covering the following: pathophysiology and differential diagnosis, preoperative evaluation and preparation, intraoperative management, and postoperative anesthetic management. The book is designed to stress essential anesthetic problems and to give the reader the opportunity to organize his own ideas of patient care. A reasonable answer with updated references follows each question.

The text reflects the opinions and the clinical experience of the Department of Anesthesiology at The New York Hospital–Cornell Medical Center. The material in this book is prepared for the education of the resident and the practicing anesthesiologist; it will also serve as a review source for continuing education of the anesthesiologist. The question-and-answer format, combined with current references, enhances its education value.

The editors would like to acknowledge the help of our colleagues at The New York Hospital–Cornell Medical Center for the expertly written chapters they contributed to this book. Without their efforts, the book would have remained a pleasant daydream in the editors' minds. We particularly thank Betty J. Malino for her excellent editorial assistance and the many hours she devoted to this book. Our sincerest thanks must be expressed to Josephine C. Chiarelli for the hours she spent typing this manuscript for publication. We greatly appreciate the help offered by Drs. Jacqueline A. Salzer and Theresa T. Kudlak in preparing this manuscript for publication. Above all, our deepest appreciation goes to our families. Their understanding, patience, and encouragement made this book possible.

Fun-Sun F. Yao, M.D.
Joseph F. Artusio, Jr., M.D.

Contents

Section One The Respiratory System

1 Asthma—Chronic Obstructive Pulmonary Disease   3
Fun-Sun F. Yao

2 Bronchoscopy and Thoracotomy   19
Fun-Sun F. Yao

3 Aspiration Pneumonitis and Acute Respiratory Failure   31
Fun-Sun F. Yao

4 Fat Embolism   51
Joseph F. Artusio, Jr.

5 Tracheoesophageal Fistula   62
Marjorie J. Topkins

Section Two The Cardiovascular System

6 Congenital Heart Disease and Profound Hypothermia   75
Marjorie J. Topkins

7 Ischemic Heart Disease and Coronary Artery
Bypass Graft 88
Fun-Sun F. Yao

8 Valvular Heart Disease 125
Marjorie J. Topkins

9 Pacemaker 137
Fun-Sun F. Yao

10 Abdominal Aortic Aneurysm 148
Vinod Malhotra

Section Three The Gastrointestinal System

11 Intestinal Obstruction 161
Joseph F. Artusio, Jr.

12 Esophageal Varices 171
Alan Van Poznak

13 Pyloric Stenosis 176
Vinod Malhotra

Section Four The Nervous System

14 Brain Tumor and Craniotomy 189
Alan Van Poznak

15 Carotid Endarterectomy 200
Alan Van Poznak

16 Spinal Cord Tumor 208
Alan Van Poznak

17 Reflex Sympathetic Dystrophy 213
Vinod Malhotra

Section Five   The Endocrine System

18 Thyrotoxicosis   223
    Joseph F. Artusio, Jr.

19 Pheochromocytoma   234
    Joseph F. Artusio, Jr.

20 Diabetes   244
    Vinod Malhotra

21 Adrenocortical Tumor   253
    Vinod Malhotra

Section Six   The Genitourinary System

22 Transurethral Resection of the Prostate   263
    Joseph F. Artusio, Jr.

23 Kidney Transplant   272
    Fun-Sun F. Yao

24 Placenta Praevia   286
    Michael Tjeuw

25 Toxemia   302
    Michael Tjeuw

26 Breech Presentation and Fetal Distress   319
    Michael Tjeuw

Section Seven   The Hematologic System

27 Sickle Cell Disease   331
    Vinod Malhotra

28 Hemophilia   338
    Michael Tjeuw

Section Eight **Miscellaneous**

29 Myasthenia Gravis — 353
Alan Van Poznak

30 Malignant Hyperthermia — 358
Vinod Malhotra

31 Prolonged Apnea — 368
Alan Van Poznak

32 Burn — 373
Michael Tjeuw

33 Trauma — 392
Michael Tjeuw

34 Porphyria — 408
Michael Tjeuw

35 Cleft Palate — 422
Marjorie J. Topkins

36 The Bleeding Tonsil — 434
Joseph F. Artusio, Jr.

37 Morbid Obesity — 441
Fun-Sun F. Yao

Index — 453

Section One
The Respiratory System

1 Asthma—Chronic Obstructive Pulmonary Disease (COPD)

Fun-Sun F. Yao

A 45-year-old man had cholelithiasis. Cholecystectomy was planned. He had a long history of asthma. He developed dyspnea with only moderate exertion. He slept on two pillows. There was no peripheral edema. Arterial blood gases showed the following: pH, 7.36; P_{CO_2}, 60 torr; P_{O_2}, 70 torr; CO_2, 36 mEq/L.

A. Medical Disease and Differential Diagnosis

1. What differential diagnosis is compatible with these symptoms?
2. How would you distinguish obstructive lung disease from restrictive lung disease by spirometry?
3. Define normal lung volumes and lung capacities and their normal values in the average adult man.
4. Define closing capacity and closing volume. What is the normal value of closing volume?
5. What are the effects of age and posture on functional residual capacity (FRC) and closing capacity (CC)?
6. What are the effects of anesthesia on FRC and CC?
7. Why is the FRC important in oxygenation?
8. Are there methods to measure FRC and closing volume?
9. Are there any other pulmonary function tests?
10. Define lung compliance, chest wall compliance, and total compliance. What are their normal values?
11. Give the equation for Q_S/Q_T and V_D/V_T. What are their normal values?
12. Interpret the following arterial blood gases: pH, 7.36; P_{CO_2}, 60; P_{O_2}, 70; CO_2, 36.
13. What is normal PaO_2 if F_IO_2 is 1.0?
14. What are the common physiologic causes of hypoxemia?
15. What is the etiology of asthma?
16. What are the predisposing factors of asthmatic attacks?

17. What are the universal findings in arterial blood gases during asthmatic attacks, hypoxemia, or CO_2 retention?
18. What changes are seen in spirometry during an asthmatic attack?

B. Preoperative Evaluation and Preparation

1. What preoperative work-up would you order?
2. Would you order any special preoperative preparations for asthmatic patients with chronic obstructive lung disease?
3. What medicines would you expect the patient to have taken in the past or be taking at the present time?
4. Would you order preoperative steroid preparation? Why?
5. What is the onset of action of intravenous steroid therapy on asthma?
6. How would you premedicate the patient? Why?

C. Intraoperative Management

1. What are the disadvantages of administering atropine to the asthmatic patient?
2. If the patient had a severe asthmatic attack in the operating room before the induction of anesthesia, would you put the patient to sleep or postpone the surgery?
3. The patient did not have an asthmatic attack in the operating room. How would you induce anesthesia?
4. Why would you use methohexital instead of thiopental?
5. What is your choice of agents for maintenance of anesthesia? Why?
6. What are the mechanisms of halothane producing bronchodilation?
7. Why would you choose an inhalational instead of an intravenous technique?
8. Is regional anesthesia better than general anesthesia in this situation?
9. Which muscle relaxants would you use? Why?
10. In the middle of surgery, the patient developed a severe wheezing attack. How do you manage it?
11. How would you administer aminophylline? How does aminophylline relieve bronchospasm? What is the mechanism of action? What are the therapeutic blood levels of aminophylline? What are the toxic effects of aminophylline?
12. How would you give isoproterenol? What problems may arise when isoproterenol is given during halothane anesthesia? What is its mechanism of action on asthma?
13. If the patient does not respond to the above treatment and becomes cyanotic, what would you do?
14. The asthmatic attack was finally relieved and the operation was completed. The patient was found to be hypoventilating. What are the common causes? Would you like to reverse the muscle relaxant?

D. Postoperative Management

1. In asthmatic patients, are narcotics contraindicated for postoperative pain control?
2. The patient was breathing well and was extubated. How much oxygen would you give to this asthmatic patient with chronic obstructive pulmonary disease (COPD) in the recovery room?

A. Medical Disease and Differential Diagnosis

A.1. What differential diagnosis is compatible with these symptoms?

The differential diagnosis of wheezing and dyspnea includes the following: bronchial asthma, acute left ventricular failure (cardiac asthma), upper airway obstruction by tumor or laryngeal edema, endobronchial disease such as foreign body aspiration, neoplasms, bronchial stenosis, carcinoid tumors, recurrent pulmonary emboli, chronic bronchitis, eosinophilic pneumonias, chemical pneumonias, and occasionally polyarteritis. To differentiate asthma from other diseases with wheezing and dyspnea is usually not difficult. The triad of dyspnea, coughing, and wheezing, in addition to a history of periodic attacks, is quite characteristic. A personal or family history of allergic diseases is valuable contributory evidence. A patient with long-standing asthma may develop chronic obstructive lung disease and suffer from exertional dyspnea and orthopnea. Cardiac asthma is a misnomer and refers to acute left ventricular failure. Although the primary lesion is cardiac, the disease manifests itself in the lung. The symptoms and signs may mimic bronchial asthma, but the findings of moist basilar rales, gallop rhythms, blood-tinged sputum, peripheral edema, and a history of heart disease allow the appropriate diagnosis to be reached.

Isselbacher KJ, Adams RD, Braunwald E et al: Harrison's Principles of Internal Medicine, 9th ed, pp 1207–1208. New York, McGraw-Hill, 1980

A.2. How would you distinguish obstructive lung disease from restrictive lung disease by spirometry?

In restrictive lung disease (*e.g.*, pulmonary fibrosis and ankylosing spondylitis) the forced vital capacity (FVC) is low because of the limited expansion of the lung or chest wall. However, the forced expiratory volume at 1 second (FEV_1) is often not reduced proportionately, because airway resistance is normal. Thus, the FEV_1/FVC percentage is normal or high.

In obstructive lung disease (*e.g.*, emphysema) the FEV_1/FVC is grossly reduced because the airway resistance is high. Maximum breathing capacity (MBC) and maximal mid-expiratory flow rate (MMEFR) are reduced early in small airway obstruction. MMEFR is obtained by dividing the volume between 75% and 25% of the vital capacity by the corresponding elapsed time.

Table 1-1. Differentiation of obstructive and restrictive lung diseases

	OBSTRUCTIVE	RESTRICTIVE
VC	N or ↓	↓
TLC	↑	↓
FEV/FVC	↓	N or ↑
MMEFR	↓	N
MBC	↓	N

N = normal; ↑ = increased; ↓ = decreased

Normally, FEV_1 is greater than 80% of FVC and vital capacity should be more than 80% of predicted value. The predicted values depend on body size, age, and sex. The total lung capacity is increased in obstructive lung disease and decreased in restrictive lung disease. But the total lung capacity cannot be obtained by routine screening spirometry.

Isselbacher KJ, Adams RD, Braunwal E et al: Harrison's Principles of Internal Medicine, 9th ed, p 1197. New York, McGraw-Hill, 1980

A.3. Define normal lung volumes and lung capacities and their normal values in the average adult man.

There are four basic "volumes" and four derived "capacities" which are combinations of these volumes.

Tidal volume (VT) is the volume of air inhaled or exhaled during normal breathing. Normal VT is 500 ml.

Inspiratory reserve volume (IRV) is the maximal volume of gas that can be inhaled following a normal inspiration while at rest. Normal IRV is 3000 ml.

Expiratory reserve volume (ERV) is the maximal volume of gas that can be exhaled following a normal expiration. Normal ERV is 1000 ml.

Residual volume (RV) is the volume of gas remaining in the lungs after a forced exhalation. Normal RV is 1500 ml.

Vital capacity (VC) is the maximal amount of gas that can be exhaled after a maximum inhalation. The vital capacity is the sum of VT, ERV, and IRV. Normal VC is 4500 ml.

Inspiratory capacity (IC) is the maximal amount of gas that can be inhaled from the resting expiratory position after a normal exhalation. It is the sum of VT and IRV. Normal IC is 3500 ml.

Functional residual capacity (FRC) is the remaining lung volume at the end of a normal quiet expiration. It is the sum of RV and ERV. Normal FRC is 2500 ml.

Total lung capacity (TLC) is the lung volume at the end of a maximal inspiration. It is the sum of VC and RV. Normal TLC is 6000 ml.

Nunn JF: Applied Respiratory Physiology, 2nd ed, pp 4–5. London–Boston, Butterworth & Co, 1977

A.4. Define closing capacity and closing volume. What is the normal value of closing volume?

Closing capacity (CC) is the lung volume at which the small airways in the dependent parts of the lung begin to close. Closing capacity is the sum of closing volume and residual volume. Closing volume (CV) is the gas volume expelled during phase IV of the single-breath nitrogen test; it denotes the lung volume from the beginning of airway closure to the end of maximal expiration. Therefore, $CV = CC - RV$.

In normal young people, the closing volume is approximately 10% of the vital capacity, or 400 ml to 500 ml. The closing volume and the closing capacity increase with age. The closing volume is increased in patients with small airway disease and in chronic smokers.

Buist AS: The single-breath nitrogen test. N Engl J Med 293:438, 1975
Editorial: Closing volume. Lancet 2:908, October 1972

A.5. What are the effects of age and posture on functional residual capacity (FRC) and closing capacity (CC)?

FRC is either independent of age in adults or increases very slightly with increasing age. CC, however, increases with age. Normally, CC becomes equal to the FRC at the age of 66 in the upright position and at the age of 44 in the supine position.

FRC increases approximately 30% by changing from the supine position to the upright position. The CC, on the other hand, is independent of body position. It is important to remember that the effects of age on CC and posture on FRC determine whether airway closure exists.

Nunn JF: Applied Respiratory Physiology, 2nd ed, pp 67–70. London–Boston, Butterworth & Co, 1977

A.6. What are the effects of anesthesia on FRC and CC?

FRC is reduced approximately 20% with spontaneous breathing and about 16% with artificial ventilation during anesthesia. However, closing capacity is not changed during anesthesia.

Bilmour I, Burnham M, Craig DB: Closing capacity measurement during general anesthesia. Anesthesiology 45:477, 1976

Nunn, JF: Applied Respiratory Physiology, 2nd ed, p 68. London–Boston, Butterworth & Co, 1977

A.7. Why is the FRC important in oxygenation?

First, when the FRC is decreased to below closing capacity (CC), airways close in the dependent parts of the lung during certain periods of normal tidal ventilation. Airway closure results in shunting of pulmonary blood flow through the unventilated alveoli. Therefore, Q_S/Q_T is increased and arterial oxygenation is decreased. Second, pulmonary circulation and alveolar gas exchange are continuous during both inspiratory and expiratory phases of respiration. Whether or not there is airway closure, blood oxygenation during the expiratory phase is mainly dependent on the remaining lung volume, which is FRC. Therefore, when the FRC is high, blood oxygenation is better and there is more time for oxygenation before hypoxemia occurs during apnea. FRC is decreased in the supine position, during general anesthesia, and in the adult respiratory distress syndrome. Positive end expiratory pressure (PEEP) increases FRC and decreases airway closure.

Nunn JF: Applied Respiratory Physiology, 2nd ed, pp 68–70. London–Boston, Butterworth & Co, 1977

A.8. Are there methods to measure FRC and closing volume?

FRC may be measured by the following three techniques: helium dilution, nitrogen wash-out, and body plethysmography. Closing volume may be determined by two techniques, the single-breath nitrogen test (residual gas technique) and the bolus technique with an inert tracer gas such as helium, xenon, or argon.

Buist AS: The single-breath nitrogen test. N Engl J Med 293:438, 1975

Nunn JF: Applied Respiratory Physiology, 2nd ed, p 6. London–Boston, Butterworth & Co, 1977

A.9. Are there any other pulmonary function tests?

Arterial blood gases, lung scan, chest x-ray, ventilation/perfusion study, diffusion capacity, Q_S/Q_T, V_D/V_T, compliance.

Nunn JF: Applied Respiratory Physiology, 2nd ed. London–Boston, Butterworth & Co, 1977

A.10. Define lung compliance, chest wall compliance, and total compliance. What are their normal values?

Lung compliance is the change in lung volume by per unit change in alveolar/intrathoracic pressure gradient. The normal value is 200 ml per cm H_2O in the upright position. Chest wall compliance is the change in lung volume by per unit change in ambient/intrathoracic pressure gradient. Its normal value is 200 ml per cm H_2O. Total compliance is the change in lung volume by per unit change in alveolar/ambient pressure gradient. Its normal value is 100 ml per cm H_2O.

Nunn JF: Applied Respiratory Physiology, 2nd ed, pp 82, 90. London–Boston, Butterworth & Co, 1977

A.11. Give the equation for Q_S/Q_T and V_D/V_T. What are their normal values?

$$Q_S/Q_T = \frac{C_{cO_2} - C_{aO_2}}{C_{cO_2} - C\bar{v}_{O_2}} \qquad V_D/V_T = \frac{P_{aCO_2} - P_{ECO_2}}{P_{aCO_2}}$$

Normal QS/QT is 4% to 5% and VD/VT is about 0.3.

Nunn JF: Applied Respiratory Physiology, 2nd ed, pp 303 and 228. London, Boston, Butterworth & Co, 1977

A.12. Interpret the arterial blood gases: pH, 7.36; P_{CO_2}, 60 torr; P_{O_2}, 70 torr; CO_2, 36 mEq/L.

The F_IO_2 is essential to evaluate PaO_2. We assume the blood is taken while the patient is breathing room air. The blood gases show respiratory acidosis, compensated by metabolic alkalosis, and mild hypoxemia. The blood gases are compatible with chronic obstructive lung disease.

A.13. What is normal PaO_2 if F_IO_2 is 1.0?

If F_IO_2 is 1.0, normal PaO_2 should be 500 torr to 600 torr. To estimate the normal PaO_2 at different values of F_IO_2, we may assume that every 10% oxygen increases 50 torr to 60 torr of PaO_2. If the F_IO_2 is 0.4, we expect the normal PaO_2 to be 200 torr to 240 torr.

Shapiro BA et al: Clinical Application of Blood Gases, 2nd ed, pp 130–131. Chicago, Year Book Medical Publishers, 1977

A.14. What are the common physiologic causes of hypoxemia?

From the shunt equation, arterial oxygen content is related to the change in pulmonary capillary oxygen content, venous oxygen content, and venous admixture. It is easier to classify hypoxemia into the following three categories:

Decreased Pulmonary Capillary Oxygen Tension
- Hypoventilation
- Low F_IO_2
- Ventilation/perfusion abnormalities from pulmonary parenchymal change
- Diffusion abnormality (rare)

Increased Shunting, Either Intrapulmonary or Cardiac

Reduced Venous Oxygen Content
- Congestive heart failure: low cardiac output
- Increased metabolism: fever, hyperthyroidism, shivering
- Decreased arterial oxygen content

Shapiro BA, Harrison RA, Walton JR: Clinical Application of Blood Gases, 2nd ed, p 90. Chicago, Year Book Medical Publishers, 1977

A.15. What is the etiology of asthma?

Asthma is a heterogeneous disease. It is difficult to define its etiology. The common denominator that underlies the asthmatic diathesis is a nonspecific hyperirritability of the tracheobronchial tree. Clinically, asthma is classified into two groups, allergic and idiosyncratic. Allergic asthma is usually associated with a personal or a family history of allergic diseases, positive skin reactions to extracts of airborne antigens, and increased levels of IgE in the serum. Immunologic mechanisms appear to be causally related to 25% to 35% of all cases and contributory in another one-third. Idiosyncratic asthma cannot be classified on the basis of immunologic mechanisms.

Isselbacher KJ, Adams RD, Braunwal E et al: Harrison's Principles of Internal Medicine, 9th ed, p 1203. New York, McGraw–Hill, 1980

A.16. What are the predisposing factors of asthmatic attacks?

- Allergens. Airborne allergens are the most common.
- Aspirin and related substances. Aspirin and indomethacin make asthma worse.
- Environmental factors. Some types of asthma, such as Tokyo–Yokohama or New Orleans asthma, tend to occur in individuals who live in heavy industrial or dense urban areas.
- Occupational factors. A variety of compounds used in industry can cause asthma in susceptible individuals. Various names have been applied to this condition, such as meat wrappers' asthma, bakers' asthma, and woodworkers' asthma.
- Infections. Respiratory infections are among the most common stimuli that evoke acute asthmatic attacks.
- Exercise. Asthma can be induced or made worse by physical exertion.
- Emotional stress also is a factor.

Isselbacher KJ, Adams RD, Braunwald E et al: Harrison's Principles of Internal Medicine, 9th ed, pp 1203–1204. New York, McGraw–Hill, 1980

A.17. What is the universal finding in arterial blood gases during asthmatic attacks, hypoxemia, or CO_2 retention?

Hypoxemia is a universal finding during asthmatic attacks. However, frank ventilatory failure with CO_2 retention is relatively uncommon because CO_2 has a diffusion capacity 20 times higher than oxygen. During acute asthmatic attacks, most patients try to overcome airway obstruction and hypoxia by hyperventilation. This results in hypocarbia and respiratory alkalosis. CO_2 retention is a late finding and indicates severe and prolonged airway obstruction, such as in status asthmaticus.

Isselbacher KJ, Adams RD, Braunwald E, et al: Harrison's Principles of Internal Medicine, 9th ed, p 1207. New York, McGraw–Hill, 1980

A.18. What changes are seen in spirometry during an asthmatic attack?

The forced vital capacity (FVC) is usually normal but may be decreased during a severe attack. The forced expiratory volume (FEV) at 1 second is sharply reduced, usually to less than 50% of FVC. The maximum mid-expiratory flow rate and maximal breathing capacity are sharply reduced as well.

Gold MI, Han YH, Helrich M: Pulmonary mechanics and blood gas tensions during anesthesia in asthmatics. Anesthesiology 27:216, 1966

B. Preoperative Evaluation and Preparation

B.1. What preoperative work-up would you order?

In addition to routine tests such as complete blood count, serum electrolytes, urinalysis, ECG, coagulation screening, special attention should be paid to cardiopulmonary function, chest x-ray, pulmonary function tests, including response to bronchodilator, and baseline arterial blood gases. A history of allergy and symptoms and signs of cardiac or respiratory failure must be checked carefully.

B.2. Would you order any special preoperative preparations for asthmatic patients with chronic obstructive lung disease?

Yes. The preoperative preparation should include the following:
- Eradication of acute and chronic infection with appropriate antibiotics
- Relief of bronchial spasm with a bronchodilator
- Chest physiotherapy to improve sputum clearance and bronchial drainage
- Reversal of uncompensated or borderline cor pulmonale with diuretics, digitalis, improved oxygenation, and correction of acidemia by more efficient ventilation
- Correction of dehydration and electrolyte imbalance
- Familiarization with respiratory therapy equipment likely to be used in the postoperative period

Heironimus TW III: The anesthetic management of the pulmonary cripple. ASA Refresher Courses in Anesthesiology 3:92–93, 1975

B.3. What medicines would you expect the patient to have taken in the past or be taking at the present time?

The asthmatic patient might take a bronchodilator such as theophylline and sympathomimetics. Special attention is required if the patient is taking glucocorticoids.

Isselbacher KJ, Adams RD, Braunwald E et al: Harrison's Principles of Internal Medicine, 9th ed, pp 1208–1209. New York, McGraw–Hill, 1980

B.4. Would you order preoperative steroid preparation? Why?

It is recommended that preoperative glucocorticoid replacement therapy be given to all patients with known or suspected adrenal insufficiency. Patients who have been treated with high-dose glucocorticoids within the previous year should also be assumed to have an unknown element of adrenocortical suppression that should be treated with full replacement therapy. The human adrenal glands normally secrete approximately 30 mg of hydrocortisone (cortisol) per day under baseline conditions; however, under stress up to 300 mg a day may be secreted. It is reasonable to replace 300 mg of hydrocortisone per day during perioperative periods. The night before surgery, 100 mg of hydrocortisone acetate may be given intramuscularly. In addition, a 100-mg dose of hydrocortisone phosphate is given intravenously before induction and during operation. Postoperatively, hydrocortisone phosphate 100 mg, IV, is given every 8 hours for 48 hours and then the steroid therapy is tapered. The biologic half-life of hydrocortisone is 8 to 12 hours. If the patient had less than 1 week of steroid therapy more than 6 months ago and there are no signs of adrenal insufficiency, routine steroid preparation is not advised. However, intravenous steroid preparations should be available in the operating room in case intractable hypotension from adrenal insufficiency occurs during surgery.

Katz J, Benumof J, Kadis LB: Anesthesia and Uncommon Diseases, Pathophysiologic and Clinical Correlations, 2nd ed, p 190. Philadelphia, WB Saunders, 1981

Vandam LD: To make the patient ready for anesthesia. In Medical Care of the Surgical Patient, p 125. Menlo Park, California, Addison–Wesley Publishing Co, 1980

B.5. *What is the onset of action of intravenous steroid therapy on asthma?*

The bronchial effects of intravenous steroids are not immediate and may not be seen for 6 hours or more after the initial administration.

Isselbacher KJ, Adams RD, Braunwald E et al: Harrison's Principles of Internal Medicine, 9th ed, p 1209. New York, McGraw–Hill, 1980

B.6. *How would you premedicate the patient? Why?*

The asthmatic patient may be premedicated with atropine and diphenhydramine alone or in combination with droperidol. Atropine is an anticholinergic drug. It decreases airway resistance, diminishes secretion-initiated airway reactivity, and prevents bronchospasm and bradycardia from vagal reflex following intubation. Diphenhydramine is a H_1-receptor blocking drug. It inhibits histamine-mediated bronchoconstriction and possesses a sedative effect. Droperidol decreases airway resistance by its alpha-adrenergic blockade. The sedative effects of droperidol and diphenhydramine may prevent bronchospasm induced by psychological stress.

Editorial views: Clinical epilog on bronchomotor tone. Anesthesiology 42:1–3, 1975

Aviado DM: Regulation of bronchomotor tone during anesthesia. Anesthesiology 42:68–80, 1975

C. Intraoperative Management

C.1. What are the disadvantages of administering atropine to the asthmatic patient?

Some physicians consider atropine relatively contraindicated because it causes drying of secretions, further plugging, and perhaps the initiation of a severe attack of asthma. This assumption has proven to be more theoretical than real in the reasonably well-managed asthmatic patient.

Editorial views: Clinical epilog on bronchomotor tone. Anesthesiology 42:1–3, 1975

C.2. If the patient had a severe asthmatic attack in the operating room before the induction of anesthesia, would you put the patient to sleep or postpone the surgery?

First of all, medical treatment should be given to relieve the asthmatic attack. Elective surgery should be postponed and the patient should be reevaluated carefully and better prepared preoperatively. If this is emergency surgery, such as acute appendicitis, the operation can be performed after the asthmatic attack is terminated with medical treatment. During surgery, the medical treatment should be continued.

C.3. The patient did not have an asthmatic attack in the operating room. How would you induce the anesthesia?

Methohexital is used for induction. Then oxygen and a potent inhalation agent, such as halothane, enflurane, or isoflurane, are administered by mask to achieve adequate depth of anesthesia before endotracheal intubation following injection of succinylcholine. Topical endotracheal spray of 80 mg to 120 mg of lidocaine through LTA kit may be used before intubation to suppress the cough reflex induced by intubation, but the introduction of lidocaine itself may cause cough reflex when the depth of anesthesia is light.

Gilman AG, Goodman LS, Gilman A: Goodman and Gilman's, The Pharmacological Basis of Therapeutics, 6th ed, p 294. New York, Macmillan, 1980

C.4. Why would you use methohexital instead of thiopental?

Thiopental is a thiobarbiturate and clinical evidence indicates that it may cause coughing and laryngospasm that may lead to bronchospasm. Methohexital is an oxybarbiturate that has no sulfa component. Clinically, both barbiturates have been used successfully in the asthmatic patient, provided that an adequate depth of anesthesia is achieved before stimulating the airway.

Converse JG, Smotrilla MM: Anesthesia and the asthmatic. Anesth Analg (Cleve) 40:336, 1961

C.5. What is your choice of agents for maintenance of anesthesia? Why?

We use inhalational agents such as halothane, enflurane, and isoflurane with nitrous oxide and oxygen. Halothane, enflurane, and isoflurane are direct bronchodilators. They are more efficacious in reducing bronchomotor tone than are diethyl ether, ketamine, and fluroxene, all of which produce a release of adrenal medullary catecholamines that is not totally dose-dependent.

Methoxyflurane is avoided because of its dose-related renal toxicity and lack of significant effect on airway resistance. Cyclopropane should be avoided because it produces bronchoconstriction. Both ether and cyclopropane are explosive agents. They are not suitable for modern surgery.

Aviado DM: Regulation of bronchomotor tone during anesthesia. Anesthesiology 42:68–80, 1975

Editorial views: Clinical epilog on bronchomotor tone. Anesthesiology 42:1–3, 1975

C.6. What are the mechanisms of halothane that produce bronchodilation?

The major component of bronchodilation elicited by halothane is mediated through beta-adrenergic receptor stimulation which is decreased by beta-blocking agents. The beta-agonistic effect works through two intracellular mechanisms. The first mechanism is direct relaxation of bronchial musculature mediated by an increase in intracellular cyclic 3', 5'-adenosine monophosphate (cAMP). Increased cAMP may bind free calcium within bronchial myoplasm and thus promote relaxation by a negative-feedback mechanism. The second mechanism may arise from the first, inasmuch as elevated levels of cAMP seem to impede antigen–antibody mediated enzyme production and release of histamine from leukocytes.

Aviado DM: Regulation of bronchomotor tone during anesthesia. Anesthesiology 42:68–80, 1975

Editorial views: Clinical epilog on bronchomotor tone. Anesthesiology 42:1–3, 1975

C.7. Why would you choose an inhalational instead of an intravenous technique?

First, inhalational agents such as halothane, enflurane, and isoflurane have dose-related direct bronchodilator effect. Ketamine has an indirect bronchodilator effect, which is not dose-related and not predictable. Large doses of morphine produce bronchoconstriction because morphine increases central vagal tone and releases histamine. Droperidol has an alpha-blocking effect that may relieve bronchospasm induced by alpha stimulation. Meperidine was shown to have a spasmolytic effect in asthmatic patients, but not in experimental dogs. Fentanyl does not have a significant effect on bronchial tone. Second, cholinesterase inhibitors can induce bronchospasm. Inhalational agents potentiate muscle relaxants; therefore, lower doses of relaxants are needed for surgery. The use of cholinesterase inhibitors to reverse the effect of muscle relaxants may be avoided or decreased.

Aviado DM: Regulation of bronchomotor tone during anesthesia. Anesthesiology 42:68–80, 1975

Editorial views: Clinical epilog on bronchomotor tone. Anesthesiology 42:1–3, 1975

C.8. Is regional anesthesia better than general in this situation?

This issue is controversial. The use of regional anesthesia avoids the possibility of bronchospasm that may be induced by endotracheal tube stimulation. However, respiratory complications were reported to be quite common (83%) in patients undergoing intraperitoneal surgery who had relatively high spinal anesthesia (T6–T4). Low spinal, epidural, and caudal anesthesia for surgery of the perineum, lower extremities, and pelvic extraperitoneal organs resulted in fewer respiratory complications than with general anesthesia.

Endotracheal general anesthesia is advantageous because it provides a controlled airway to deliver the desirable oxygen concentration, but the endotracheal tube may also induce bronchospasm during light anesthesia.

Gold MI, Helrich M: A study of the complications related to anesthesia in asthmatic patients. Anesth Analg 42:283–293, 1963

C.9. Which muscle relaxants would you use? Why?

Pancuronium is the preferred relaxant because the histamine released is insignificant. D-tubocurarine can cause bronchospasm by histamine release. Metocurine and succinylcholine also cause histamine release, but to a lesser extent. Gallamine has minimal histamine release, but has been reported to cause bronchospasm in patients.

Gilman AG, Goodman LS, Gilman A: Goodman and Gilman's, The Pharmacological Basis of Therapeutics, 6th ed, pp 2, 8, 10. New York, Macmillan, 1980

C.10. In the middle of surgery, the patient developed a severe wheezing attack. How do you manage it?

First, deepen the level of anesthesia and increase F_IO_2. Remember that the patient is under anesthesia and surgery. Therefore, medical intervention, such as aminophylline administration, is not the first choice of treatment. The most common cause of asthmatic attack during surgery is inadequate anesthesia. The asthmatic patient has an extremely sensitive tracheobronchial tree. When the level of anesthesia is too light, he may develop bucking, straining, or coughing due to the foreign body (endotracheal tube) in his trachea, and go on to bronchospasm. First of all, the blood pressure is taken to make sure it is normal or high. Then anesthesia is deepened by increasing the concentration of inhalational agents such as halothane, enflurane, or isoflurane, which are direct bronchodilators, as well. At the same time, oxygenation can be improved by increasing the oxygen concentration and decreasing the nitrous oxide. The patient should be continuously ventilated with a volume-cycled ventilator.

Second, relieve mechanical stimulation. Pass a catheter through the endotracheal tube to suction secretions and to determine whether there is any obstruction or kinking of the tube. The cuff of the endotracheal tube can be deflated, the tube moved back 1 cm to 2 cm, and the cuff reinflated. Occasionally, the endotracheal tube slips down and stimulates the carina of the trachea, causing severe bronchospasm during light anesthesia. Surgical stimulation, such as traction on the mesentery, intestine, or stomach, should be stopped temporarily, since it causes vagal reflex and can cause bronchospasm.

Third, medical intervention is necessary if the above treatment cannot break the bronchospasm, or anesthesia cannot be increased because of hypotension. Aminophylline, a beta–adrenergic stimulant such as isoproterenol, and a corticosteroid may be administered in sequence. The refractory asthmatic patient may even require atropine and alpha-receptor blockade for relief of severe bronchospasm.

Editorial views: Clinical epilog on bronchomotor tone. Anesthesiology 42:1–3, 1975

Isselbacher KJ, Adams RD, Braunwald E et al: Harrison's Principles of Internal Medicine, 9th ed, p 1209. New York, McGraw–Hill, 1980

C.11. How would you administer aminophylline? How does aminophylline relieve bronchospasm? What is the mechanism of action? What are the therapeutic blood levels of aminophylline? What are the toxic effects of aminophylline?

The usual loading dose is 5.6 mg/kg, IV, slowly, followed by 0.9 mg/kg/hr in young adults; 0.7 mg/kg/hr in patients over 40 years old; and 0.45 mg/kg/hr in patients with liver failure or congestive heart failure.

Aminophylline increases intracellular cyclic AMP through inhibition of the enzyme phosphodiesterase (PDE), which inactivates cyclic AMP. The therapeutic plasma levels of aminophylline range from 10 μg/ml to 20 μg/ml. The common side-effects of aminophylline include nervousness, nausea, vomiting, anorexia, and headache; cardiac arrhythmias and seizures occur with high plasma levels.

Vandam LD: To make the patient ready for anesthesia. In Medical Care of the Surgical Patient, pp 32–33. Menlo Park, CA, Addison–Wesley Publishing Co, 1980

C.12. How would you give isoproterenol? What problem may arise when isoproterenol is given during halothane anesthesia? What is its mechanism of action on asthma?

Isoproterenol, 1 mg in 100 or 250 ml of dextrose in water, may be titrated by intravenous drip to relieve bronchospasm. Halothane anesthesia sensitizes the myocardium to catecholamines and arrhythmias may ensue. It is better to use enflurane or isoflurane as the anesthetic agent. Adrenergic stimulants produce bronchodilation through action on beta-adrenergic receptors. Beta-agonists increase intracellular cAMP by activating adenylcyclase, which produces cAMP from ATP. Terbutaline, having more beta-2 selective effects, may be administered subcutaneously.

Vandam LD: To make the patient ready for anesthesia. In Medical Care of the Surgical Patient, p 33. Menlo Park, CA, Addison-Wesley Publishing Co, 1980

C.13. If the patient does not respond to the above treatment and becomes cyanotic, what would you do?

The values of arterial blood gases should be determined immediately. In a severe, prolonged asthmatic attack, there will be combined respiratory and metabolic acidosis due to CO_2 retention and lactic acidosis from tissue hypoxia. $NaHCO_3$ should be given to correct the acidosis, because aminophylline and beta-agonists are not effective in severe acidosis. At the same time, bronchodilator therapy should be continued or increased. Consultation with senior staff or physician in pulmonary medicine may be necessary.

Kampschulte S, Marcy J, Safar P: Simplified physiologic management of status asthmaticus in children. Crit Care Med 1:69–74, 1973

C.14. The asthmatic attack was finally relieved and the operation was completed. The patient was found to be hypoventilating. What are the common causes? Would you like to reverse the muscle relaxant?

The following are common causes of apnea or hypoventilation at the end of surgery:

- Respiratory center depression by inhalational anesthetics, narcotics, or hyperventilation
- Peripheral blockade by muscle relaxants

Since the patient is a severe asthmatic, it is better to avoid the use of an anticholinesterase, such as neostigmine, to reverse a nondepolarizing relaxant. Neostigmine may trigger bronchospasm. It is advisable to use inhalational agents to potentiate relaxants and use less relaxants for surgery. If spontaneous respiration is not adequate, artificial ventilation should be continued.

Editorial views: Clinical epilog on bronchomotor tone. Anesthesiology 42:1–3, 1975

Dripps RD et al: Introduction to Anesthesia: The Principles of Safe Practice, 5th ed, p 213. Philadelphia, WB Saunders, 1977

D. Postoperative Management

D.1. In asthmatic patients, are narcotics contraindicated for postoperative pain control?

Narcotics should be used very carefully because prolonged respiratory depression may further compromise the airway. Morphine is avoided because of possible histamine release and increased central vagal tone which may cause bronchospasm. Meperidine may be a better choice for postoperative analgesia because of its spasmolytic action. Narcotics should be titrated carefully to control pain and not depress respiration. Poor pain control may compromise respiration due to splinting of the thoracic cage.

Aviado DM: Regulation of bronchomotor tone during anesthesia. Anesthesiology 42:77, 1975

D.2. The patient was breathing well and was extubated. How much oxygen would you give to this asthmatic patient with chronic obstructive pulmonary disease (COPD) in the recovery room?

Forty percent oxygen by mask is usually used postoperatively in the recovery room. However, for patients with COPD, the hypoxic drive might be taken away by increased F_IO_2. It is important to watch the patient's respiration very carefully during oxygen therapy. Venturi masks with F_IO_2 of 0.24 to 0.4 may be used for patients with COPD. It should be emphasized that high oxygen concentration should be used in the presence of hypoxemia. Hypoventilation can be assisted or controlled by artificial ventilation.

Heironimus TW III: The anesthesic management of the pulmonary cripple. ASA Refresher Courses in Anesthesiology 3:97, 1975

2 Bronchoscopy and Thoracotomy

Fun-Sun F. Yao

A 60-year-old man has suffered from cough, hemoptysis, and weight loss for 2 months. He has smoked one pack of cigarettes per day for 40 years. Chest x-ray film showed right middle lobe infiltrate. The infiltrate did not respond to antibiotic therapy. He was scheduled for fiberoptic bronchoscopy and thoracotomy for possible lobectomy or pneumonectomy.

A. Medical Disease and Differential Diagnosis

1. What is your tentative diagnosis?
2. How many types of bronchogenic carcinoma are there?
3. What are the uncommon metabolic manifestations of bronchogenic carcinoma?
4. How would you diagnose bronchogenic carcinoma?
5. The patient has a long history of cigarette smoking. What does it mean to you?

B. Preoperative Evaluation and Preparation

1. How would you evaluate the patient preoperatively?
2. What are the pulmonary function guidelines that indicate high risk of morbidity and mortality in major general surgery?
3. How do you know the patient can tolerate lobectomy or pneumonectomy?
4. How would you premedicate the patient? Why?

C. Intraoperative Management

1. How would you monitor the patient?
2. What kind of anesthesia would you give for fiberoptic bronchoscopy?
3. How many types of bronchoscopes are there?
4. Are there other anesthetic techniques for bronchoscopy?

5. After bronchoscopy, the surgeon decided to perform a thoracotomy. How would you maintain the anesthesia?
6. Why was the muscle jumping during electrocautery and cutting even after a paralyzing dose of d-tubocurarine was given? How would you prevent muscle twitching during electrocautery?
7. The patient was put in the lateral decubitus position for thoracotomy. Describe the circulatory and respiratory effects of the lateral position in the anesthetized patient.
8. Would you control respiration or let the patient breathe spontaneously? Why?
9. Would you consider one-lung anesthesia for lobectomy? Why?
10. What are the indications for one-lung anesthesia?
11. How could you achieve one-lung anesthesia if it is indicated?
12. Could you use double-lumen endotracheal tubes in pediatric patients?
13. How could you improve oxygenation during one-lung anesthesia?
14. Are there any advantages of high frequency positive pressure ventilation (HFPPV) for thoracotomy?
15. Right middle lobectomy was performed. Would you extubate the patient or leave the patient on the respirator at the end of the procedure?

D. Postoperative Management

1. What are the immediate life-threatening complications that follow lobectomy or pneumonectomy?
2. How would you prevent postoperative atelectasis? Would you order intermittent positive pressure breathing (IPPB) or incentive spirometry?
3. Why is it important to control postoperative pain? How would you control it?

A. Medical Disease and Differential Diagnosis

A.1 What is your tentative diagnosis?

Any pulmonary infiltrate not responding to antibiotic therapy should suggest carcinoma. The differential diagnosis of atypical pneumonia includes mycoplasmas, mycobacteria, fungi, Q fever, psittacosis, adenovirus, influenzal pneumonia, and pulmonary infarction. Sputum cytology, culture, skin test, and biopsy are necessary to make a definite diagnosis.

Krupp MA, Chatton MJ: Current Medical Diagnosis and Treatment, pp 129–138. Los Altos, CA, Lange Medical Publications, 1981

A.2. How many types of bronchogenic carcinoma are there?

According to the World Health Organization classification, the principal histoligic types include the following:

- Epidermoid (squamous cell)
- Small cell anaplastic: fusiform cell type, polygonal cell type, lymphocyte-like ("oat-cell") type
- Adenocarcinoma: bronchogenic, acinar, papillary
- Bronchiolo-alveolar
- Large cell
- Combined epidermoid and adenocarcinomas

Krupp MA, Chatton MJ: Current Medical Diagnosis and Treatment, p 136. Los Altos, CA, Lange Medical Publications, 1981

A.3. What are the uncommon metabolic manifestations of bronchogenic carcinoma?

The recognized metabolic manifestations are symptoms that resemble those of myasthenia gravis; peripheral neuritis involving both motor and sensory components; Cushing's syndrome; carcinoid syndrome; hypercalcemia not due to osseous metastasis; and hyponatremia due to inappropriate excessive secretion of antidiuretic hormone.

Krupp MA, Chatton MJ: Current Medical Diagnosis and Treatment, p 137. Los Altos, CA, Lange Medical Publications, 1981

A.4. How would you diagnose bronchogenic carcinoma?

The symptoms of nonproductive cough, hemoptysis, and the unresolved lung infiltrate suggest carcinoma. However, some laboratory tests are needed to confirm the diagnosis. They include sputum cytology, bronchoscopy and brush biopsy, biopsy of palpable nodes in the neck or axilla, mediastinoscopy, needle aspiration biopsy, and exploratory thoracotomy biopsy. Prior to thoracotomy, a search should be made for metastases that would contraindicate surgery.

Krupp MA, Chatton MJ: Current Medical Diagnosis and Treatment, pp 136–137. Los Altos, CA, Lange Medical Publications, 1981

A.5. The patient has a long history of cigarette smoking. What does it mean to you?

The patient may develop chronic bronchitis and emphysema from cigarette smoking. He may also develop cor pulmonale and pulmonary hypertension from long-standing pulmonary disorders. Preexisting pulmonary and cardiac disorders increase operative risk and postoperative complications. Heavy smokers have an increased closing volume that may cause postoperative atelectasis.

Tisi GM: Preoperative evaluation of pulmonary function: Validity, indications, and benefits. Am Rev Respir Dis 119:293, 1979

B. Preoperative Evaluation and Preparation

B.1. How would you evaluate the patient preoperatively?

All preoperative evaluations should include a complete systemic history, physical examination, and laboratory tests. Special attention should be paid to the respiratory and circulatory function in this patient. A history of smoking, cough, sputum production or dyspnea are hallmarks of respiratory disease. Assessment of exercise tolerance, such as climbing stairs, can anticipate the patient's response to the stress of anesthesia and surgery.

A physical examination should include the character of respiration and any signs of right ventricular failure and pulmonary hypertension such as right ventricular heave, palpable pulmonary artery pulsation, hepatojugular reflux, distended jugular veins, and peripheral edema. Laboratory tests should include the following:

Routine Tests
- ECG, chest x-ray, complete blood count, prothrombin time, partial thromboplastin time, urinalysis, electrolytes, BUN, creatinine, and blood sugar

Pulmonary Function Tests
- Arterial blood gases
- Spirometry, including vital capacity (VC), forced expiratory volume in the first second (FEV_1), and maximum breathing capacity (MBC)
- Xenon scanning
- Pulmonary artery pressure with balloon occlusion

Lebowitz PW: Clinical Anesthesia Procedures of the Massachusetts General Hospital, p 118. Boston, Little, Brown & Co, 1978

B.2. What are the pulmonary function guidelines that indicate high risk of morbidity and mortality in major general surgery?

Spirometry
- MBC less than 50% of predicted value, FEV_1 less than 2 liters or 50% of forced VC

Arterial Blood Gases
- Arterial PCO_2 greater than 45 torr
- Arterial PO_2 less than 50 torr

Pulmonary Vasculature
- Pulmonary artery pressure during unilateral occlusion greater than 30 torr

Tisi GM: Preoperative evaluation of pulmonary function: Validity, indications, and benefits. Am Rev Respir Dis 119:293, 1979

B.3. How do you know the patient can tolerate lobectomy or pneumonectomy?

The patient should be evaluated carefully, especially his cardiopulmonary status. The above mentioned pulmonary function tests should be performed; of particular importance are differential xenon scanning and unilateral pulmonary artery pressure measurement.

If pulmonary function tests suggest that a patient will be at high risk for major extrathoracic surgery, then he should be considered unsuitable for major thoracic surgery. If differential xenon scan suggests that the pulmonary resection will remove "useful" lung, the surgical procedure will be less acceptable than it would be if it were designed to remove the "bad part" of the lung. If the scans reveal gross abnormalities throughout the lung fields, then any pulmonary surgery will entail a high risk. If the mean pulmonary artery pressure during unilateral pulmonary artery occlusion exceeds 22 torr, the patient can be considered as being at risk for resection. If the pulmonary artery pressure in the "good" lung rises to above 35 torr on exercise, then the resection is contraindicated.

Ayers LN, Whipp BJ, Ziment I: A Guide to the Interpretation of Pulmonary Function Tests, 2nd ed, pp 51–53. New York, Roerig, Pfizer Pharmaceuticals, 1978

B.4. *How would you premedicate the patient? Why?*

Atropine, 0.4 mg, and pentobarbital, 100–150 mg, are given for premedication. Atropine is given to eliminate excessive airway secretions and possibly to prevent bradycardia induced by intubation. Pentobarbital is an intermediate-acting barbiturate sedative to eliminate anxiety.

C. Intraoperative Management

C.1. *How would you monitor the patient?*

Circulatory Monitoring
- Electrocardiogram to monitor heart rate, rhythm, and ischemia, using a V_5, CM_5 or CB_5 lead
- Blood pressure cuff
- Arterial line, if frequent blood gases determinations or serious cardiac problems are anticipated
- Central venous pressure, to evaluate circulatory volume and cardiac performance
- Swan–Ganz catheter, only when there is documented left ventricular dysfunction, severe pulmonary hypertension, or cor pulmonale
- Intake and output
- Capillary refill

Respiratory Monitoring
- Esophageal stethoscope or precordial stethoscope over the dependent lung
- Inspired oxygen concentration
- End-tidal CO_2, if available
- Arterial blood gases, when indicated
- Airway pressure

Temperature
Urine Output, to evaluate circulatory and renal function

C.2. What kind of anesthesia would you give for fiberoptic bronchoscopy?

Since bronchoscopy is followed by thoracotomy, I recommend general anesthesia for both procedures. Anesthesia is induced with thiopental sodium, deepened with oxygen and an inhalation agent such as isoflurane, enflurane, or halothane. Endotracheal intubation is facilitated with succinylcholine. Prior to intubation, 2 ml of 4% lidocaine is sprayed to the larynx and tracheobronchial tree by means of the LTA Kit to prevent bucking and coughing during intubation and bronchoscopy. Anesthesia is maintained with oxygen and a potent inhalation agent to maintain adequate oxygenation during bronchoscopy. The fiberoptic bronchoscope can be introduced by means of a swivel adapter into the endotracheal tube and ventilation can be assisted or controlled during bronchoscopy.

C.3. How many types of bronchoscopes are there?

There are three types of bronchoscopes in current use: flexible fiberoptic, rigid ventilating, and rigid venturi (Sanders injector).

The fiberoptic bronchoscope is often used in the sedated patient under local anesthesia. This bronchoscope can be used with endotracheal intubation while the patient is under general anesthesia. The patient can be ventilated through a swivel adapter.

The rigid ventilating bronchoscope has a side-arm adapter that can be attached to the anesthesia machine. A variable air leak usually exists around the bronchoscope, so high flow rates of inspired gases are needed.

The rigid venturi-effect bronchoscope relies on an intermittent (10–12/min), high pressure oxygen jet to entrain air and insufflate the lungs with an air–oxygen mixture. The jet is delivered through a reducing valve into a 16– or 18–gauge needle inside and parallel to the lumen of the bronchoscope. The major disadvantage of this bronchoscope is lack of control of the inspired oxygen concentration.

Miller RD: Anesthesia, p 1298. New York, Churchill Livingstone, 1981

C.4. Are there other anesthetic techniques for bronchoscopy?

There are five anesthetic techniques for bronchoscopy. They can be used separately or in combination.

Local Anesthesia with Intravenous Sedation
Local anesthesia is accomplished by lidocaine spray through a nebulizer with a long nozzle or an LTA Kit under direct laryngoscopy, or a bilateral superior laryngeal nerve block; or a transtracheal block. Intravenous sedation is supplemented with increments of diazepam, 2.5 mg, until the patient is calm and cooperative but not obtunded and obstructed.

General Anesthesia with an Inhalation Agent
Halothane is the agent of choice. Isoflurane and enflurane can also be used smoothly and successfully. Only oxygen and a potent inhalation agent are used to provide a high oxygen concentration. Respiration may be assisted or controlled. Succinylcholine drip may be used for muscle relaxation.

Balanced General Anesthesia with Nitrous Oxide, Oxygen, Thiopental Sodium, Narcotics, and Succinylcholine Drip
This technique is useful only for short procedures by experienced surgeons. Hypoxemia may ensue because nitrous oxide decreases the inspired oxygen concentration and alveolar hypoventilation is not unusual during the procedure.

Apneic Oxygenation
Following pre-oxygenation and induction of anesthesia with thiopental sodium, the patient is paralyzed, and oxygen is insufflated by a small catheter placed above the carina, or through the side-arm of a rigid bronchoscope, or a swivel adapter to the endotracheal tube. The period of apnea should be limited to less than 5 minutes because carbon dioxide accumulates at a rate of 3 to 6 torr/min, and thus, respiratory acidosis and cardiac arrhythmias may ensue.

General Anesthesia with High Frequency Positive Pressure Ventilation (HFPPV)
A ventilatory frequency of 60/min and a relative insufflation time of 22% of the ventilatory cycle are used. By utilizing HFPPV and a pneumatic valve principle, it is possible to ventilate the patient safely through an open bronchoscope.

Eriksson I, Sjostrand U: Effects of high frequency positive pressure ventilation (HFPPV) and general anesthesia on intrapulmonary gas distribution in patients undergoing diagnostic bronchoscopy. Anesth Analg (Cleve) 59:585–593, 1980

Miller RD: Anesthesia, pp 1297–1298. New York, Churchill Livingstone, 1981

C.5. After bronchoscopy, the surgeon decided to perform a thoracotomy. How would you maintain the anesthesia?

I maintain anesthesia with a potent inhalation agent such as insoflurane, enflurane, or halothane. Nitrous oxide may be added to decrease the concentration of a halogenated agent. Oxygen concentration should be kept at 50% or more to minimize the risk of hypoxemia from compression and packing of the nondependent lung. A nondepolarizing muscle relaxant, such as d-tubocurarine, or pancuronium, is given to facilitate surgical exposure.

C.6. Why was the muscle jumping during electrocautery and cutting even after a paralyzing dose of d-tubocurarine was given? How would you prevent muscle twitching during electrocautery?

D-tubocurarine is a nondepolarizing relaxant which blocks neuromuscular transmission at the neuromuscular junction. It cannot block direct muscle stimulation. Succinylocholine is a depolarizing relaxant which keeps the muscle depolarized and not responding to direct muscle stimulation.

Gilman AG, Goodman LS, Gilman A: Goodman and Gilman's The Pharmacological Basis of Therapeutics, 6th ed, pp 223–226. New York, MacMillan, 1980

C.7. The patient was put in the lateral decubitus position for thoracotomy. Describe the circulatory and respiratory effects of the lateral position in the anesthetized patient.

Circulatory Effect

Pooling of blood in the dependent half of the body can result in decreased venous return and a subsequent fall in cardiac output. This effect is intensified by raising the kidney bar or hyperextending the table.

Respiratory Effects
- The lateral position causes mechanical interference with chest movement and, therefore, limitation of lung expansion.
- Mismatching of ventilation and perfusion in the lateral position is another effect. The lower lung is compressed by the mediastinum and abdominal contents. If the patient is awake, the lower diaphragm is able to contract more efficiently during spontaneous respiration and preferential ventilation to the lower lung matches the increased perfusion by gravity. In the patient who is anesthetized, with or without paralysis, most ventilation is preferentially switched from the lower lung to the upper lung. This preferential ventilation of the upper lung, coupled with the greater perfusion of the lower lung, results in an increased degree of mismatching of ventilation and perfusion.

   The ventilation–perfusion ratio increases in the upper lung, resulting in an increased physiologic dead space and CO_2 retention. The ventilation–perfusion ratio decreases in the lower lung, resulting in an increased intrapulmonary shunt and hypoxemia. The application of positive end-expiratory pressure to both lungs restores ventilation to the lower lung.

Rheder K, Katch DJ, Sessler AD et al: The function of each lung of anesthetized and paralyzed man during mechanical ventilation. Anesthesiology 37:16, 1972

C.8. Would you control respiration or let the patient breathe spontaneously? Why?

Controlled positive-pressure ventilation is the only practical way to provide adequate ventilation during thoracotomy. Spontaneous breathing is usually inadequate because of depressed ventilation from anesthesia and muscle relaxants. Moreover, spontaneous respiration in the open-chest patient with lateral position causes mediastinal shift and paradoxical respiration. During inspiration, negative pressure in the intact lower hemithorax causes the mediastinum to move downward. During expiration, relative positive pressure in the intact lower hemithorax causes the mediastinum to move upward. During inspiration, movement of air into the open hemithorax and movement of gas from the exposed lung into the intact lung cause collapse of the exposed lung. During expiration, the reverse occurs, and the exposed lung expands.

Tarhan S, Muffitt EA: Principles of thoracic anesthesia. Surg Clin North Am 53:813, 1973

C.9. Would you consider one-lung anesthesia for lobectomy? Why?

No. Lobectomy can be done easily with regular endothracheal two-lung anesthesia. Although one-lung anesthesia may provide better operating conditions for a surgeon, there are certain disadvantages and complications associated with one-lung anesthesia and the use of double-lumen endotracheal tubes. A large and variable alveolar-to-arterial oxygen pressure difference ($P(A-a)O_2$) is a necessary consequence, because there is continued perfusion to the nondependent, nonventilated lung, creating an increase in transpulmonary shunt.

The increased $P(A-a)O_2$ often results in systemic hypoxemia. Severe hypoxemia and hypercarbia may be caused by incorrect positioning of double-lumen tubes. Other complications include traumatic laryngitis and traumatic tracheobronchial rupture.

Miller RD: Anesthesia, pp 945–951. New York, Churchill Livingstone, 1981

C.10. What are the indications for one-lung anesthesia?

Absolute Indications:
- Isolation from spillage or contamination
  - Infection-bronchiectasis and lung abscess
  - Massive hemorrhage
- To control the distribution of ventilation
  - Bronchopleural fistula
  - Bronchopoleural cutaneous fistula
  - Giant unilateral lung cyst

Relative Indications:
- Facilitation of surgical exposure—high priority
  - Thoracic aortic aneurysm
  - Pneumonectomy
- Facilitation of surgical exposure—low priority
  - Esophageal resection
  - Lobectomy

The advantages of one-lung anesthesia should be weighed against its disadvantages.

Miller RD: Anesthesia, p 939. New York, Churchill Livingstone, 1981

C.11. How could you achieve one-lung anesthesia if it is indicated?

There are three techniques available for providing one-lung anesthesia: bronchial blockers, endobronchial tubes, and double-lumen endotracheal tubes. Currently, the Robertshaw, Carlens, and White (right-sided Carlens) double-lumen tubes are most commonly used. They allow simultaneous ventilation of both lungs, as well as selective ventilation of either lung.

Miller RD: Anesthesia, pp 939–944. New York, Churchill Livingstone, 1981

C.12. Could you use double-lumen endothracheal tubes in pediatric patients?

No. Children's tracheas are too small to allow passage of double-lumen endotracheal tubes. The Robertshaw tubes come in three sizes: small, medium, and large, which correspond to internal diameters of 8 mm, 9.5 mm, and 11 mm, respectively. The Carlens and White tubes are available in four sizes: 35, 37, 39, and 41 French catheter gauge (size in French equals 3.14 times external diameter or 4 times internal diameter plus 2).

Miller RD: Anesthesia, pp 939–944. New York, Churchill Livingstone, 1981

C.13. How could you improve oxygenation during one-lung anesthesia?

The following could be done to improve oxygenation:

- Use high oxygen concentrations.
- Maintain two-lung ventilation as long as possible.
- Use high tidal volume (14 ml/kg) to ventilate the lower lung.
- Utilize oxygen insufflation with 10 cm H_2O PEEP to the upper deflated lung while the lower lung is ventilated with zero end-expiratory pressure.
- Clamp, temporarily, the pulmonary artery to the nonventilated lung.

Capan LM, Turndorf H, Patel C, et al: Optimization of arterial oxygenation during one-lung anesthesia. Anesth Analg (Cleve) 59:847–851, 1980

Miller RD: Anesthesia, p 950. New York, Churchill Livingstone, 1981

Katz JA, Laverne KG, Fairly B et al: Pulmonary oxygen exchange during endobronchial anesthesia: Effect of tidal volume and PEEP. Anesthesiology 56:164–171, 1982

C.14. Are there any advantages of HFPPV for thoracotomy?

During volume-controlled HFPPV with a fixed frequency of 60/min and a relative insufflation time of 22%, the exposed lung is moderately expanded and exhibits only minor movements during insufflation. Repeated blood gas analyses during surgery showed normocarbia and good oxygenation, even during compression of the exposed lung. After compression, the lung can readily be re-expanded with the aid of a brief period of positive end-expiratory pressure. Thus, even relatively low intrapulmonary pressures during volume-controlled HFPPV without PEEP are adequate to keep the open-chest lung expanded during thoracotomy. This creates optimal conditions for the surgeons.

Malina JR, Nordstrom SG, Sjostrand UH et al: Clinical evaluation of high frequency positive-pressure ventilation (HFPPV) in patients scheduled for open-chest surgery. Anesth Analg (Cleve) 60:324–330, 1981

C.15. Right middle lobectomy was performed. Would you extubate the patient or leave the patient on the respirator at the end of the procedure?

It is our practice to have an awake, comfortable, extubated patient at the end of the procedure. However, if the patient cannot maintain adequate oxygenation and ventilation, mechanical ventilation is indicated. Extubation avoids the potential hazards of postoperative positive-pressure ventilation on fresh bronchial stump suture lines. It is important to re-expand both the collapsed upper lung and the compressed lower lung before closing the chest to prevent atelectasis.

Lebowitz PW: Clinical Anesthesia Procedures of the Massachusetts General Hospital, pp 136–137. Boston, Little, Brown & Co, 1978

D. Postoperative Management

D.1. What are the immediate life-threatening complications that follow lobectomy or pneumonectomy?

The serious complications include massive hemorrhage caused by loosening of a ligature from a pulmonary vessel, bronchopleural fistula from blowout of a bronchial stump, and herniation of the heart following radical pneumonectomy by the intrapericardial approach.

Miller RD: Anesthesia, pp 951–952. New York, Churchill Livingstone, 1981

D.2. How would you prevent postoperative atelectasis? Would you order intermittent positive pressure breathing (IPPB) or incentive spirometry?

Before the chest is closed, both the collapsed upper lung and the compressed lower lung must be re-expanded by deep positive pressure breaths. Chest tubes have to be positioned properly and connected to constant negative pressure suction (about 15 to 20 cm H_2O).

Postoperatively, the following are recommended: chest physiotherapy, including incentive spirometry, deep breathing, encouragement to cough; mobilization of secretions; early ambulation; and proper pain control. We recommend incentive spirometry instead of IPPB for post-lobectomy patients. The ideal respiratory maneuver is one in which a high alveolar-inflating pressure is sustained for a relatively long period of time, and this can only be achieved with a large inhaled volume. A high inhaled volume can be achieved passively by proper IPPB or actively by incentive spirometry. Recently, IPPB lost its popularity, because, as usually performed, the inflating volume is not measured and the tidal volume is limited by the peak airway pressure. In addition, the use of IPPB may lead to cross-contamination from the equipment, pneumothorax or blowout of a bronchial stump from high airway pressure, and decreased cardiac output by decreasing the venous return to the heart. Moreover, the cost of using IPPB is ten times that of using incentive spirometry.

Miller RD: Anesthesia, pp 954–955. New York, Churchill Livingstone, 1981

D.3. Why is it important to control postoperative pain? How would you control it?

Postoperative pain control is important not only for patient comfort but also to minimize pulmonary complications by enabling the patient to breathe deeply without splinting, to cough, and to ambulate. Systemic administration of narcotics is employed most often to control postoperative pain. We titrate small doses of morphine in 2-mg increments to achieve adequate pain relief and avoid excessive sedation and respiratory depression. Intercostal nerve blocks and thoracic epidural analgesia using local anesthetics are alternatives to narcotic treatment. Transcutaneous electrical stimulation and epidural morphine injection are under investigation. Their ultimate use awaits further studies.

Miller RD: Anesthesia, p 956. New York, Churchill Livingstone, 1981

3 Aspiration Pneumonitis and Acute Respiratory Failure

Fun-Sun F. Yao

A 20-year-old full-term pregnant woman was rushed to the operating room for emergency caesarean section because of fetal distress. After rapid induction with thiopental and succinylcholine, the patient vomited and aspirated.

A. Management of Aspiration

1. What would you do right away?
2. What is Mendelson's syndrome?
3. What is the critical pH value of aspirate to cause Mendelson's syndrome?
4. Would you give prophylactic antibiotics to the patient? Why or why not?
5. Would you give steroid therapy? Why or why not?
6. Would you irrigate the bronchial tree with bicarbonate or saline solution?

B. Oxygen Therapy

The patient was extubated in the recovery room. Chest x-ray films showed questionable mottled density. She was sent back to her floor. Six hours later, she was found dyspneic and cyanotic. Arterial blood gases showed pH 7.46, P_{CO_2} 30 torr, P_{O_2} 55 torr, HCO_3 20 mEq/L on room air.

1. Interpret the blood gases.
2. What is adult respiratory distress syndrome (ARDS)?
3. What are the common causes of ARDS?
4. What oxygen therapy would you order?
5. How many liters of air are entrained into a venturi mask or venturi humidifier when one liter of oxygen is used to deliver 50% oxygen?
6. Are there other ways to give oxygen?
7. Is it possible to give 100% F_IO_2 to the patient through a face mask?

32 · Anesthesiology

C. Mechanical Ventilation

The patient did not improve after receiving 50% oxygen through face mask. Arterial blood gases showed pH 7.25, P_{CO_2} 50 torr, P_{O_2} 55 torr, CO_2 content 22 mEq/L. Respiratory rate was 40 per minute.

1. What would you do now?
2. What are the criteria for mechanical ventilation?
3. What kind of ventilator would you order?
4. What are the advantages and disadvantages of pressure-cycled ventilators?
5. What are the advantages and disadvantages of volume-cycled or volume-limited ventilators?
6. How would you set the volume-cycled ventilator?
7. Would you set sigh volume? How much? How often?
8. How do you know the ventilator settings are right?
9. What are the effects of intermittent positive pressure ventilation (IPPV) on the cardiovascular system?
10. What are the complications of mechanical ventilation?
11. What are the disadvantages of hyperventilation?
12. How do you normalize $PaCO_2$?

D. Continuous Positive Pressure Ventilation

The patient did not improve clinically. The arterial blood gases on F_IO_2 0.7 showed pH 7.30; P_{CO_2} 40 torr; P_{O_2} 57 torr; CO_2 content 18 mEq/L.

1. What would you do to improve the oxygenation?
2. What are the major factors governing oxygen toxicity?
3. What is the mechanism of oxygen toxicity?
4. What is the pathology of pulmonary oxygen toxicity?
5. How do you improve oxygenation without increasing F_IO_2?
6. What are your criteria to start PEEP?
7. What are PEEP, CPAP, CPPV, EPAP, IPAP, and ZEEP?
8. How does PEEP improve arterial oxygenation?
9. What are prophylactic, conventional, and high PEEP?
10. What is best PEEP or optimal PEEP?
11. How would you monitor the level of PEEP?
12. What are the cardiovascular effects of PEEP?
13. How would you correct hypotension during mechanical ventilation with PEEP?
14. What are the complications of CPPV?

E. Weaning from Ventilatory Support

The patient's condition improved after respiratory support with 20 cm H_2O PEEP. Arterial blood gases showed: pH 7.45; P_{CO_2} 35 torr ; P_{O_2} 150 torr; F_IO_2 0.75.

1. What would you do now? Lower F_iO_2 or lower PEEP?
2. The patient continued to improve. When would you consider weaning the patient from the respirator? Discuss the criteria for weaning.
3. How would you wean the patient from the respirator?
4. What are IMV, IAV, and IDV?
5. What are the advantages of IMV over controlled or assisted ventilation?

F. Special Techniques of Respiratory Support

1. What is differential or selective PEEP? What are the indications?
2. What are the indications and contraindications of extracorporeal membrane oxygenation (ECMO)? How many ways can ECMO be used?
3. What is HFPPV? What are the characteristics of HFPPV? What are the indications?
4. What are the frequencies used in HFPPV, high frequency oscillation, and high frequency jet ventilation (HFJV)?

A. Management of Aspiration

A.1. What would you do right away?

The operating table is rapidly tilted to a 30° head down position to have the larynx at a higher level than the pharynx and to allow gastric content to drain to the outside. The mouth and pharynx should be suctioned as rapidly as possible. Endotracheal intubation should be done immediately and the cuff inflated to prevent further aspiration. Quickly suction through the endotracheal tube before administrating 100% oxygen by positive pressure ventilation. This is to prevent pushing aspirated material beyond your reach. Suction should be brief to avoid cardiac arrest from hypoxia. Give 100% oxygen both before and after suctioning. Once the patient is intubated and suctioned, the table can be straightened and surgery should be continued to save the fetus.

A nasogastric tube should be inserted to empty the stomach. The *p*H of the gastric content should be determined. Tracheobronchial aspirate is collected for culture and sensitivity test. Auscultation of chest will determine if there are diminished breathing sounds, wheezing, rales, and rhonchi. Aminophylline may be given to relieve bronchospasm.

Abouleish E, Grenvik A: Vomiting, regurgitation, and aspiration in obstetrics. Pa Med 77:45–58, 1974

A.2. What is Mendelson's syndrome?

Acute chemical aspiration pneumonitis was first described by Mendelson in 1946. The triphasic sequence of immediate respiratory distress with bronchospasm, cyanosis, tachycardia, and dyspnea, followed by partial recovery and a final phase of gradual return of respiratory dysfunction is characteristic of Mendelson's syndrome. No signs of mediastinal shift are seen, but chest x-ray films usually show irregular mottled densities. This syndrome is due to the irritative action of gastric hydrochloric acid that produces bronchiolar spasm and a peribronchiolar exudate and congestive action.

Mendelson CC: The aspiration of stomach contents into the lungs during obstetric anesthesia. Am J Obstet Gynecol 52:191–205, 1946

A.3. What is the critical pH value of aspirate to cause Mendelson's syndrome?

The critical pH value is 2.5. Above pH 2.5 the response is similar to that of distilled water. Maximum pulmonary damage is achieved at an aspirate pH of 1.5.

Hedley–Whyte J, Burgess GE, Feeley TW et al: Applied Physiology of Respiratory Care, p 343. Boston, Little, Brown & Co, 1976

Teabeault JR: Aspiration of gastric contents, experimental study. Am J Pathol 28:51–67, 1952

A.4. Would you give prophylactic antibiotics to the patient? Why or why not?

We usually do not give prophylactic antibiotics to the patient unless there are signs of infection such as fever, leukocytosis, and positive cultures. The initial aspirate, excluding feculent aspirate, is usually sterile and remains so for the first 24 hours. Thereafter, cultures demonstrate gram-positive or gram-negative superinfection or both, usually with *Escherichia, Klebsiella Staphylococcus, Pseudomonas,* and *Bacterioides,* or anaerobes. No prophylactic antibiotic has been shown to improve mortality or reduce secondary infection rates. It is important to take cultures as soon as possible after aspiration and thereafter as clinically indicated. The antibiotic therapy is given according to the sensitivity test. Prophylactic use of broad-spectrum antibiotics may develop drug-resistant bacterial and fungal superinfection, too. However, if there is a possibility of intestinal obstruction, antimicrobial drugs, such as pencillin plus an aminoglycoside, are sometimes administered without waiting for evidence of progressive pulmonary infection. They can be discontinued if there is no laboratory or clinical evidence of infection.

Hedley–Whyte J, Burgess GE, Feeley TW et al: Applied Physiology of Respiratory Care, p 348. Boston, Little, Brown & Co, 1976

Krupp MA, Chatton MJ: Current Medical Diagnosis and Treatment, pp 128–129. Los Altos, CA, Lange Medical Publications, 1981

A.5. Would you give steroid therapy? Why or why not?

The value of systemic steroids is controversial. The effectiveness of steroid therapy seems to be related to the pH of aspirates. When the pH of aspirate is less than 1.5, the pulmonary parenchymal damage is maximal. Therefore, steroid therapy is not effective. When the pH of aspirate is above 2.5, the response is similar to that of water. Therefore, steroids are not necessary. Steroid therapy may be beneficial in acid aspiration pneumonitis when the pH of aspirate material is in the narrow range of 1.5 to 2.5. Dexamethasone 0.08 mg/kg every 6 hours decreased pulmonary water content significantly starting at 24 hours, with return to the normal range by 72 hours. The use of steroids may decrease the patient's resistance to infection.

Downs JB, Chapman RL Jr, Modell JH et al: An evaluation of steroid therapy in aspiration pneumonitis. Anesthesiology 40:129–135, 1974

Dudley WR, Marshall BE: Steroid treatment for acid-aspiration pneumonitis. Anesthesiology 40:136–141, 1974

Hedley–Whyte J, Burgess GE, Feeley TW et al: Applied Physiology of Respiratory Care, p 348. Boston, Little, Brown & Co, 1976

A.6. Would you irrigate the bronchial tree with bicarbonate or saline solution?

No. In acid aspiration pneumonitis, Bannister and associates demonstrated that pulmonary lesions were aggravated by irrigation with sodium bicarbonate, normal saline, and sodium hydroxide. This was explained on the basis that (a) the large volume of fluid served to push the hydrochloric acid deeper into the lungs; (b) mixing of the acid and treatment solution was impossible because of the minute size of the interface; (c) hydrochloric acid probably causes damage within a very short time; (d) if equal volumes of hydrochloric acid (*e.g.* with a pH of 1.6) and sodium chloride are mixed together, the pH only increases to 1.8; and (e) neutralization of hydrochloric acid with sodium bicarbonate produces heat and a thermal burn of the bronchial mucosa may occur.

Bronchial irrigation is indicated only in the obstructive type of aspiration. Five to ten milliliters of normal saline are instilled into the tracheobronchial tree, followed immediately by suction. It is preceded and followed by oxygenation. The sequence is repeated until the aspirate fluid is clear.

Bannister WK, Sattilaro AJ, Otis RD: Therapeutic aspects of aspiration pneumonitis in experimental animals. Anesthesiology 22:440–443, 1961

B. Oxygen Therapy

The patient was extubated in the recovery room. Chest x-ray films showed questionable mottled density. She was sent back to her floor. Six hours later, she was found dyspneic and cyanotic. Arterial blood gases showed **pH 7.46, P_{CO_2} 30 torr, P_{O_2} 55 torr, HCO_3 20 mEq/L** *on room air.*

B.1. Interpret the blood gases.

pH 7.46 means mild alkalosis. P_{CO_2} 30 torr means alveolar hyperventilation to compensate for hypoxemia. P_{O_2} 55 torr on room air means moderate hypoxemia due to aspiration pneumonitis. P_{CO_2} of 30 torr alone normally increases the pH to 7.50. Now the pH is 7.46. It means there is mild metabolic acidosis. HCO_3 20 mEq/L correlates with mild metabolic acidosis due to hypoxemia.

B.2. What is adult respiratory distress syndrome (ARDS)?

ARDS is a term given to a disorder resulting from diffuse injury to the alveolar capillary membranes. It encompasses a clinical syndrome which was previously labeled "post-traumatic pulmonary insufficiency," "Da Nang lung," "shock lung," and "congestive atelectasis." It can follow almost any injury. Although the onset may be acute, there is usually a latent period of hours or days during which respiratory damage is minimal or slowly progressing. Then, progressive, severe respiratory failure develops, and usually advances rapidly to the point of requiring tracheal intubation, mechanical ventilation, and use of positive end-expiratory pressure (PEEP). The physiological changes are characterized by hypoxemia, reduced functional residual capacity and compliance, increased intrapulmonary shunting, and radiologically, by pulmonary interstitial infiltrate.

Collina JA: The acute respiratory distress syndrome. Adv Surg 11:171, 1977

Wilson JW: Diffuse alveolar damage in the adult respiratory distress syndrome. ASA Refresher Courses in Anesthesiology 3:183–190, 1974

B.3. What are the common causes of ARDS?

The common causes of ARDS include multiple trauma, massive blood transfusion, septic shock, fat embolism, disseminated intravascular coagulation, aspiration pneumonitis, fluid overload, burns, smoke or gas inhalation, viral and mycobacterial pneumonia. The following conditions are also associated with ARDS: acute renal failure, oxygen toxicity, drug overdose, radiation, immunosuppression, neurogenic pulmonary edema, acute vasculitis, and Goodpasture's syndrome.

Pontoppidan H, Wilson RS, Rie MA, Schneider RC: Respiratory intensive care. Anesthesiology 47:96, 1977

B.4. What oxygen therapy would you order?

We run oxygen at 10–15 liters per minute through a venturi humidifier to deliver 50% oxygen with mist to the patient. It is important to specify a high oxygen flow rate in order to satisfy the patient's inspiratory flow rate.

The F_IO_2 depends on the patient's inspiratory flow rate and the flow rate and the concentration of delivered oxygen. The inspiratory flow rate is usually 30 to 40 liters/min. If the delivered flow rate is lower than inspiratory flow rate, air will be breathed in to mix with the delivered oxygen and the F_IO_2 will be lowered.

B.5. How many liters of air are entrained into a venturi mask or venturi humidifier when one liter of oxygen is used to deliver 50% oxygen?

1.67 liters of air are entrained. It is important to remember that air contains 20% oxygen. Let A be the amount of air. Total oxygen delivered = 1 liter × 100% + A liter × 20% = (1 + A) liter × 50%, then 1 + 0.2 A = (1 + A) 0.5. A = 1.67 liters. The general formula is: 1 + 0.2 A = (1 + A) × F_IO_2. The total oxygen from 100% oxygen and air is equal to the oxygen in the mixed gas. Let oxygen flow rate be 1 L/min. When F_IO_2 is set at 0.3, 0.4, 0.5, and 0.6, the air entrained will be 7, 3, 1.67, and 1 L/min, respectively.

Gibson RL et al: Actual tracheal oxygen concentrations with commonly used oxygen equipment. Anesthesiology 44:71–73, 1976

Nakamara Y, Jebson P: Inspired oxygen concentrations using a humidifier/tracheostomy T-piece system. Br J Anesth 44:61–65, 1961

B.6. Are there other ways to give oxygen?

Oxygen may be administered through a face mask, nasal catheter, nasal cannula, face hood, face tent, face mask with a reservoir bag, venturi-mask, and a T-piece for endotracheal tube.

Barton GG, Gee GN, Hodgkin JE: Respiratory Care, pp 395–398. Philadelphia, JB Lippincott, 1977

B.7. Is it possible to give 100% F_IO_2 to the patient through a face mask?

The wall oxygen meter can only deliver oxygen up to 10 to 15 liters per minute. It is not enough to satisfy our normal inspiratory flow rate, which is usually 30 to 40 liters per minute. (Inspiratory flow rate is different from minute volume.) Therefore, air has to be breathed in to mix with oxygen to meet the inspiratory flow rate. Usually, the oxygen mask can only deliver 40% to 50% oxygen to the airway. If a high concentration of oxygen is needed, a nonrebreathing face mask with reservoir bag and one-way valve has to be used. Clinically, it is not used very often, because mechanical ventilation is usually indicated when high concentrations of oxygen are needed.

C. Mechanical Ventilation

The patient did not improve after receiving 50% oxygen through face mask Arterial blood gases showed pH 7.25, PCO_2 50 torr, PO_2 55 torr, CO_2 content 22 mEq/L. Respiratory rate was 40 per minute.

C.1. What would you do now?

The patient should be intubated and mechanical ventilation should be started.

C.2. What are the criteria for mechanical ventilation?

The physiologic criteria for mechanical ventilation are as follows:

Mechanics
- Respiratory rate of more than 35/min

- Vital capacity of less than 15 ml/kg
- Inspiratory force less than 25 cm H_2O

Oxygenation
- PaO_2 less than 70 torr on mask oxygen
- $P(A-a)DO_2$ more than 350 torr on 100% F_1O_2

Ventilation
- $PaCO_2$ more than 55 torr, except in patients with chronic hypercarbia
- V_D/V_T more than 0.60

The trend of values is of utmost importance. The numerical guidelines should not be followed to the exclusion of clinical judgment.

Pontoppidan H, Geffin B, Lowenstein E: Acute respiratory failure in the adult. N Engl J Med 287:743–751, 1972

C.3. What kind of ventilator would you order?

I recommend using a volume-cycled ventilator, such as the Bennett MA-I, MA-II, Bourns, Engstrom, or Ohio 560.

C.4. What are the advantages and disadvantages of pressure-cycled ventilators?

The pressure-cycled or pressure-limited ventilators deliver gas until a preset pressure has been reached, at which point inspiration stops and passive expiration starts. The advantages are that these ventilators can compensate for mild leakage in the system and deliver the same amount of gas to the patient, provided the compliance is not changed. Also, the instruments are smaller and cheaper than volume-cycled ventilators. The main disadvantage is that the tidal volume varies with the patient's total compliance. When airway resistance increases, tidal volume decreases, resulting in hypoventilation. Therefore, frequent measurement of the expired tidal volume is necessary.

Barton GG, Gee GN, Hodgkin JE: Respiratory Care: A Guide to Clinical Practice, pp 589–592. Philadelphia, JB Lippincott, 1977

C.5. What are the advantages and disadvantages of volume-cycled or volume-limited ventilators?

The volume-cycled ventilators deliver a preset volume of inflation gas regardless of the pressure required to do so. The main advantage is that the tidal volume does not change with total pulmonary compliance or airway resistance. The disadvantages are that there is no compensation for leaks in the system and airway pressure may reach very high levels when the resistance is high. There is usually a pressure limit control to prevent excessive airway pressure. But this device will not maintain delivery of a constant tidal volume to the patient.

Barton GG, Gee GN, Hodgkin JE: Respiratory Care: A Guide to Clinical Practice, pp 591–592. Philadelphia, JB Lippincott, 1977

C.6. How would you set the volume-cycled ventilator?

It is most important to set tidal volume, respiratory rate, inspiratory flow rate, and F_IO_2. Normal tidal volume is 7 ml per kg of body weight. For patients with respiratory failure, the tidal volume is usually set at 10–12 ml per kg of body weight because of increased physiologic dead space (VD/VT.) Respiratory rate is usually set at 10 to 15 per minute. Inspiratory flow rate is usually set at 30 to 40 liters per minute. Slow inspiratory flow rate allows more even distribution of inspired gas, but may compromise venous return because of prolonged inspiratory phase. F_IO_2 is set at 50% to 60% oxygen. The settings are changed according to blood gases.

C.7. Would you set sigh volume? How much? How often?

When tidal volume is more than 10 ml/kg, it is not necessary to set sigh volume. Normal tidal volume, 7 ml/kg, needs occasional sighs to prevent atelectasis. Sigh volume is usually set at twice the tidal volume and 3 to 6 per hour.

Pontoppidan H, Laver MB, Geffin B: Acute respiratory failure in the surgical patient. Advances in Surgery, Vol 4. Chicago, Year Book Medical Publishers, 1970

C.8. How do you know the ventilator settings are right?

Arterial blood gas determinations and clinical evaluation of the patient's conditions are the only ways to tell whether the settings are right or not.

C.9. What are the effects of intermittent positive pressure ventilation (IPPV) on the cardiovascular system?

The initiation of IPPV is associated with a decrease in cardiac output and arterial blood pressure in patients without significant lung consolidation. Cardiac output and stroke volume decrease as the peak airway pressure increases. There is also a fall in cardiac output with increasing inspiratory-to-expiratory ratios. IPPV increases intrathoracic pressure, resulting in decreased venous return and cardiac output. Patients with normal lungs behave differently from patients with significant cardiopulmonary disease. When pulmonary compliance decreases, the transmission of airway pressure to intrathoracic pressure decreases. Patients with more rigid lungs can tolerate higher airway pressures.

IPPV decreases transmural pulmonary artery pressure, as well. There is no change in pulmonary vascular resistance. The systemic vascular resistance increases slightly when IPPV is begun. The fall in cardiac output during IPPV is rarely of any clinical significance because it is compensated by an increase in peripheral vascular resistance in non-anesthetized patients. When patients are hypovolemic, the decrease in blood pressure can be significant.

Grenvik A et al: Circulatory effects of mechanical ventilation. ASA Refresher Courses in Anesthesiology 5:99–110, 1977

Hedley–Whyte J et al: Applied Physiology of Respiratory Care, p 348. Boston, Little, Brown & Co, 1976

C.10. What are the complications of mechanical ventilation?

Physiological Complications
- Decreased cardiac output due to increased intrathoracic pressure
- Respiratory alkalosis from hyperventilation
- Increased venous admixture (Q_S/Q_T) from prolonged low tidal volume ventilation

Pulmonary Complications
- Infection
- Barotrauma-pneumothorax, mediastinal, interstitial, and subcutaneous emphysema in 10% to 15% of adults
- Oxygen toxicity if the inspired oxygen concentration is more than 60%
- Atelectasis due to immobilization, ineffective humidification, and low tidal volume ventilation

Complications from Endotracheal Intubation
- Problems with tubes: bronchial intubation, kinking or obstruction, leaking cuffs
- Nasal intubation: nose bleeding, fractured turbinates, septal perforation, partial loss of alae nasae, nasal synechiae
- Laryngeal damage: edema, vocal cord paresis and granulomata, laryngotracheal membranes, subglottic fibrotic stenosis
- Tracheal damage: tracheal erosion, tracheoesophageal fistula, tracheomalacia, tracheal stenosis

Fairley HB: Management of respiratory failure. ASA Refresher Courses in Anesthesiology, 41–55, 1973

C.11. What are the disadvantages of hyperventilation?

- Decreased cardiac output due to increased intrathoracic pressure and decreased sympathetic stimulation and catecholamine release from hypocarbia
- Respiratory alkalosis
- Left shift of oxygen dissociation curve and inceased oxygen affinity to hemoglobin
- Decreased cerebral blood flow, decreasing 2% by every torr decrease in $PaCO_2$ when $PaCO_2$ ranges from 20 torr to 80 torr
- Hypokalemia and cardiac arrhythmias from alkalosis
- Decreased ionized calcium and tetany from alkalosis
- Decreased PaO_2
- Increased oxygen consumption

Breivik H, Grenvik A et al: Normalizing low arterial CO_2 tension during mechanical ventilation. Chest 63:525–531, 1973

C.12. *How do you normalize $PaCO_2$?*
- Decrease the rate or tidal volume of the ventilator or both
- Add mechanical dead space to the ventilator tubing
- Add 1% to 3% CO_2 mixture to the inspired gases
- Use intermittent mandatory ventilation (IMV)

Breivik H et al: Normalizing low arterial CO_2 tension during mechanical ventilation. Chest 63:525–531, 1973

D. Continuous Positive Pressure Ventilation

The patient did not improve clinically. The arterial blood gases on F_IO_2 0.7 showed: pH 7.30; PCO_2 40 torr; PO_2 57 torr; CO_2 content 18 mEq/L.

D.1. *What would you do to improve the oxygenation?*

PaO_2 may be improved by increasing the F_IO_2 or applying positive end-expiratory pressure (PEEP). Diuresis may improve oxygenation if there is interstitial or frank pulmonary edema.

D.2. *What are the major factors governing oxygen toxicity?*

Oxygen toxicity is governed by the oxygen partial pressure during exposure, the duration of exposure, and the susceptibility of the individual to pulmonary oxygen injury. The degree of toxicity is related to the partial pressure, but not to the percentage of oxygen inspired, as shown by toleration of 100% oxygen for 2 to 4 weeks at a tension of 250 mmHg during U.S. space flights. Systemic oxygen toxicity is related to arterial oxygen tension, whereas pulmonary oxygen toxicity depends on alveolar oxygen tension. Retrolental fibroplasia in the premature neonate has been reported after exposure to PaO_2 of more than 150 torr for a few hours. Pulmonary toxicity can develop after prolonged exposure to oxygen at concentrations between 0.5 and 1.0 atmospheres. It must be emphasized that generally the adult patient can tolerate one atmosphere of oxygen partial pressure for at least 24 hours. Moreover, there is no evidence that clinically relevant pulmonary oxygen toxicity occurs in humans at inspired partial pressures below 0.5 atmospheres. Moreover, no patients should ever experience life-threatening levels of hypoxemia in order to avoid possible oxygen toxicity.

Hedley–Whyte J, Burgess GE, Feeley TW et al: Applied Physiology of Respiratory Care, pp 397–406. Boston, Little, Brown & Co, 1976

Winter PM: Pulmonary oxygen toxicity. ASA Refresher Courses in Anesthesiology 2:163–177, 1974

D.3. *What is the mechanism of oxygen toxicity?*

The so-called free radical theory of oxygen toxicity proposed in the early 1960s has garnered a great deal of recent experimental support and is now accepted as the most probable molecular level explanation for oxygen toxicity. Various highly reactive and potentially cytotoxic free radical products of oxygen are generated metabolically in the cell. These short-lived O_2 metabolites, including superoxide anion (O_2^-), hydroxyl radical (OH), hydrogen peroxide (H_2O_2), and singlet oxygen (O_2) have been shown to be capable of effects such as inactivation of sulfhydryl enzymes, interaction with and disruption of DNA, and peroxidation of unsaturated membrane lipids with resultant loss of membrane integrity. The cell is also equipped with an array of antioxidant defenses, including the enzymes superoxide dismutase (SOD), catalase, and glutathione peroxidase, vitamin E, and ascorbate. Under hyperoxia, the intracellular generation and influx of free radicals is believed to increase markedly and may overwhelm the detoxifying capacity of the normal complement of antioxidant defenses, with resultant cytotoxicity.

Frank L, Massaro D: The lung and oxygen toxicity. Arch Intern Med 139:347–350, 1979

D.4. What is the pathology of pulmonary oxygen toxicity?

The pathology of oxygen toxicity is nonspecific and consists of atelectasis, edema, alveolar hemorrhage, inflammation, fibrin deposition, and thickening and hyalinization of alveolar membanes. There are exudative and proliferative phases. Capillary endothelium is damaged early and plasma leaks into interstitial and alveolar spaces. Pulmonary surfactant may be altered. Type I alveolar lining cells are injured early and bronchiolar and tracheal ciliated cells can be damaged by 80% to 100% oxygen. Resolution of exudative changes, hyperplasia of alveolar type II cells, fibroplastic proliferation, and interstial fibrosis occur with recovery or with the development of tolerance to oxygen. Total resolution is possible if the initial hyperoxia is not overwhelming.

Deneke SM, Fanbarg BL: Normobaric oxygen toxicity of the lung. N Engl J Med 303:76–86, 1980

D.5. How do you improve oxygenation without increasing F_IO_2?

Positive end-expiratory pressure (PEEP) may be applied to improve oxygenation.

D.6. What are your criteria to start PEEP?

If PaO_2 is less than 60 torr with F_IO_2 of 0.60 or more, PEEP is indicated.

Down JB, Modell JH: Patterns of respiratory support aimed at pathophysiologic conditions. ASA Refresher Courses in Anesthesiology 71–84, 1977

D.7. What are PEEP, CPAP, CPPV, EPAP, IPAP, and ZEEP?

PEEP refers to positive end-expiratory pressure. CPAP denotes continuous positive airway pressure. CPPV signifies continuous positive pressure ventilation. EPAP means expiratory positive airway pressure. IPAP stands for inspiratory positive airway pressure. ZEEP denotes zero end-expiratory pressure. The terminology is not standardized. In order to understand the literature, it is important to know the airway pressure patterns during inspiration and expiration. Respiration may be categorized into the following three types: spontaneous breathing (SB); mechanical ventilation (MV); and intermittent mandatory ventilation (IMV), which is the combination of SB and MV. Mechanical ventilation with IPAP and ZEEP is called intermittent positive pressure ventilation (IPPV). Mechanical ventilation with PEEP is equal to CPPV. Therefore, CPPV = IPPV + PEEP. Both CPPV and CPAP have positive airway pressure during both inspiratory and expiratory phases (IPAP + EPAP). CPPV is usually used with mechanical ventilation, whereas CPAP is usually used with spontaneous breathing. PEEP is often referred to as CPPV. However, "spontaneous PEEP" has been used to describe a different respiratory pattern. In spontaneous PEEP, the inspiratory airway pressure can be positive, zero, or negative, depending on the inspiratory efforts and the level of PEEP. When PEEP is low and inspiratory effort is strong, the inspiratory airway pressure tends to reach levels below zero. PEEP or EPAP only describes the airway pressure during expiration and is not equivalent to CPAP or CPPV.

Ashbough DG et al: Continuous positive-pressure breathing (CPPV) in adult respiratory distress syndrome. J Thorac Cardiovasc Surg 57:31–41, 1969

Gillick JS: Spontaneous positive end-expiratory pressure (SPEEP). Anesth Analg (Cleve) 56:627–632, 1977

Gregory GA et al: Treatment of the idiopathic respiratory distress syndrome with continuous positive airway pressure. N Engl J Med 284:1333–1340, 1971

Sturgeon CL, Douglas ME, Downs JB: PEEP and CPAP: Cardiopulmonary effects during spontaneous ventilation. Anesth Analg (Cleve) 56:633-641, 1977

D.8. How does PEEP improve arterial oxygenation?

The mechanism is related to an increase in the functional residual capacity (FRC). The FRC expands linearly with increases in the end-expiratory pressure, usually at a rate of 400 cc or more for each 5 cm H_2O end-expiratory pressure. This increase in FRC represents alveoli that remain open and available for gas exchange during all phases of respiratory cycle. The increase in FRC improves the relationship between FRC and closing capacity and therefore decreases intrapulmonary shunt or venous admixture.

Abbound N, Rehder K, Rodarte JR et al: Lung volume and closing capacity with continuous positive airway pressure. Anesthesiology 42:138–142, 1975

Hedley–Whyte J, Burgess GE, Feeley TW et al: Applied Physiology of Respiratory Care, pp 18–19. Boston, Little, Brown & Co, 1976

D.9. What are prophylactic, conventional, and high PEEP?

The ranges of PEEP can be divided into the following three groups:

- Prophylactic PEEP—1–5 cm H_2O, used to increase FRC to more than closing capacity, to prevent atelectasis and decrease shunting
- Conventional PEEP—6–20 cm H_2O, indicated if PaO_2 is less than 60 torr with F_IO_2 more than 60%
- High PEEP—over 20 cm H_2O, used in extreme hypoxemia when there is no response to conventional PEEP

D.10. What is best PEEP or optimal PEEP?

Best *conventional* PEEP was described by Suter and associates in 1975. The best PEEP is defined as the level of PEEP with the highest oxygen transport, which is the product of cardiac output and oxygen content. This PEEP correlates with the highest total respiratory compliance, the highest mixed venous oxygen tension, and the lowest V_D/V_T. Arterial oxygen tension and intrapulmonary shunt are not good indicators of the best conventional PEEP. They continue to improve even after this level has been reached. Oxygen transport decreases after the best PEEP is reached, because the cardiac output decreases.

Optimal *high* PEEP was described by Civetta in 1975. It is defined as the level of PEEP with the lowest intrapulmonary shunt and without compromising cardiac output. The PEEP used in Civetta's report is so-called high or super PEEP, over 25 cm H_2O, while the PEEP in Suter's article is conventional PEEP, ranging 5 to 20 cm H_2O.

Civetta JM, Barnes TA, Smith LO: Optimal PEEP and intermittent mandatory ventilation in the treatment of acute respiratory failure. Respiratory Care 20:551–557, 1975

Suter PM, Fairley HB, Isenberg MD: Optimum end-expiratory airway pressure in patients with acute pulmonary failure. N Engl J Med 292:284–288, 1975

D.11. How would you monitor the level of PEEP?

The level of PEEP needed depends on the severity of pulmonary injury and the response of the individual patient. It is important to titrate the levels of PEEP individually to maximize oxygen transport without compromising cardiac output. When low levels of PEEP (less than 10 cm H_2O) are used, PaO_2, total respiratory compliance, $P\bar{v}O_2$, $A-aDO_2$, and Q_S/Q_T have to be monitored. When high levels of PEEP are used, cardiac output measurement is necessary because excessive PEEP decreases cardiac output.

Hedley–Whyte J, et al: Applied Physiology of Respiratory Care, pp 21–22. Boston, Little, Brown & Co, 1976

D.12. What are the cardiovascular effects of PEEP?

The cardiovascular effects of PEEP depend on the severity of respiratory failure, the level of PEEP, the intravascular volume, the contractility of the heart, and the pulmonary vasculature. In normal subjects without respiratory failure, PEEP decreases cardiac output because of increased intrathoracic pressure resulting in decreased venous return. In persons with respiratory failure, PEEP, up to optimal levels, usually increases or does not change cardiac output because of an increase in oxygenation with resultant improvement of cardiac performance. Cardiac output falls when PEEP exceed the individuals optimal PEEP. Hypovolemia increases hypotension during PEEP therapy.

Hedley–Whyte J et al: Applied Physiology of Respiratory Care, pp 20–23. Boston, Little, Brown & Co, 1976

D.13. How would you correct hypotension during mechanical ventilation with PEEP?

Hypovolemia has to be corrected first. When the patient is normovolemic, hypotension and low cardiac output from PEEP may be corrected by either expansion of the blood volume or infusion of dopamine. When there is some degree of cardiac failure, hypervolemia can be dangerous. Therefore, dopamine is preferred in cardiac patients. However, dopamine produces a substantial increase in pulmonary shunt.

Berk JL, Hagen JF, Tongirk, Maly GI: The use of dopamine to correct the reduced cardiac output resulting from positive end-expiratory pressure: A two-edged sword. Crit Care Med 5:269–271, 1977

Quist J, Pontoppidan H, Wilson RS et al: Hemodynamic responses to mechanical ventilation with PEEP: The effect of hypervolemia. Anesthesiology 42:45–55, 1975

D.14. What are the complications of CPPV?

CPPV has the same complications as IPPV. Because of higher mean and peak airway pressures with CPPV, the incidences of barotrauma and hypotension are greater with CPPV. IPPV increases urinary output and decreases plasma antidiuretic hormone (ADH). CPPV decreases urinary output and increases plasma ADH.

Baratz RA, Philbin DM, Patterson RW: Plasma antidiuretic hormone and urinary output during continuous positive pressure breathing in dogs. Anesthesiology 34:510–513, 1971

Hedley–Whyte J et al: Applied Physiology of Respiratory Care, pp 23–26. Boston, Little, Brown & Co, 1976

E. Weaning from Ventilatory Support

The patient's condition improved after respiratory support with 20 cm H_2O PEEP. Arterial blood gases showed: pH, 7.45; PCO_2 35 torr; PO_2 150 torr; F_IO_2 0.75.

E.1. What would you do now? Lower F_IO_2 or lower PEEP?

Because PaO_2 is 150 torr, F_IO_2 should be lowered gradually to prevent oxygen toxicity. When F_IO_2 is lowered to less than 0.5 or 0.6, PEEP level should be lowered gradually to avoid increased barotrauma and decreased cardiac output associated with excessive PEEP. The suggested criteria to lower PEEP level are a stable, nonseptic patient; $PaO_2/F_IO_2 > 200$; effective compliance > 25 ml/cm H_2O; $A-aDO_2 < 200$ at F_IO_2 0.5. PEEP should not be decreased by more than 5 cm H_2O during a trial. At least 6 hours should elapse before undertaking a further attempt at lowering the PEEP level.

Luterman A, Horovitz JH, Carrico CJ et al: Withdrawal from PEEP. Surgery 39:328–332, 1978

E.2. The patient continued to improve. When would you consider weaning the patient from the respirator? Discuss the criteria for weaning.

The criteria for discontinuance of mechanical ventilation are essentially the converse of the criteria for the institution of mechanical support and are as follows:

- Clear consciousness with adequate gag and cough reflex
- Cardiovascular stability
- Stable metabolic state without hypothermia, hyperpyrexia, metabolic acidosis, or alkalosis
- Adequate pulmonary function
  Mechanics
  - A vital capacity of more than 10 ml per kg or more than twice the normal tidal volume
  - A maximum inspiratory force of at least -20 to -30 cm H_2O

  Oxygenation
  - PaO_2 more than 80 torr with F_IO_2 0.4
  - $A-aDO_2$ less than 300 torr with F_IO_2 1.0
  - Q_S/Q_T less than 15%

  Ventilation
  - $PaCO_2$ less than 45 torr
  - V_D/V_T less than 0.6

Hedley–Whyte J et al: Applied Physiology of Respiratory Care, pp 133–137. Boston, Little, Brown & Co, 1976

E.3. How would you wean the patient from the respirator?

There are two methods for weaning the patient from the respirator: (1) the conventional T-piece technique and (2) the intermittent mandatory ventilation technique.

Conventional T-Piece Technique

When the patient meets the criteria for weaning, a T-piece adaptor and heated nebulizer are connected to the patient's endotracheal tube. The patient should be in a semi-sitting or sitting position. The inspired oxygen concentration is set at a level 5% to 10% higher than the patient was receiving during mechanical ventilation. The vital signs and cardiac rhythm are monitored carefully every 5 to 10 minutes. Arterial blood gases are determined 15 minutes after weaning is begun and then every hour. The patient who tolerates the T-piece very well is extubated after 2 to 4 hours. Oxygen is then administered, through a face mask with a heated nebulizer, at the same inspired oxygen concentration as during the T-piece trial.

Intermittent Mandatory Ventilation Technique

Weaning is accomplished by a gradual decrease in the IMV rate that the ventilator delivers, allowing the patient slowly to take over spontaneous ventilation. This system allows the patient to breathe spontaneously between the preset mechanical ventilation. This system assures intermittent hyperinflation of the lung. IMV has been reported to be helpful in weaning when conventional methods have failed.

Spontaneous PEEP can be applied to both weaning techniques. PEEP is especially useful in patients in whom rapid alveolar collapse and hypoxemia develop during weaning. Five cm H_2O PEEP during weaning minimizes alveolar collapse and improves the relationship between the closing capacity and functional residual capacity.

Feeley TW, Hedley–Whyte J: Weaning from controlled ventilation and supplemental oxygen. N Engl J Med 292:903–906, 1975

E.4. What are IMV, IAV, and IDV?

IMV refers to intermittent mandatory ventilation. IMV is comprised of breaths controlled by the ventilator as well as breaths supplied spontaneously by the patient. The same inspired oxygen concentration is used for both forms of ventilation. The air-oxygen mixture is led to a reservoir bag and connected to the ventilator tubing by a one-way valve immediately before the humidifier. Although IMV was originally introduced as a weaning technique, it is now used by some groups as a primary means of ventilatory support, especially in combination with high levels of PEEP, throughout the entire course of a patient's illness. Because the ventilator cycles are independent of the patient's breathing phase, airway and intrapleural pressure may increase when IMV inflations come at the end of spontaneous inhalation.

IAV stands for intermittent assisted ventilation, which is also called synchronized IMV (SIMV). Each mechanical ventilation is triggered by the patient. Both IMV and IAV rates are set by the operator.

IDV means intermittent demand ventilation. Each mechanical ventilation is triggered by the patient, as in IAV. The operator sets the IDV/spontaneous breathing ratio rather than the IDV rate. Therefore, the total IDV rate varies with the spontaneous breathing rate.

E.5. What are the advantages of IMV over controlled or assisted ventilation?

- There is selective application of mechanical support in accord with the individual patient's need.
- It's more comfortable for the patient. There is less need for sedatives or narcotics.

- There is a higher cardiac output because of lower intrathoracic pressure.
- There is decreased incidence of barotrauma because of lower airway pressure.
- There is less discoordination on spontaneous breathing because the respiratory center is activated and the patient uses his respiratory muscles.
- There is less psychologic dependence on ventilator.

Kirby RR: Intermittent Mandatory Ventilation. ASA Refresher Courses in Anesthesiology 7:169–188, 1979

F. Special Techniques on Respiratory Support

F.1. What is differential or selective PEEP? What are the indications?

By using a Carlens double-lumen endobronchial tube, both lungs can be ventilated simultaneously and separately with different levels of PEEP to each lung. Two ventilators have to be synchronized by a controller to prevent mediastinal movement and cardiovascular instability. A modified circuit has been described by Power and associates to permit independent ventilation from a single ventilator. Selective PEEP is indicated when there is a severe unilateral pulmonary disorder such as pneumonia or atelectasis, because certain PEEP levels may be too high for the normal lung and too low for the pathologic lung.

Power DJ, Eross B, Grenvik A: Differential lung ventilation with PEEP in the treatment of unilateral pneumonia. Crit Care Med 5:170–172, 1977

Trew GF, Warren BR, Potter WA: Differential ventilation of the lungs in man. Crit Care Med 4:112, 1976

F.2. What are the indications and contraindications of extracorporeal membrane oxygenation (ECMO). How many ways can ECMO be used?

ECMO should be used for patients in severe acute respiratory failure with reversible lung disease, who are dying of severe hypoxemia despite maximal conventional ventilatory care as defined here (tracheal intubation, mechanical ventilation with 10 to 15 cm H_2O PEEP, diuresis, chest physical therapy, antibiotics, normothermia or mild hypothermia, sedation, paralysis, and increased oxygen concentration). National Institute of Health indications are as follows: A PaO_2 less than 50 torr for more than 2 hours with F_1O_2 of 1.0 and conventional PEEP; and a PaO_2 less than 50 torr for more than 12 hours with F_1O_2 of more than 0.6 and conventional PEEP. Active bleeding is the only absolute contraindication to use of the artificial lung. There are three routes for ECMO (1) venovenous perfusion from the inferior vena cava by way of the femoral vein to the oxygenator and then to the supeior vena cava, (2) venoarterial perfusion from the femoral vein to the oxygenator and then to the femoral artery, and (3) venovenous arterial perfusion from the femoral vein to the oxygenator and then to both the internal jugular vein and the femoral artery. The mortality is high with ECMO. The IMV/high PEEP therapy has about the same result.

Hedley–Whyte J, Burgess GE, Feeley TW et al: Applied Physiology of Respiratory Care, pp 407–410. Boston, Little, Brown & Co, 1976

F.3. What is HFPPV? What are the characteristics of HFPPV? What are the indications?

HFPPV signifies high frequency positive pressure ventilation. The major characteristics of the ventilatory pattern of volume-controlled HFPPV are as follows:

- A ventilatory frequency of about 60–100/min and an inspiration expiration ratio of less than 0.3
- Smaller tidal volumes and therefore lower maximal and mean airway and transpulmonary pressures, yet a higher FRC than in conventional IPPV/CPPV
- Positive intratracheal and negative intrapleural pressures throughout the ventilatory cycle
- Less circulatory interference than in IPPV/CPPV
- Reflex suppression of spontaneous respiratory rhythmicity during normoventilation
- Decelerating inspiratory flow without an end-inspiratory plateau
- More efficient pulmonary gas distribution than in IPPV/CPPV

The indications for HFPPV include the following:

- Respiratory failure with bronchopleural fistula, tracheoesophageal or bronchioesophageal fistula, barotrauma, pulmonary fibrosis, and pulmonary hemorrhage, because of low airway pressure with HFPPV
- Anesthesia for bronchoscopy, laryngoscopy, and microlaryngeal surgery
- Open chest surgery because of moderately expanded lung and minimal respiratory movement with HFPPV

Carlon GC, Kahn RC, Howland WS et al: Clinical experience with high frequency jet ventilation. Crit Care Med 9:1–6, 1981

Malina JR, Nordstrom SG, Sjostrand UH et al: Clinical evaluation of high frequency positive pressure ventilation in patients scheduled for open-chest surgery. Anesth Analg (Cleve) 60:324–330, 1981

Sjostrand U: High frequency positive-pressure ventilation (HFPPV): A review. Crit Care Med 8:345–364, 1980

Eng UB, Eriksson I, Sjostrand U: HFPPV: A review based on its use during bronchoscopy and for laryngoscopy and microlaryngeal surgery under general anesthesia. Anesth Analg (Cleve) 59:594–603, 1980

F.4. What are the frequencies used in HFPPV, high frequency oscillation, and high frequency jet ventilation (HFJV)?

The respiratory rate described in HFPPV is 40–200/min. In ventilation by high frequency oscillation, the rate is 15–50 Hz, (900–3000/min), and tidal volume is 1.5 to 3.0 ml/kg of body weight. In HFJV, a frequency of up to 200–900/min is used.

Butler WJ, Bohn DJ, Bryan AC et al: Ventilation by high frequency oscillation in humans. Anesth Analg (Cleve) 59:577–584, 1980

Klain M, Smith B: High frequency percutaneous transtracheal jet ventilation. Crit Care Med 5:280–287, 1977

4 Fat Embolism

Joseph F. Artusio, Jr.

A 63-year-old woman was admitted to the hospital with a mid-shaft compound comminuted fracture of the femur sustained in an automobile accident. No other injuries were found. The day following the trauma, she was scheduled for an open reduction and internal fixation of the femur. Preoperative evaluation showed a restless, dyspneic patient. Blood pressure 105/65, pulse 112/m, respiration 36/m, temperature 40°C.

A. Medical Disease and Differential Diagnosis

1. Define the terms dyspnea, tachypnea, and eupnea?
2. What are the causes of dyspnea and tachypnea?
3. Can we distinguish a fat embolus from a blood embolus?
4. How do we distinguish atelectasis from pneumothorax?
5. What are the signs and symptoms of aspiration of gastric contents into the tracheobronchial tree?
6. How do we make a diagnosis of fat embolism?
7. If a diagnosis of fat embolism is made, what treatment would you institute?
8. What is meant by a V/Q abnormality?
9. What is a right to left shunt? How do you measure the extent of a pulmonary shunt? What is the shunt equation?
10. What is the significance of an increased V_D/V_T ratio?
11. Why does airway obstruction increase the work of breathing?

B. Preoperative Evaluation and Preparation

1. Is there any way to prepare this patient to better withstand the fixation of her femur?
2. How would you premedicate the patient?

C. Intraoperative Management

1. What are the essential intraoperative monitors that should be used and followed?
2. What anesthetic regimen would you choose—regional or general?

D. Postoperative Management

1. Would you expect any ventilatory problems in the postanesthesia period?
2. Is tracheostomy ever necessary in these patients and in what situation would you recommend it?

A. Medical Disease and Differential Diagnosis

A.1. Define the terms dyspnea, tachypnea, and eupnea?

Dyspnea is the subjective feeling of difficulty in breathing experienced by the conscious subject. Tachypnea is increased rate of respiration. Eupnea is easy, free respiration—the type observed in the normal subject under resting conditions.

Stedman's Medical Dictionary, 22nd ed, pp 387, 439, and 1251. Baltimore, Williams & Wilkins, 1973

A.2. What are the causes of dyspnea and tachypnea?

The general causes of dyspnea and tachypnea are as follows:

Airway Obstruction
- Extrathoracic—aspiration of food or a foreign body, angioneurotic edema of the glottis, tumors of the airway, fibrotic stenosis
- Intrathoracic—asthma, chronic bronchitis, bronchiectasis, emphysema

Diffuse Parenchymal Lung Diseases
- Infection—viruses, bacteria, fungi, parasites
- Occupational causes—mineral dusts, and chemical fumes
- Neoplasm—primary or metastatic cancer, cystic fibrosis, congenital or familial causes
- Metabolic causes—uremic pneumonitis
- Physical agents—postirradiation fibrosis, thermal injury, oxygen toxicity, blast injury
- Immunologic causes—hypersensitivity pneumonia, drug reactions, collagen disease
- Unknown origin—sarcoidosis, histiocytosis, hemosiderosis, alveolar proteinosis

Pulmonary Vascular Occlusive Diseases
- Pulmonary thromboembolism, fat embolism

Disease of the Chest Wall or Respiratory Muscles
- Severe kyphoscoliosis, pectus excavatum, polio, myasthenia gravis

Anxiety Neurosis or Pain
Heart Disease
- Congenital or acquired heart disease with congestive heart failure

Other Causes
- Hypoxemia, shock, acidosis, sepsis, fever, residual effect of muscle relaxant, high spinal anesthesia.

For this patient, the most probable causes of dyspnea are pain, infection, fat embolism, chest injury, and aspiration pneumonitis.

Isselbacher KJ et al: Harrison's Principles of Internal Medicine, 9th ed, pp 163, 164, and 1242. New York, McGraw–Hill, 1980

A.3. Can we distinguish a fat embolus from a blood embolus?

An embolus is a detached intravascular mass (solid or gaseous) that is carried by the blood to a site distant from its point of origin. Inevitably, these lodge in vessels too small to permit their further passage, resulting in partial or complete occlusion of the vessel. Ninety-nine percent of all emboli arise in thrombi (rare forms include fragments of bone or bone marrow, bits of tumor, foreign bodies such as bullets, and bubbles of air or nitrogen). Fat embolism is the occlusion of small vessels of the microcirculation by fat globules. It is encountered most often in patients suffering from severe traumatic injuries to fat-laden tissues, such as fractures of bones containing fatty marrow, or extensive damage to subcutaneous fat deposits. Rupture of small venules occurs and fat globules enter the circulation. Another theory is based on physiochemical changes in the circulating blood lipids. This theory postulates that the normal emulsion of fat within the plasm is altered to allow coalescence of the chylomicrons into larger fat droplets, with subsequent embolization. Clinically, blood embolization may present with similar findings, but usually occurs later. A friction rub is more common, and evidence of venous thrombosis may be apparent. The classic physical finding of fat embolism is the appearance of petechial hemorrhages in the capillary plexus of the dermis. They may also be noted in the subconjunctival region and on the palate because fat emboli may pass through the pulmonary filter to reach the circulation and lodge in the vessels of the skin, causing petechiae.

Robbins: Pathologic Basis of Disease, pp 337–338. Philadelphia, WB Saunders, 1974

Schwartz S et al: Principles of Surgery, 3rd ed, pp 509–510. New York, McGraw–Hill, 1974

A.4. How do we distinguish atelectasis from pneumothorax?

Atelectasis usually develops in the first 24 hours after an operation and rarely appears after 48 hours. There is often a sudden onset of fever and tachycardia. Early findings include rales located posteriorly in the bases, diminished breath sounds, and bronchial breathing. There is dullness to percussion on the affected side. With massive involvement there may be a shift of the trachea, mediastinum, and heart to the involved side, but this does not present with the more common subsegmental lesions. Pronounced dyspnea or cyanosis are relatively uncommon. Roentgenograms may demonstrate areas of consolidation. Blood gas determinations indicating intrapulmonary shunting of blood provide the diagnosis. Characteristically with atelectasis and significant shunting, the arterial PaO_2 is decreased, whereas the arterial $PaCO_2$ may be normal or decreased. The ventilation is normal or increased. Pneumothorax is spontaneous, traumatic, or iatrogenic—"closed" when the chest wall is intact, "open" when a breach in the chest wall exists. When the visceral and parietal pleuras are not adherent, pressure in the pleural space may be sufficient to displace the mediastinum to the opposite side (tension pneumothorax). Symptoms are chest pains, shortness of breath, cough, and shoulder pain; 5% show no symptoms at all. Severe cases may be associated with syncope, nausea, vomiting, or shock. Physical findings include evidence of diminished ventilation of the affected lung and hyperresonance, percussion reveals a tympanitic quality. The diagnosis may elude the examiner unless a chest x-ray is obtained. Tension pneumothorax may produce mediastinal shift and tracheal displacement away from the affected side with neck vein distention, cyanosis, and shock. Chest x-ray shows area of air without lung markings.

Schwartz S et al: Principles of Surgery, 3rd ed, pp 502, 651–654. New York, McGraw–Hill, 1979

A.5. What are the signs and symptoms of aspiration of gastric contents into the tracheobronchial tree?

The pulmonary consequences of aspiration relate to both the volume and the character of the material aspirated. Large amounts of fluid will inundate the lungs, while particulate matter may result in obstruction at any level—either will cause varying degrees of asphyxiation. Depending on the amount of material aspirated, patients may have acute respiratory distress with cyanosis and cardiac arrest, or may exhibit a milder, chronic course leading to lobar pneumonitis and lung abscess. Pathogenic bacteria and colonic bacilli in stagnant secretions or feculent matter will produce infection, but perhaps the most serious consequences result from the relative acidity of gastric secretions. Aspiration of material with a *p*H less than 2.5 results in a chemical burn and causes an immediate intense bronchoconstriction with dyspnea, tachypnea, and cyanosis. There is also destruction of the tracheal mucosa. This clinical picture is referred to as Mendelson's syndrome. Within hours, a spreading and patchy pneumonitis appears as a fluffiness or "whiteout" on chest x-ray. As a result of obstruction and atelectasis, a major degree of shunting of arteriolar blood occurs, with a widening of the alveolar-arterial oxygen gradient. Pulmonary edema may develop as a consequence of the chemical insult alone, or secondary to heart failure. Eventually, the full-blown pathogenic picture resembles that of the so-called adult respiratory distress syndrome. In severe cases, cardiac arrest may develop. Immediate therapy includes oxygen, endotracheal suctioning, methyl prednisolone given IV, and broad-spectrum antibiotics. Bronchoscopy is indicated if particulate matter is found in the vomitus or if signs of obstructive atelectasis develop. (Tracheobronchial lavage with large volumes of saline solution is no longer recommended.)

Dripps RD, Eckenoff JE, Vandam LD: Introduction to Anesthesia: The Principles of Safe Practice, 5th ed, pp 427–428. Philadelphia, WB Saunders, 1977

Schwartz S et al: Principles of Surgery, 3rd ed, p 227. New York, McGraw–Hill, 1979

A.6. *How do we make a diagnosis of fat embolism?*

- Cardiopulmonary effects are tachycardia, hypotension, fullness of the superficial veins secondary to increased venous pressure. Acute heart failure may occur. The direct pulmonary effects may be manifested by dyspnea, cyanosis not relieved by oxygen, bubbly rales, and blood-tinged tracheobronchial secretions.
- Primary symptoms are frequently cerebral in origin and include confusion, disorientation, delirium, and acute psychosis, progressing to coma and stupor. Local weakness, spasticity, or decerebrate rigidity also may be noted. Incontinence occurs relatively frequently and most patients are febrile, with temperatures as high as 107°F.
- The classic finding for fat embolism is the appearance of petechial hemorrhages in the capillary plexus of the dermis. They occur in a distinctive pattern over the shoulders, chest, and axilla. Rarely, they occur in the abdominal wall and extremities and also in the subconjunctival region and on the palate. Emboli may appear within the retinal vessels, and there may be streaks of hemorrhage throughout the retina as well as macular edema.
- A sudden and precipitous drop in hemoglobin may occur, related to hemorrhage within the pulmonary parenchyma.
- The x-ray pattern is that of unevenly distributed areas of radiodensity, congestive hilar shadows, and increased bronchovascular markings, with dilation of the right side of the heart.
- Serial measurement of PaO_2 offer a better index of the degree of pulmonary involvement.
- The EKG may reveal changes which reflect myocardial ischemia and right ventricular strain. A prominent S wave in lead I and prominent Q waves in lead III may appear as may right bundle branch block, arrhythmias, inverted T waves, and ST depression.
- Lipuria occurs in the first few days following injury and is usually associated with a serious degree of fat embolism. Sudan III stain → orange; Scuderi "sizzle" test—wire loop with patient's blood over flame will sizzle if fat is contained.
- Biopsy of petechiae and frozen section

56 · Anesthesiology

- Needle biopsy of the kidney to demonstrate fat globules
- Serum lipase level elevation is apparent in approximately 50% of cases (maximum level on day 7–8). Elevation greater than 1 ml is significant. Favorable outcome is expected with elevation not greater than 2 ml.
- Fat in cryostat reaction of clotted blood (Hauman) involves fat staining serial frozen sections on a clot of the patient's blood. In addition, a fat particle count is done on the plasma (size and number). This test requires serial examinations. There are little data on its reliability.

Schwartz S et al: Principles of Surgery, 3rd ed, pp 510–511. New York, McGraw–Hill, 1979

Zauder H: Anesthesia for Orthopedic Surgery, p 165. Philadelphia, F.A. Davis, 1980

A.7. If a diagnosis of fat embolism is made, what treatment would you institute?

- Prophylaxis—gentle handling of the patient and early splinting of fractures
- Vigorous resuscitative measures to correct shock
- Pulmonary manifestations are treated by the following: oxygen therapy, intermittent positive pressure breathing, positive end-expiratory pressure, and rapid digitalization.
- Intensive endotracheal suctioning to minimize accumulation of secretions
- Maintain PaO_2 (through arterial blood gases) between 89 torr and 100 torr
- Corticosteroids 100 mg q 6 hr in conjunction with assisted ventilation
- Cerebral manifestations should be treated with sedation and anti-convulsive therapy
- Heparin (not in anticoagulant doses) will clear lipemic plasma and stimulate lipase activity. (25 mg q 6 hr IV)
- Low molecular weight dextran IV to counteract intravascular thrombosis when there is an increased erythrocyte sedimentation rate
- Ethyl alcohol may decrease the rate of hydrolysis of neutral fat and slow the release of toxic free fatty acids. It also dilates the pulmonary capillaries.

Schwartz S et al: Principles of Surgery, 3rd ed, p 511. New York, McGraw–Hill, 1979

A.8. What is meant by a V/Q abnormality?

V/Q abnormality occurs in an alveolar capillary unit that has either a poorly ventilated alveolus, an excessive rate of blood flow, or an impedance to oxygen diffusion. Inequality of ventilation in relation to blood flow causes impairment of both oxygen and carbon dioxide transfer. The ratio is reduced by obstructing ventilation, leaving blood flow unchanged. The ratio is increased by obstructing blood flow leaving ventilation unchanged. A lung with ventilation/perfusion inequality is not able to transfer as much oxygen and carbon dioxide as a lung that is uniformly ventilated and perfused; moreover, the lung cannot maintain as high an arterial PO_2 or as low an arterial PCO_2 as a homogeneous lung.

West J: Respiratory Physiology: The Essentials, 2nd ed, pp 58–66. Baltimore, Williams & Wilkins, 1979.

A.9. What is a right to left shunt? How do you measure the extent of a pulmonary shunt? What is the shunt equation?

A right to left shunt usually requires either an obstructive lesion at some point in the right-sided circulation (i.e., tricuspid stenosis or atresia, pulmonary valvular or infundibular stenosis, elevated pulmonary vascular resistance), or an obligatory mixing of systemic venous and arterial blood (i.e., total anomalous pulmonary venous drainage, a single atrium or ventricle, or a persistent truncus arteriosus).

To measure the extent of a pulmonary shunt we must note that the physiologic shunt is composed of three parts. The first part is anatomic shunting. Normally, 2% to 4% of cardiac output goes directly from the right to the left heart without entering the pulmonary vasculature by way of bronchial, pleural, and thebesian veins. Abnormal pulmonary arteriovenous fistulas and vascular lung tumors also increase anatomic shunt. The second part is capillary shunting. Blood entering a pulmonary capillary that is adjacent to an unventilated alveolus will not exchange with alveolar air. The third component is perfusion in excess of ventilation (venous admixture, shunt effect), also known as V/Q abnormality, see above. The sum of anatomic and capillary shunting is termed true shunting, because it will be the same at 100% inspired oxygen concentration as it is at room air. True shunting is unaffected by oxygen therapy.

Shunt Equation $\dfrac{Q_S}{Q_T} = \dfrac{C_cO_2 - C_aO_2}{C_cO_2 - C_{\bar{v}}O_2}$

C_cO_2, end-pulmonary capillary oxygen content
C_aO_2, arterial oxygen content
$C_{\bar{v}}O_2$, mixed venous oxygen content

Oxygen Content = oxygen in hemoglobin (Hb) + oxygen in plasma.
= $1.34 \times O_2$ saturation $\times$ Hb + $0.003 \times P_{O_2}$

When PaO_2 is over 150 torr, the hemoglobin is 100% saturated. We usually use 100% oxygen to ventilate the patient for 15 minutes. The shunt equation is represented in the following:

Clinical Shunt Equation $\dfrac{Q_S}{Q_T} = \dfrac{(P_AO_2 - PaO_2) \times 0.003}{(C_aO_2 - C_vO_2) + (P_AO_2 - PaO_2)}$

Alveolar Oxygen $P_AO_2 = F_IO_2 (P_B - 47) - \dfrac{PaCO_2}{0.8}$

Barometric Pressure P_B

Clinically, 3.5 ml per 100 ml of blood is used for arterial-venous oxygen difference in critically ill patients.

Isselbacher KJ et al: Harrison's Principles of Internal Medicine, 9th ed, p 1078. New York, McGraw–Hill, 1980.

Shapiro B et al: Clinical Application of Blood Gases, 2nd ed, pp 83–84, 88–90, 221–225. Chicago, Year Book Medical Publishers, 1977

A.10. What is the significance of an increased V_D/V_T ratio?

V_D/V_T Ratio

$$\frac{V_D}{V_T} = \frac{\text{dead space}}{\text{tidal volume}}$$

The total dead space ventilation is usually termed the "physiological dead space" ventilation, and is equal to the sum of the anatomic dead space ventilation (volume of gas that ventilates the conducting airways and, therefore, does not take part in effective gas exchange), and the "alveolar dead space" ventilation (volume of gas that does not take part in effective gas exchange at the alveolar level). An increased V_D/V_T ratio occurs when the quantity of ventilation delivered to the alveoli exceeds that required to arterialize the pulmonary capillary blood flow. Ventilation to such alveoli cannot take part in gas exchange, and so behaves as if it were ventilating a dead space.

Factors Influencing Physiological Dead Space

- Age—ratio increases (V_D increases 1 ml per year)
- Body size—larger in larger people
- Posture—average V_D/V_T 34% in upright position, 30% in supine position
- Increasing duration of inspiration causes decreased V_D
- Smoking—highly significant increase in V_D/V_T
- Pulmonary disease—pulmonary embolus, pulmonary hypoperfusion, emphysema—highly increased V_D/V_T; increases more with anesthesia
- Anesthesia—increasing V_D/V_T
- Artificial ventilation—variations in respiratory pressures and phasing, minimized by the optimal value of PEEP

An increased physiological dead space results in reduced alveolar ventilation unless there is a compensatory increase in minute volume. Alveolar PCO_2 will rise and alveolar PO_2 will fall. The ratio is an index of efficiency of ventilation. In health it does not exceed 0.3. As it increases, less ventilation takes an effective part in gas exchange (*e.g.*, 70% dead space = 30% effective ventilation).

Nunn JF: Applied Respiratory Physiology, 2nd ed, pp 228–230. London–Boston, Butterworth & Co, 1977

Wylie WD, Churchill–Davidson H: A Practice of Anaesthesia, 4th ed, pp 70–71. Philadelphia, WB Saunders, 1979

A.11. Why does airway obstruction increase the work of breathing?

During spontaneous respiration, the work of breathing is accomplished by the patient's respiratory muscles. The work is normally performed during inspiration. Expiration is powered by the potential energy stored in the tissues that have been distorted from their resting position during inspiration. During inspiration, active muscular contraction provides the force necessary to overcome elastic recoil of the lungs and thorax, the force required to overcome frictional resistance during movement of the tissues of the lung and thorax, and the force necessary to overcome frictional resistance to the air flow through the hundreds of thousands of fine tubes and ducts of the tracheobronchial tree. Airway obstruction will reduce the radius of the airway, increase air flow resistance, and thus increase the work of breathing. According to Poiseulle's Law, the resistance is inversely proportional to the fourth power of the radius.

Nunn JF: Applied Respiratory Physiology, 2nd ed, pp 195–201. London–Boston, Butterworth & Co, 1977

B. Preoperative Evaluation and Preparation

B.1. Is there any way to prepare this patient to better withstand the fixation of her femur?

Yes. The four main considerations are as follows:
- Assessment of blood loss and replacement is important, especially in the very young or very old patient. Albumin improves the circulation and helps bind the free fatty acids. Poor perfusion can result in altered lipid metabolism and coagulation abnormalities, both of which can contribute to the effects of the fat embolism syndrome.
- Immobilization of the fracture is essential. The risk of developing fat embolism is higher in patients in whom this is not done than in those who are splinted adequately.
- Vigorous respiratory care and close monitoring of arterial blood gases will maintain adequate oxygenation.
- Heparin therapy. Heparin has a clearing effect on lipemic serum and this effect improves metabolic oxidation of the embolic fat. Moreover, heparin has an anticoagulant effect which prevents platelet aggregation and subsequent serotonin release. However, care must be taken not to cause excessive bleeding at the wound site.

Zauder: Anesthesia for Orthopaedic Surgery, pp 170–171. Philadelphia, F.A. Davis, 1980

B.2. How would you premedicate the patient?

Consider preanesthetic suppression of pain according to the patient's general physical condition. Be careful not to depress cardiac or respiratory function. If the patient is unconscious or disoriented, give no premedication.

Atropine is useful because it suppresses undesirable reflexes of cardiac rhythm and depresses the secretory function of glands in the airway. However, we would not use atropine in the presence of tachycardia secondary to shock.

Shires T: Care of the Trauma Patient, 2nd ed, pp 83–84. New York, McGraw–Hill, 1979

C. Intraoperative Management

C.1. What are the essential intraoperativce monitors that should be used and followed?

- ECG—for signs of arrhythmias, myocardial ischemia and anoxia, and electrolyte disturbances
- Central venous pressure monitor
- Arterial line for continuous monitoring of blood pressure, as well as for arterial pH, P_{CO_2}, and P_{O_2}. This information will warn of the onset of metabolic acidosis, and will provide guidance in therapy and ventilatory adequacy.
- Repeated auscultation with a fixed precordial or esophageal stethoscope to assess intensity and rhythm of heart sounds
- Urine output
- Esophageal temperature

Shires T: Care of the Trauma Patient, 2nd ed, pp 93–94. New York, McGraw–Hill, 1979

C.2. What anesthetic regimen would you choose—regional or general?

The best anesthetic approach is a regional technique such as a femoral–sciatic block for lower extremity work. This technique can be used if the patient is cooperative or if his physiologic state is such that he may be sedated without undue adverse effect. A spinal or epidural anesthetic may be used (1) if the CNS is not involved, (2) if blood volume has been replaced or is at a normal level, and (3) if the patient is not intoxicated. Local anesthesia may be used in poor risk patients; however, large amounts of local anesthetic can further depress blood pressure, pulse, respiration, and level of consciousness.

Use general anesthesia if the patient is hypoxemic and, therefore, requires a high percentage of oxygen. Thiopental is a strong myocardial depressant, especially for a patient with hypovolemic shock. Morphine and thiopental both decrease the responsiveness of the microcirculation to epinephrine and norepinephrine, thereby causing decreased effectiveness of compensatory mechanisms. Many anesthetic agents can abolish these circulatory reflexes, which are already weakened by trauma and blood loss; therefore, extreme care must be taken if these agents are used. We prefer to use an inhalation anesthetic such as isoflurane or enflurane and N_2O–O_2 technique.

Goodman LS, Gilman AG: The Pharmacological Basis of Therapeutics, 6th ed, p 293 and 503. New York, MacMillan, 1980

Shires T: Care of the Trauma Patient, 2nd ed, pp 84–85. New York, McGraw–Hill, 1979

D. Postoperative Management

D.1. Would you expect any ventilatory problems in the postanesthesia period?

Ventilatory problems in the postanesthetic period can be expected to occur as a result of embolism (*i.e.*, the problems of continued secretions, congestive heart failure, cyanosis, and cerebral effects). If a general anesthetic is used, hypoventilation can result from one or a combination of several conditions secondary to delayed emergence from anesthesia, anesthetic overdose, excess of narcotics given for postoperative pain relief, fluid overload, shock, overdose of muscle relaxant, upper or lower airway obstruction, pneumothorax, hemothorax, or pain.

Shires T: Care of the Trauma Patient, 2nd ed, pp 102–103. New York, McGraw–Hill, 1979

D.2. Is tracheostomy ever necessary in these patients, and in what situation would you recommend it?

Patients with severe preoperative chronic bronchitis and emphysema, or those who develop extensive post-atelectatic bronchopneumonia may require prolonged endotracheal intubation to prevent them from drowning in their secretions or dying from hypoxia, carbon dioxide retention, and respiratory failure. Tracheostomy will be required if it is believed that extubation cannot be tolerated soon, and 5 to 7 days have already passed. If bronchial toilet is adequate and the decrease in dead space afforded by the tracheostomy fail to arrest the respiratory failure, then assisted or controlled ventilation on a mechanical ventilator must begin.

Dripps R, Echenhoff J, Vandam L: Introduction to Anesthesia. In The Principles of Safe Practice, 4th ed, pp 515–517. Philadelphia, WB Saunders, 1977

5 Tracheoesophageal Fistula

Marjorie J. Topkins

A 12-hour-old neonate born after 37 weeks of gestation and weighing 2200 grams, had frothing about the nose and mouth. The child regurgitated the first feeding almost immediately. Coughing and mild cyanosis were associated with the regurgitation.

A. Medical Disease and Differential Diagnosis

1. What is the working diagnosis?
2. What information is needed to confirm the diagnosis? What information is obtained from each of the following?
   - Radiopaque catheter
   - Barium swallow or instillation
   - Chest x-ray
   - Flat plate of abdomen
3. Classify tracheoesophageal (t-e) fistulae or atresia.
4. What other congenital anomalies are associated with t-e fistulae or atresia?
5. What is the embryology of t-e fistulae?

B. Preoperative Evaluation and Preparation

1. What problems concern you and what laboratory data do you need to evaluate these problems?
2. Discuss the classification of patients with t-e fistulae or atresia according to Waterston or Calverley. What is the implication for this patient?
3. Discuss fluid replacement in this patient.
4. What is the role of antibiotics preoperatively or postoperatively?
5. Discuss the role of gastrostomy in the management of t-e fistulae.
6. What premedication is indicated in this patient?

C. Intraoperative Management

1. Discuss transportation of the neonate to the operating room.
2. Discuss the problems of induction and intubation. Would you put the endotracheal tube above or beyond the fistula?
3. In what position will surgery be performed? Is this important?
4. What problems can be anticipated during surgery? How can you maintain a stable mediastinum? Is there a role for muscle relaxants?
5. What type of monitoring will you use?
6. What emergency drugs should be available?

D. Postoperative Management

1. When can this infant be extubated?
2. What are the dangers of extubating an infant who is depressed, cold, or asleep?
3. What are the complications seen following tracheoesophageal fistulae repair?
4. Discuss the management of postoperative pneumonia or atelectasis. Are these anesthetic complications?

A. Medical Disease and Differential Diagnosis

A.1. What is the working diagnosis?

The presence of frothing about the nose and mouth suggests tracheoesophageal pathology. A history of polyhydramnios in the mother, supplied by the obstetrician, should alert the physician to the possibility of tracheoesophageal pathology or other gastrointestinal atresias. Whether or not a catheter passes easily into the stomach is important. In some institutions it is standard practice to pass a catheter into the stomach at birth, increasing the likelihood of early diagnosis. This is important to prevent pulmonary complications that can occur from feeding or from reflux. Early diagnosis offers the surgeon and anesthesiologist the opportunity to operate on the neonate before pulmonary complications occur.

Redo SF: Principles of Surgery in the First Six Months of Life, p 59. Hagerstown, Harper & Row, 1976

Smith RM: Anesthesia for Infants and Children, p 309. St. Louis, C.V. Mosby, 1980

A.2. What information is needed to confirm the diagnosis? What information is obtained from each of the following?

- Radiopaque catheter
- Barium swallow or instillation
- Chest x-ray
- Flat plate of abdomen

A radiopaque catheter passed into the esophagus stops abruptly 10 cm to 12 cm or less from the nares. An x-ray will show the curled catheter in the upper pouch. A small amount of water-soluble contrast may be used; however, it is better to avoid this method for fear that either the contrast will be aspirated into the lung from overflow or material will enter the lung through a fistulous tract. A chest x-ray will determine the presence of pneumonia, especially of the right upper lobe, and may give some information concerning associated cardiac lesions. A flat plate of the abdomen will show the presence or absence of air in the gastrointestinal tract. The absence of air is pathognomonic for esophageal atresia, though not necessarily associated with a fistula. The presence of air, however, does not rule out atresia. Air may enter the GI tract through a fistula between the trachea and a lower esophageal segment. This is present in the Type C (Gross Classification), the most frequently seen type of t-e fistula.

Redo SF: Principles of Surgery in the First Six Months of Life, p 60. Hagerstown, Harper & Row, 1976

A.3. Classify tracheoesophageal (t-e) fistulae or atresia. Gross enumerated five types of atresia with or without fistulae.

- Type A—esophageal atresia with no fistula
- Type B—esophageal atresia, the upper segment communicating with the trachea
- Type C—esophageal atresia with a blind upper pouch and the lower segment communicating with the trachea
- Type D—esophageal atresia with both upper and lower segments communicating with the trachea
- Type E—no atresia present, but a communication exists between the esophagus and the trachea, the so-called H type, or more precisely the N type, since the tracheal opening is usually more cephalad than the esophageal opening

The most common type is C, a blind upper pouch and a lower fistulous segment, accounting for almost 87% of all cases. Atresia alone, Type A, accounts for approximately 8% of cases. Type E, the H or N type, accounts for 4% to 5%. This type is frequently missed, and the diagnosis often is not made until frequent pulmonary problems present, often months after birth. The other two types, Type B and Type D, account for less than 1% each.

Redo SF: Principles of Surgery in the First Six Months of Life, p 61. Hagerstown, Harper & Row, 1976

A.4. What other congenital anomalies are associated with tracheoesophageal fistulae or atresia?

Associated anomalies occur in approximately 30% to 50% of atresias in reported large series. The most common are cardiovascular, genitourinary, imperforate anus and other intestinal atresias, neurologic and orthopedic anomalies. The VATER association is an acronym for a group of associated defects identified by Quan and Smith, which include **V**ascular **V**ertebral defects, **A**nal atresia or other GI atresias, **T**rachea-**E**sophageal fistulae, **R**enal and **R**adial anomalies. The most common cardiac anomalies include ventricular septal defect, coarctation of the aorta, tetrology of Fallot, and atrial septal defect. Patent ductus arteriosus was seen frequently in one series. The incidence of cardiac anomalies associated with t-e fistula is approximately 14% to 15%. Approximately one-half the patients with t-e fistula have some other congenital anomaly.

Quan L, Smith DW: The VATER association, vertebral defect, anal atresia, t-e fistula with esophageal atresia, radial and renal dysplasia. A spectrum of associated defects. J Pediatr 82:104, 1973

Smith RM: Anesthesia for Infants and Children, pp 307–313. St Louis, C.V. Mosby, 1980

Stroedel WE et al: Esophageal atresia. Arch Surg 114:523–527, 1979

Thein RMH, Epstein BS: General Surgical Procedures in the Child with a Congenital Anomaly. In Stehling LC and Zauder HL (eds): Anesthetic Implications of Congenital Anomalies in Children, pp 90–95. New York, Appleton-Century-Crofts, 1980

A.5. *What is the embryology of t-e fistulae?*

The esophagus is developed from the first part of the primitive gut; the upper part of the esophagus from the retropharyngeal segment, the lower part of the esophagus from the pregastric segments. As the neck differentiates and the heart, lungs, and stomach move caudad, the esophagus elongates rapidly. Vacuoles appear in the epithelium to form a lumen by the eighth week. By the fourth week, the laryngotracheal groove develops to become the larynx, trachea, and primordia of the lungs. Two furrows develop along the sides of the respiratory primordia, move inward, separating the respiratory portion from the esophagus. Tracheoesophageal fistula results from an imperfect division of this foregut into the anterior larynx and trachea and the posterior esophagus. The incidence of t-e fistula appears in approximately 1:3000 live births, with a somewhat greater incidence in males (60:40, males to females).

Thein RMH, Epstein BS: General Surgical Procedures in the Child with a Congenital Anomaly. In Stehling LC and Zauder HL (eds): Anesthetic Implications of Congenital Anomalies in Children, pp 90–91. New York, Appleton-Century-Crofts, 1980

B. Preoperative Evaluation and Preparation

B.1. *What problems concern you and what laboratory data do you need to evaluate these problems?*

Infants who have tracheoesophageal fistula may have pneumonia or atelectasis secondary to aspiration of secretions that cannot be swallowed, or to reflux from the stomach through the fistula. To evaluate this condition, a chest x-ray is mandatory. This infant was admitted early and the diagnosis was made promptly; therefore extensive pulmonary complications are not expected. If the diagnosis is delayed, aspiration pneumonia, and atelectasis, with or without bacterial pneumonitis, may result in sepsis, shunting, hypoxia, and hypercarbia. Metabolic acidosis secondary to dehydration may be added to the already existing respiratory acidosis.

Blood gases may be helpful in differentiation of acidosis. A complete blood count and urinalysis is needed. Most deaths or serious complications occur in infants with other congenital anomalies, especially cardiovascular anomalies. If cyanosis is prominent, it could be due to cardiac anomalies or respiratory complications secondary to the t-e fistula, with atelectasis or gastric distention and elevation of the diaphragm. The absence of obvious pulmonary complications should alert the physician to the possible existence of congenital heart disease. Prematurity adds an increased risk if associated with severe anomalies. A complete physical examination is essential, as well as the pre- and perinatal maternal history.

Calverley RK, Johnston AE: The anaesthetic management of the tracheooesophageal fistula: A review of ten years' experience. Can Anaesth Soc J 19:270–282, 1972

Smith RM: Anesthesia for Infants and Children, pp 309–310. St Louis, C.V. Mosby, 1980

Thein RMH, Epstein BS: General Surgical Procedures in the Child with a Congenital Anomaly. In Stehling LC and Zauder HL (eds): Anesthetic Implications of Congenital Anomalies in Children, pp 91–92. New York, Appleton-Century-Crofts, 1980

B.2. Discuss the classification of patients with t-e fistulae or atresia according to Waterston or Calverley. What is the implication for this patient?

The classification according to the criteria of Waterston includes five groups.

- Group A—birth weight more than 2500 grams and well
- Group B_1—birth weight 1800–2500 grams and well
- Group B_2—higher birth weight (> 2500 gm) moderate pneumonia and congenital anomaly
- Group C_1—birth weight less than 1800 grams
- Group C_2—higher birth weight and severe pneumonia and severe congenital anomaly

In Calverley's 10 year report, 100% of groups A, B_1, and B_2 survived. Survival rate was 22% in group C_1 and 59% in C_2. On the basis of this classification, our infant, weighing 2200 grams and with an early diagnosis, has an excellent chance of survival, assuming there is no severe congenital anomaly. Smith noted an association of t-e fistula exceeding 50% in infants weighing less than 2500 grams.

Calverley RK, Johnston AE: The anaesthetic management of tracheooesophageal fistula: A review of ten years' experience. Can Anaesth Soc J 19:270–282, 1972

Smith RM: Anesthesia for Infants and Children, p 309. St Louis, C.V. Mosby, 1980

B.3. Discuss fluid replacement in this patient.

Unless dehydration is obviously apparent, which should not be the case in this infant, fluid replacement should be conservative. Approximately 4 ml/kg/hr should be sufficient, with allowances for suction and gastric drainage and blood loss. Because of the high incidence of congenital cardiac disease (15%) associated with t-e fistula, special care is required to prevent overload. The diagnosis of congenital cardiac disease cannot always be made early and should remain suspect until ruled out. A solution of dextrose 5% in 1/4 strength normal saline, may be used at the rates suggested above. The use of a Halter pump will prevent administration of excessive fluid.

Smith RM: Anesthesia for Infants and Children, p 312. St. Louis, C.V. Mosby, 1980

B.4. What is the preoperative or postoperative role of antibiotics?

It is standard practice to use antibiotics to control pulmonary infection. Specifically, a broad spectrum antibiotic is used. Postoperatively, antibiotics are used for the same purpose. In addition, antibiotics are used to control infection if there is anastomotic leak. The presence of chemical pneumonitis secondary to reflux is more serious.

Redo F: Surgery in the First Six Months of Life, p 67. Hagerstown, Harper & Row, 1976

Smith RM: Anesthesia for Infants and Children, p 310. St Louis, C.V. Mosby, 1980

B.5. Discuss the role of gastrostomy in the management of t-e fistulae.

Gastrostomy may be performed as a first step. The presence of a functioning gastrostomy will decrease the possibility of gastric distention and prevent reflux of gastric contents into the lungs. It is necessary to maintain proper nutrition in the pre- or post-repair period. If gastrostomy is not undertaken as a first step, it will be performed during the definitive repair, for all of the above mentioned reasons.

In some cases, as in acute distention of the stomach with elevation and immobilization of the diaphragm, gastrostomy may be a life-saving maneuver. In premature or critically ill infants, it is the first step undertaken in a staged repair, which is later followed by ligation of the fistula. Still later, when the condition of the infant has improved sufficiently, the esophageal atresia will be repaired.

Calverley RK, Johnston AE: The anesthetic management of tracheoesophageal fistula: A review of ten years' experience. Can Anaesth Soc J 19:270–282, 1972

Redo FS: Principles of Surgery in the First Six Months of Life, p 64. Hagerstown, Harper & Row, 1976

B.6. What premedication is indicated in this patient?

Atropine is indicated, to decrease secretions and to prevent the bradycardia associated with halothane anesthesia. Bradycardia also may occur during traction on the hilum or the vagus during mobilization of the esophagus. The dose of atropine has been variously given as 0.01 to 0.02 mg/kg intramuscularly. Sedation is not required preoperatively, but anti-

68 · Anesthesiology

biotics should be given preoperatively and postoperatively to prevent or control pulmonary infection.

Calverley RK, Johnston AE: The anesthetic management of tracheoesophageal fistula: A review of ten years' experience. Can Anaesth Soc J 19:272–280, 1972

Smith RM: Anesthesia for Infants and Children, p 312. St Louis, C.V. Mosby, 1980

Thein RMH: Epstein BS: General Surgical Procedures in the Child with a Congenital Anomaly. In Stehling LC and Zauder HL (eds): Anesthetic Implications of Congenital Anomalies in Children, p 74. New York, Appleton-Century-Crofts, 1980

C. Intraoperative Management

C.1. Discuss the problems associated with transporting the neonate to the operating room.

Every effort must be made to prevent or control the aspiration of secretions from the blind upper pouch, secretions of which may cause pneumonia or atelectasis, and to prevent reflux of gastric contents through the fistula into the trachea and lungs. The chemical pneumonia produced from reflux can be serious. For this reason, the blind upper pouch is placed on continuous suction, utilizing a sump tube, and the infant is maintained and transported in the semi-sitting position. Koop and associates favor a head up but face down position for better control of tracheal secretions.

Koop CE et al: Esophageal atresia and tracheoesophageal fistula: Supportive measures that affect survival. Pediatrics 54:558, 1974

Smith RM: Anesthesia for Infants and Children, p 310. St Louis, C.V. Mosby, 1980

C.2. Discuss the problems of induction and intubation. Would you put the endotracheal tube above or beyond the fistula?

During induction, gastric distention and immobilization of the diaphragm (causing respiratory embarrassment) is always a potential problem. Bradycardia and severe cardiac depression have been reported secondary to gastric dilatation in cases of t-e fistula. For this reason, spontaneous respiration is preferred to assisted or controlled respiration during induction or until the fistula is ligated. Frequently, the infant can be intubated while awake after preoxygenation, but a struggling infant can regurgitate from the stomach into the trachea by way of the distal fistulous tract. If a prior gastrostomy has been performed, anesthetic gases may pass out of the lungs to the stomach. Partial clamping of the gastrostomy tube may be necessary.

The endotracheal tube should be large enough to permit easy suctioning, and a small leak around the endotracheal tube is recommended by many anesthesiologists (Smith RM, Calverley RK). This will also prevent gastric distention when assisted or controlled ventilation is employed. Salem advocates using an endotracheal tube without a Murphy eye, placed first into the right main stem bronchus and then withdrawn until breath sounds are heard bilaterally, but not over the stomach. The endotracheal tube is placed with the bevel facing anteriorly and down. The tracheal opening of the fistula is blocked by the endotracheal tube. This supposes that the fistula is above the carina and posterior. This is not a substitute for gastrostomy.

Another technique involves passing the endotracheal tube beyond the fistulous opening until the fistula is ligated, at which time the tube is withdrawn to ensure ventilation of both lungs. In this case, using a Murphy eye endotracheal tube will ensure adequate ventilation on the left side even if the endotracheal tube enters the right stem bronchus. If a gastrostomy has been performed previously, it will permit decompression of the stomach and will decrease the problem of distention and reflux. Secretions from an infected right upper lobe can enter the trachea or endotracheal tube and must be removed. Retraction of the right lung can cause obstruction of the endotracheal tube and impairment of ventilation to the dependent lower lung.

Calverley RK, Johnston AE: The anesthetic management of tracheoesophageal fistula: A review of ten years' experience. Can Anaesth Soc J 19:270, 1972

Salem MR et al: Prevention of gastric distention during anesthesia for newborns with tracheoesophageal fistulas. Anesthesiology 38:83, 1973

Smith RM: Anesthetic Management of Tracheoesophageal Atresia in Anesthesia for Infants and Children, p 313. St Louis, C.V. Mosby, 1980

C.3. In what position will surgery be performed? Is this important?

Gastrostomy is performed in the 45° head-up position, but the definitive repair requires that the infant be placed in the left lateral position and the thoracotomy performed under the right scapula in the fourth or fifth interspace. Secretions from the right upper lobe, in particular, can be a problem in this position, draining into the trachea and dependent lung. Frequent suctioning may be needed to prevent obstruction of the endotracheal tube by these secretions or by blood.

Traction on the upper lung is common during surgery and may kink the main bronchus of the dependent lung. A stethoscope placed in the dependent axilla will aid in the diagnosis of airway obstruction due to blood, mucus, purulent exudate or kinking.

Calverley RK, Johnston AE: The anesthetic management of tracheoesophageal fistula: A review of ten years' experience. Can Anaesth Soc J 19:270, 1972

Redo SF: Principles of Surgery in the First Six Months of Life, p 65. Hagerstown, Harper & Row, 1976

C.4. What problems can be anticipated during surgery? How can you maintain a stable mediastinum? Is there a role for muscle relaxants?

The problems anticipated during surgery have been discussed before. Prior to opening the chest, the infant breathes spontaneously to avoid over distention of the stomach. When the chest has been opened, respirations are gently assisted until the fistula is ligated. During repair of the esophagus, an absolutely stable mediastinum is essential for a good result. Pancuronium, metocurine, or d-tubocurarine can be used for muscle relaxation. Controlled ventilation is used, and a small amount of continuous positive airway pressure (CPAP) may be needed to maintain mediastinal stability.

Endobronchial intubation can occur at any time during the procedure and must be corrected. Blood or mucus can obstruct the endotracheal tube and must be suctioned. Surgical manipulation can also obstruct the endotracheal tube or the trachea itself. Bradycardia may occur from traction and requires treatment with atropine in doses of 0.01 to 0.02 mg/kg. Frequent expansion of the collapsed or retracted lung during surgical manipulation is advocated by some anesthesiologists. This must be done in consultation with the surgeon so that it does not interfere with the repair. A degree of trespass may be necessary to accomplish the surgery.

Smith RM: Anesthesia for Infants and Children, pp 312–313. St Louis, C.V. Mosby, 1980

C.5. What type of monitoring will you use?

An ECG for rate and rhythm and a reliable blood pressure monitor. In children with complicated cardiac lesions, an intra-arterial cannula will permit frequent blood gas sampling as well as blood pressure monitoring. A precordial stethoscope under the left chest wall will monitor both respiratory and cardiac rates and quality. It will also detect the presence of secretions. An esophageal stethoscope is not indicated because of the danger of perforating the blind upper pouch.

Hypothermia can be dangerous. Temperature must be monitored throughout. In addition, the anesthesiologist must be careful to maintain normothermia by using overhead heaters, warm rooms, and a thermal mattress. Fluids and blood should be warmed prior to administration. Blood loss should be measured accurately by weighing sponges promptly and collecting suction in graduated containers.

Smith RM: Anesthesia for Infants and Children, p 312. St Louis, C.V. Mosby, 1980

C.6. What emergency drugs should be available?

- Atropine, diluted to 0.04 mg/ml. Give 3 to 4 ml or 0.12 to 0.16 mg
- Calcium chloride, 20 mg/kg
- Epinephrine, 1 mg/ml diluted to 0.1 mg/ml. Give 0.1 ml/kg.
- Phenylephrine 0.1 to 1 Mg (microgram)

Atropine is given for bradycardia, to remove any vagal component. Calcium and epinephrine are used as inotropic agents. Phenylephrine is utilized to produce peripheral vasoconstriction.

D. Postoperative Management

D.1. When can this infant be extubated?

If nondepolarizing relaxants have been used, they must be reversed. The anesthetic, most commonly halothane (with or without nitrous oxide), must be discontinued early enough to permit spontaneous respiration. Most infants can be extubated at the end of the procedure. The endotracheal tube must be suctioned and the lungs inflated with oxygen prior to extubation. Be careful to avoid stress on the suture line. If pulmonary complications are present, postoperative mechanical ventilation may be needed.

Smith RM: Anesthesia for Infants and Children, p 313. St Louis, C.V. Mosby, 1980

Thein RMH, Epstein BS: General Surgical Procedures in the Child with a Congenital Anomaly. In Stehling LC and Zauder HL (eds): Anesthetic Implications of Congenital Anomalies in Children, p 94–95. New York, Appleton-Century-Crofts, 1980

D.2. What are the dangers of extubating an infant who is depressed, cold, or asleep?

Apnea can ensue. Infants are allowed to wake up, move their extremities, and open their eyes before the endotracheal tube is removed. They are kept warm and are observed for a period of time in the operating room until it is safe to take them to an intensive care unit or recovery room.

Smith RM: Anesthesia for Infants and Children, p 303. St Louis, C.V. Mosby, 1980

D.3. What are the complications seen following tracheoesophageal fistulae repair?

Complications can be divided into the following two categories:
- Complications that existed prior to surgery, such as continuing pneumonia, and problems related to other congenital anomalies, especially cardiovascular.
- Complications that occur as a result of surgery, such as pneumothorax, atelectasis, anastomotic leaks, esophageal stricture, subcutaneous emphysema, recurrent laryngeal nerve injury, and recurrent fistula.

The principal causes of death are pulmonary complications (62%), associated anomalies (43%), and anastomotic leaks (21%).

Redo SF: Principles of Surgery in the First Six Months of Life, pp 66–69. Hagerstown, Harper & Row, 1976

D.4. Discuss the management of postoperative pneumonia or atelectasis. Are these anesthetic complications?

Pulmonary complications are treated with antibiotics, suctioning, high humidity, chest physiotherapy, and promotion of crying. These are probably not anesthetic complications but are the result of traction on the lung during surgery or preexisting infection from reflux or aspiration. Care must be taken at the end of surgery to reinflate the lungs and suction the trachea adequately.

Redo SF: Principles of Surgery in the First Six Months of Life, pp 66–67. Hagerstown, Harper & Row, 1976

Section Two
The Cardiovascular System

6 Congenital Heart Disease and Profound Hypothermia

Marjorie J. Topkins

This four-week-old infant was profoundly cyanotic at birth. A Raskind balloon septostomy was performed at one day and some improvement was noted. The patient is scheduled for a Mustard repair under profound hypothermia. Weight, 3200 g; temperature, 37°C; respiration, 50/min; pulse, 140/min; BP, 60/30 torr.

A. Medical Disease and Differential Diagnosis

1. What is the diagnosis?
2. Describe the pathology in transposition of the great arteries (TGA).
3. What is a Raskind balloon septostomy? Why is it performed?
4. What is the embryologic mechanism for the production of TGA?
5. What is the most common form of TGA?
6. What is corrected transposition?
7. What is a Mustard procedure?
8. What effect would the coexistence of a ventricular septal defect have on this patient?
9. If a ventricular septal defect or atrial septal defect coexists with complete TGA, in which direction is the shunt?

B. Preoperative Evaluation and Preparation

1. What preoperative information or preparation do you want?
2. What premedication do you want?

C. Intraoperative Management

1. What emergency drugs will you have available?
2. What monitoring will you prepare?
3. What laboratory data will you collect?

76 · Anesthesiology

4. How will you anesthetize this infant? What agents will you use?
5. How do you establish hypothermia?
6. What is profound hypothermia?
7. How do you classify hypothermia? How long can patients tolerate arrest during hypothermia?
8. What is the rationale for combined surface and core cooling for profound hypothermia?
9. Discuss the physiologic and pathologic changes associated with hypothermia.
10. What effect does this technique have on anesthetic time and pump time?
11. Discuss arrhythmias during hypothermia.
12. How is warming accomplished?

D. Postoperative Management

1. Discuss postoperative ventilation.
2. How do you manage postoperative secretions?
3. What are some of the complications that might be expected in this case?

A. Medical Disease and Differential Diagnosis

A.1. What is the diagnosis?

The Raskind balloon septostomy is performed at the time of cardiac catheterization in infants with transposition of the great arteries. Therefore, the presumptive diagnosis is transposition. Tricuspid atresia similarly may require a septostomy, but the incidence of atresia is 1/3 to 1/4 that of transposition. Other diagnostic criteria include an egg-shaped heart on PA chest x-ray with a narrow base and indistinct pulmonary artery.

Krovetz LJ, Gesner IH, Schrebler GL: Handbook of Pediatric Cardiology, p 230. New York, Hoeber Medical Division, Harper & Row, 1969

A.2. Describe the pathology in transposition of the great arteries (TGA).

In the most common form, the aorta arises from the right ventricle and the pulmonary artery arises from the left ventricle. No mixing of blood occurs unless an atrial or ventricular septal defect exists or is created. A life-threatening condition exists without venous–arterial mixing. A second component of TGA is the transposed positions of the aorta and pulmonary artery. In the normally developed heart, the aorta is posterior and to the left, and the pulmonary artery is anterior and to the right. In TGA, however, this relationship is reversed. The aorta is anterior and to the right, and the pulmonary artery is posterior and to the left. Physiologically, the normal pulmonary and systemic circulations are in series—the blood flows from right atrium to right ventricle to pulmonary artery and back from the lungs through the pulmonary veins to the left atrium, left ventricle and then out to the body by way of the aorta. In transposition of the great arteries, the pulmonary and systemic circulations are parallel. The blood passes from the right side of the heart to the aorta back to the right side, and the blood from the left side goes to the lung back to the left side. In the absence of a naturally occurring defect, one must be created to permit arteriovenous mixing.

TGA is the seventh or eighth most common congenital heart condition. The incidence is approximately 5% of all congenital heart disease and approximately 19% of autopsies in infants under one month of age at Boston Childrens' Hospital. The incidence in males is 3 times that of females.

Nadas AS, Fyler DC: Pediatric Cardiology, p 608. Philadelphia, WB Saunders, 1972

A.3. *What is a Raskind balloon septostomy? Why is it performed?*

A Raskind septostomy is performed by passing a balloon tipped catheter into the left atrium by way of the foramen ovale and pulling the distended balloon sharply back into the inferior vena cava creating a functional atrial septal defect. It is performed whenever an obligatory shunt is needed to establish a site of venous–arterial mixing.

Nadas AS, Fyler DC: Pediatric Cardiology, p 123. Philadelphia, WB Saunders, 1972

A.4. *What is the embryologic mechanism for the production of TGA?*

In the three-week-old embryo, the primitive cardiac tube is a ventricle structure consisting of five chambers. Most caudad is the sinus venosus from which the posterior portion of the right and left atria will arise. Next is the atrial canal which will produce the atrial appendage, then the ventricular canal which will become the left ventricle. Proceeding cephalad is the bulbus cordis which will contribute the right ventricular inflow and outflow tracts. Most cephalad is the truncus arteriosus which gives rise to the aorta and pulmonary arteries.

This original straight tube undergoes changes, usually looping to the right at about the third week and swinging of the apex from the right to the left (D-loop) at about the fifth week. When this occurs, the right ventricle is on the right and the left ventricle is on the left. If looping occurs to the left, the right ventricle is on the left (L-loop). Previously, researchers thought that transposition occurred because of a straight-line division of the bulbar trunk instead of the usual spiraling division. Now researchers assume that transposition is the result of disturbances of differential conal growth.

The current hypothesis postulates that in the straight tube stage, the aorta is anterior and the pulmonary artery posterior. If looping to the right occurs, the aorta is anterior and to the right; if looping to the left occurs, the aorta is anterior and to the left. In the normal heart, there is overdevelopment of the subpulmonary conus and underdevelopment of the subaortic conus and the pulmonary valve is lifted above the level of the aortic valve. In transposition, the subaortic conus is overdeveloped and the subpulmonary conus is underdeveloped; the aortic valve remains anterior to the pulmonary valve. Because true circulation is established in the four-week-old embryo and the ventricular septum is fully developed by the end of the seventh week, we can assume that congenital heart alterations develop by the eighth week.

Nadas AS, Fyler DC: Pediatric Cardiology, pp 609–611. Philadelphia, WB Saunders, 1972

A.5. What is the most common form of TGA?

The most common form of complete transposition is D-loop, with the right ventricle on the right and the aorta anterior and to the right of the pulmonary artery. Blood flows from the cavae to the right atrium, by way of the tricuspid valve to the right ventricle, out the anterior aorta to the body, and back to the right atrium. The blood exits the left ventricle through a posterior pulmonary artery to the lungs and back again to the left side of the heart. The two parallel circuits never mix unless there is a septal defect, a patent foramen ovale, or a patent ductus arteriosus.

Krovetz LJ, Gessner IH, Schiebler GL: In Chapter 18 of Handbook of Pediatric Cardiology, p 228. New York, Hoeber Medical Division, Harper & Row, 1969

A.6. What is corrected transposition?

Many variations of transposition occur. The vessels can be anatomically transposed in their anteroposterior relationship but physiologically normal, or normal in the anteroposterior relationship and physiologically transposed. In corrected transposition, there is looping to the left so that the right ventricle is on the left. The aorta is anterior to the pulmonary artery and on the left. The resulting transposition is physiologically normal. Blood flows from the cavae to the right atrium through a mitral valve to the left ventricle, out the pulmonary artery to the lungs, back to the left atrium of the heart through the pulmonary veins, through the tricuspid valve to the right ventricle situated on the left. The blood exits from this right ventricle to the body by way of the anterior aorta. The flow is physiologic. No surgical correction is needed.

Braunwald E: Heart Disease, p 1034. Philadelphia, WB Saunders, 1980

A.7. What is a Mustard procedure?

A Mustard procedure is a technique used for total correction of transposition of the great arteries. It consists of excision of the atrial septum and the creation of a tunnel or baffle (from pericardium) which directs blood returning to the right atrium from the vena cavae to the mitral valve and the left ventricle. From the left ventricle, the blood passes to the pulmonary artery. Blood returning from the lung through the pulmonary veins passes around this tunnel exiting the atrium by way of the tricuspid valve to the right ventricle and out the aorta. The left ventricle has, therefore, become the supplier of the lesser circulation (pulmonary) and the right ventricle has become the systemic ventricle.

Braunwald E: Heart Disease, p 1033. Philadelphia, WB Saunders, 1980

A.8. What effect would the coexistence of a ventricular septal defect (VSD) have on this patient?

Infants with transposition and VSD present with congestive failure but without the profound cyanosis present in TGA without the VSD. If there is some degree of pulmonic obstruction, the VSD will allow mixing without undue pulmonary vascular overload. This will buy some time and allow the neonate to grow before surgery is needed. If there is increased pulmonary blood flow, the infant is at greater risk, and without surgery the infant will probably not survive beyond 5 months of age. Pulmonary artery banding will protect the pulmonary vasculature if complete correction cannot be performed.

Nadas AS, Fyler DC: Pediatric Cardiology, pp 621–627. Philadelphia, WB Saunders, 1972

A.9. If a ventricular septal defect or atrial septal defect coexists with complete TGA, in which direction is the shunt?

The shunt is bidirectional; the left to right flow is equal to the right to left flow.

Nadas AS, Fyler DC: Pediatric Cardiology, pp 617–619. Philadelphia, WB Saunders, 1972

B. Preoperative Evaluation and Preparation

B.1. What preoperative information or preparation do you want?

The history and physical examination, a summary of the cardiac catheterization data, the chest x-ray (posteroanterioral and lateral), and the electrocardiogram are needed. Laboratory data must be checked. A complete blood count, urine analysis, blood sugar, and urea nitrogen are recorded. The following electrolytes are obtained: sodium, potassium, calcium, chloride, and bicarbonate. A blood coagulation profile that consists of prothrombin time, partial thromboplastin time, and the platelet count is also obtained. The patient's blood should be typed and cross matched, and an adequate supply of blood must be available. Plans should be made to obtain a unit of fresh blood drawn the morning of surgery. Studies of arterial blood gases are useful and should be obtained if not previously done. From the gases, the degree of metabolic imbalance can be assessed and treated prior to the onset of anesthesia.

Bland JW, Williams WH: Anesthesia for treatment of congenital heart defects. In Kaplan, JA (ed): Cardiac Anesthesia, pp 290–291. New York, Grune & Stratton, 1979

B.2. What premedication do you want?

Infants this small and sick do not need sedation, but atropine, 0.01 mg/kg, intramuscularly may be given approximately 1 hour prior to induction. Infants respond to hypoxia with bradycardia, which is treated with atropine and oxygen. Whether given preoperatively or not, atropine must be available for emergency use.

Kaplan JA: Cardiac Anesthesia, p 504. New York, Grune & Stratton, 1979

C. Intraoperative Management

C.1. What emergency drugs will you have available?

- Atropine diluted to 0.04 mg/ml
- Sodium bicarbonate 1 mEq/ml
- Vasopressor
   Phenylephrine diluted to 0.1 mg/ml; give 50-mcg bolus
   Calcium chloride, 100 mg/ml; give 20 mg/kg, IV
- Lidocaine 1%; give 0.5 to 1.0 mg/kg, IV
- Chlorpromazine diluted to 1 mg/ml

Propranolol and dopamine should be available, but not mixed. We maintain a cart with all drugs that might conceivably be used. This cart has storage for needles, syringes, fluid administration sets, and fluids.

Kaplan JA: Cardiac Anesthesia, pp 333–337. New York, Grune & Stratton, 1979

C.2. What monitoring will you prepare?

For induction, we use the following monitors: precordial stethoscope, a means of determining blood pressure (Infrasonde or Doppler), electrocardiogram, oxygen analyzer for F_IO_2. For maintenance, we monitor as follows: intra-arterial line, central venous catheter and pressure, esophageal stethoscope, temperature—two sites (esophageal or nasopharyngeal and rectal), electrocardiogram, Foley catheter in bladder, and oxygen analyzer for F_IO_2.

A precordial stethoscope permits the continuous monitoring of both heart beat and respirations. Early detection of myocardial depression, respiratory obstruction, or apnea is possible. Moreover, early detection is necessary to anticipate and avoid complications.

The use of a reliable blood pressure monitor may be needed for 20 or 30 minutes if the cut down on the tiny radial artery is prolonged. The electrocardiogram will pick up arrhythmias or give evidence of ischemia. A rhythm strip taken prior to anesthesia provides a printed reference against which subsequent tracings may be compared. The arterial line and central venous pressure will monitor the cardiac performance and permit sampling of blood for gases. The esophageal stethoscope provides the same information as the precordial stethoscope which has now been removed from the operative field.

The urinary catheter gives evidence of adequate tissue perfusion (at least the kidney perfusion) and monitors urinary output both in the operating room and in the intensive-care unit. If the smallest Foley will not pass, a small polyethylene feeding tube placed in the bladder will serve the same purpose.

Esophageal or nasopharyngeal temperature reflects the core temperature and is used during the cooling period. Rectal temperature lags behind esophageal temperature during warming and is used to determine when cardiopulmonary bypass may be discontinued.

New York Hospital Protocol for Profound Hypothermia.
Kaplan JA: Cardiac Anesthesia, pp 296–306. New York, Grune & Stratton, 1979

C.3. What laboratory data will you collect?

The following laboratory data should be obtained:

- Blood gases—pH, P_{CO_2}, P_{O_2}, oxygen saturation and bicarbonate
- Hematocrit
- Activated clotting time
- Urinary output
- Sodium and potassium
- Ionized calcium if available

Blood gases are obtained to determine the level of oxygenation and the presence of acidosis. The activated clotting times will be necessary for anticoagulation as well as reversal.

Kaplan JA: Cardiac Anesthesia, pp 303–306. New York, Grune & Stratton, 1979

C.4. How will you anesthetize this infant? What agents will you use?

At the New York Hospital, after a blood pressure is obtained by using the Infrasonde or the Doppler technique, and the electrodes for electrocardiography have been placed on the extremities or back, the infant is induced using halothane, nitrous oxide, and oxygen and a modified Jackson–Rees nonrebreathing system. The F_IO_2 is kept at approximately 40% to 50% to avoid the possibility of retrolental fibroplasia. Two short (1¼-inch) 18 gauge intravenous catheters are placed in a vein in the hands or in the feet. Simultaneously, a cut down is performed on the left wrist and the radial artery is cannulated for both pressures and blood samples. Fluids are 5% dextrose in 1/4 strength normal saline. Intubation is accomplished when the intravenous catheter is present usually without the use of muscle relaxants, but occasionally utilizing succinylcholine, 1 mg/kg. Once intubated with a suitable endotracheal tube, the infant is ventilated using a modified Jackson–Rees technique. The Bloomquist pediatric circle has been used in the past with equally satisfactory results. A central venous pressure line is then placed by way of the external or internal jugular veins, if possible. Other institutions have utilized Ketamine for induction with muscle relaxants.

Kaplan JA: Cardiac Anesthesia, p 294. New York, Grune & Stratton, 1979

Radney PA: Anesthetic Consideration for Pediatric Cardiac Surgery, p. 109. Boston, Little, Brown & Co, 1980

C.5. How do you establish hypothermia?

Once intubated, thermistor probes are placed in the rectum and esophagus, and a urinary catheter placed in the bladder. The hands and feet are wrapped in cotton batting and the genitalia are similarly protected. From the time of intubation until all the lines are in place, ice bags are used in conjunction with the cooling mattress to begin the cooling process. When all of the preliminary work is accomplished, the infant is positioned and the operative site is washed; the entire skin surface is then covered with gauze. A large ice-filled plastic bag is placed on the infant and cooling continues until the esophageal temperature is 30°C. At this time, heparin, 300 IU/kg, is administered intravenously and cooling continued until the temperature reaches 25° to 27°C. Usually, 1 mg of chlorpromazine is given empirically to prevent vasoconstriction during the cooling process. When the esophageal temperature has reached 25° to 27°C, the ice bags are removed. The infant, already positioned, need only be prepped with Betadine and draped. Surgery is begun.

Further cooling to approximately 15°C is accomplished after cardiopulmonary bypass is established. In the infant less than 6 months or under 6 to 7 kg, the Mustard procedure is carried out utilizing circulatory arrest. In older or bigger children more conventional perfusion techniques are utilized with flows appropriate to the lowered temperature. Antibiotics are administered intravenously once an intravenous line has been established, and again after coming off pump.

During cooling, the anesthetic concentration is gradually decreased, but spontaneous ventilation has been observed at temperatures as low as 22°. It is not necessary to add carbon dioxide to the inspired gases, as reported by the Toronto group, but ventilation is decreased progressively as the temperature is lowered. Blood gases are followed to determine the metabolic state of the infant.

Arrhythmias are rare; the major ECG change has been sinus bradycardia and a prolonged QT interval. The rectal and esophageal temperatures are followed, but surgery is not begun until the esophageal temperature is 25° to 27°C. The rectal temperature declines more rapidly than the esophageal temperature during surface cooling.

Engle MA: Pediatric Cardiovascular Disease, p 343. Philadelphia, F.A. Davis, 1981

Johnston et al: Acid-base and electrolyte changes in infants undergoing profound hypothermia. Can Anaesth Soc J 21:23, 1974

C.6. What is profound hypothermia?

Profound hypothermia, the reduction of core temperature to approximately 15°C and subsequent circulatory arrest, is utilized in the correction of congenital cardiac lesions, especially in young infants. The hypothermia is accomplished by a combination of surface cooling and cooling during cardiopulmonary bypass. When the temperature reaches 15°C, the cannulae are removed and the repair is accomplished under circulatory arrest. At 15°C, the safe circulatory arrest time is approximately 1 hour. The advantages of this method include decreased oxygen demand by all organs, more uniform cooling of the entire body, preservation of myocardium and, most important, with a quiet relaxed heart and no cannulae interfering, the surgical correction is facilitated.

Disadvantages of this technique include prolongation of anesthetic time, the possibility of neurologic sequelae secondary to tissue hypoxia, postoperative bleeding from coagulation problems, possible cold injury to the skin and extremities, metabolic acidosis, and the possibility of ventricular fibrillation as the temperature decreases below 26° to 27°C.

Kaplan JA : Cardiac Anesthesia, pp 321–324. New York, Grune & Stratton, 1979

C.7. How do you classify hypothermia? How long can patients tolerate arrest during hypothermia?

Mild hypothermia is a reduction of temperature to 30°C. Moderate hypothermia is observed when the temperature is between 30° and 25°C. Deep hypothermia is a further reduction of temperature to between 25° and 20°C. Profound hypothermia involves temperature between 20° and 10°C.

Metabolism is reduced 40% to 50% at 30°C, 60% at 25°C, 75% at 20°C, and 85% at 10°C. At temperature greater than 32°C, 3 to 9 minutes of circulatory arrest is tolerated. Between 32° and 28°C, arrest can be prolonged to 9 to 15 minutes. Further cooling to 28° to 18°C will permit arrest periods from 15 to 45 minutes. Below 18°C, arrest can be tolerated up to one hour. Infants show higher tolerance to hypothermia with circulatory arrest than do older children and adults.

Benazon D: Hypothermia, in Scientific Foundations of Anaesthesia, pp 334–357, Chicago, Year Book Medical Publishers, 1974

Rodney PA: Anesthetic Considerations for Pediatric Cardiac Surgery, pp 133–147. Boston, Little Brown & Co, 1980

C.8. What is the rationale for using combined surface and core cooling for profound hypothermia?

Hypothermia, established by a combination of surface cooling and cardiopulmonary bypass, permits slower cooling and, we hope, uniform cooling of the patient. Rapid cooling might be nonuniform. Insufficiently cooled areas would suffer severe hypoxia when circulatory arrest was instituted. If these areas were in the brain, serious complications would ensue.

Barrett–Boyes BG, Simpson M, Nentz JM: Intracardiac surgery in neonates and infants using deep hypothermia with surface cooling and limited cardiopulmonary bypass. Circulation: Suppl I to Vol 43 and 44, 125–130, 1971

C.9. Discuss the physiologic and pathologic changes associated with hypothermia.

Metabolism parallels the fall in temperature provided shivering is prevented. Both shivering and vasoconstriction can be prevented with nondepolarizing muscle relaxants and chlorpromazine. The oxygen dissociation curve is shifted to the left during hypothermia and this inhibits the release of oxygen from hemoglobin. The solubility of oxygen in plasma is increased with cold, as is the solubility of carbon dioxide and anesthetic gases. There is some increase in the viscosity of the blood due to hemoconcentration. This increased viscosity increases the oxygen carrying capacity, but can lead to sludging. This danger can be minimized by giving heparin when the core temperature reaches 30°C. The dose of heparin administered is 300 IU/kg. Additionally, hemodilution with priming solution is achieved during cardiopulmonary bypass. Metabolic acidosis can occur if perfusion is nonuniform. Frequent blood gas determinations will establish this diagnosis. Metabolic acidosis is treated by increasing perfusion blood flow and administering sodium bicarbonate using the formula: $0.3 \times$ wt in kg $\times$ base deficit. One half of the calculated dose is given to prevent immediate over-correction.

Arterial blood pressure falls progressively with increased cooling as does the heart rate. The electrocardiogram shows progressive prolongation of the PR, QT, and QRS intervals. ST and T wave changes are seen as well. A consistent finding is the so-called J wave, a small positive wave on the downstroke of the R wave occurring at about 30°C. Cardiac output decreases as hypothermia and bradycardia ensue, but stroke volume is not significantly altered down to 25°C. Hepatic function is depressed by cold. Glucose and citrate are not metabolized. Function returns on rewarming. Renal plasma flow is decreased as temperature and cardiac output fall. Selective reabsorption decreases owing to cold depression of transport mechanisms. Isosmotic reabsorption continues. Urinary output is, therefore, maintained down to 20°C; below this urine flow ceases.

ACTH, epinephrine, and adrenal cortical steroid excretion are increased during hypothermia indicating that hypothermia produces physiologic stress. Cold prolongs the prothrombin and bleeding times due to a decrease in platelets and depression of the fibrinogen activity. A rise in serum potassium has been reported, but has not been seen in our population owing possibly to the use of chlorpromazine and a nondepolarizing muscle relaxant.

Hypothermia produces an increase in the anatomical dead space (70%–90% increase at 28°C). The respiratory rate is decreased by decreasing oxygen consumption. Alveolar and arterial carbon dioxide tensions are normal. Respirations cease at 20°C.

Benazon D: Hypothermia. In Scientific Foundations of Anaesthesia, pp 334–357. Chicago, Year Book Medical Publishers, 1974

Rodney PA: Anesthetic Considerations for Pediatric Cardiac Surgery, pp 133–147. Boston, International Anesthesiology Clinics, Little, Brown & Co, 1980

C.10. What effect does this technique have on anesthetic time and pump time?

Surface cooling is time consuming and usually requires more than 1 hour to obtain 25°C. In recent years, at the New York Hospital, surgery begins when the core temperature is 28° to 30°C. This modification has reduced the anesthetic time. Because the surgery is performed under total circulatory arrest, the total pump time is reduced.

C.11. Discuss arrhythmias during hypothermia.

During induction of hypothermia, arrhythmias are a potential problem. Ventricular fibrillation is particularly dangerous. In our experience, ventricular fibrillation has occurred in only a few cases, at temperatures of 22° to 23°C and only when the heart was manipulated. At this low temperature and with the heart exposed, the patients were simply put on cardiopulmonary bypass and cooling continued. Sinus bradycardia does occur with cooling and is progressive as the temperature declines. Small doses of atropine can be used to ameliorate this bradycardia if desired.

Steward DJ, Sloan IA, Johnston AE: Anesthetic management of infants undergoing profound hypothermia for surgical correction of congenital heart defects. Can Anaesth Soc J 21:15–22, 1974

C.12. How is warming accomplished?

Rewarming to 33°C rectally is accomplished by cardiopulmonary bypass. The esophageal temperature is usually two to three degrees higher. The mattress previously used for cooling is warmed to approximately 40° to 41°C. This will prevent loss of heat until the chest wound is closed. As warming takes place, the peripheral circulation improves. At this time, a metabolic acidosis may be seen due to a wash out of the acid metabolites from the tissues.

Rodney PA: Anesthetic Considerations for Pediatric Cardiac Surgery, p 142. Boston, International Anesthesiology Clinics, Little, Brown & Co, 1980

Smith RM: Anesthesia for Infants and Children, pp 378–379. St Louis, C.V. Mosby, 1980

D. Postoperative Management

D.1. Discuss postoperative ventilation.

At the New York Hospital, we reverse the muscle relaxant if necessary. We permit the infant to wake up and extubate in the operating room. The infant is observed for several minutes. If the infant's color remains good and respiration is unlabored, the infant is transported to the ICU in an oxygen atmosphere. If the infant's color is not good or respiration appears labored, the infant is reintubated in the operating room and placed on a ventilator in the ICU. Most infants are extubated immediately. The problems of obstructed endotracheal tubes are thus eliminated.

There is some disagreement about whether or not postoperative ventilation is desirable for this group of patients. Some physicians including those at the New York Hospital, feel that there are fewer pulmonary complications when the endotracheal tube is removed early. Others feel that 12 to 24 hours of mechanical ventilation is desirable.

Kaplan JA: Cardiac Anesthesia, p 319. New York, Grune & Stratton, 1979

Smith RM: Anesthesia for Treatment of Congenital Heart Disease, p 376. St Louis, C.V. Mosby, 1980

D.2. *How do you manage postoperative secretions?*

Infants do not cough well and secretions can be a genuine problem. All our patients are seen twice daily by the chest physiotherapist, more often if necessary. If indicated, the infant can be reintubated and the trachea and bronchi can be suctioned with the aid of small amounts of saline instilled into the endotracheal tube. Large plugs and inspissated material are often obtained. The endotracheal tube is removed following the tracheobronchial toilet. Only rarely is an infant reintubated and placed on a ventilator. Tracheostomy also is rarely indicated.

D.3. *What are some of the complications that might be expected in this case?*

Complications can be divided into those possibly produced by the hypothermia and circulatory arrest, and those that are the result of surgical repair.

Local complications consist of thermal injuries to the skin, fingers, toes, and genitalia. These can be prevented by meticulous care during the cooling period. The extremities are wrapped in cotton and the genitalia are covered. Direct contact with the ice is avoided. Neurologic sequelae have been seen. Many infants have had focal seizures postoperatively which were treated with phenobarbital and diphenylhydantoin. In most cases, seizure activity had ceased by the time the patient was seen by the cardiologist for the first postdischarge visit. Medications were discontinued.

Temporary central blindness or deafness was noted in three patients. In one case, the blindness took almost a year to resolve. When development has been studied, patients treated with profound hypothermic arrest appear to grow not unlike their nonimpaired siblings. Hematologic complications of hypothermia can cause excessive bleeding secondary to a prolonged coagulation time. Fresh whole blood administered post pump replaces clotting factors destroyed during the procedure. Thromboembolic phenomena due to the increased hematocrit and viscosity can also produce neurologic sequelae.

Arrhythmias secondary to the repair have been the major complication not of the cooling, but of surgical placement of the baffle. Atrioventricular dissociation and particularly atrial flutter have been a problem. Superior vena caval obstruction has been another surgical complication and is due to the baffle that obstructs the inflow from the superior vena cava.

Ebert PA, Gay WH, Engle MA: Correction of transposition of great arteries. Am Surg 180:433–438, 1974

Engle MA: Pediatric Cardiovascular Disease, p 343. Philadelphia, F.A. Davis, 1981

Nagashima H: Hypothermia. In Radney PA (ed): Anesthetic Considerations for Pediatric Cardiac Surgery, p 144. Boston, International Anesthesiology Clinics, Little, Brown & Co, 1980

Topkins MJ: Complications of profound hypothermia utilized for the correction of congenital heart disease. Report in Progress for Bull NY Acad Med, 1980

7 Ischemic Heart Disease and Coronary Artery Bypass Graft

Fun-Sun F. Yao

A 57-year-old man with triple coronary artery disease was scheduled for coronary artery bypass graft (CABG). He had a myocardial infarction 7 months ago. He was taking nitroglycerin, digoxin, propranolol, isosorbide dinitrate (Isordil), and nifedipine. His blood pressure was 120/80 torr. His heart rate was 60/m.

A. Medical Disease and Differential Diagnosis

1. What is triple vessel coronary artery disease (CAD)? Name the branches of the coronary arteries.
2. What are the indications for coronary artery bypass graft?
3. What is the incidence of perioperative reinfarction for noncardiac surgery at 0–3 months, 4–6 months, and over 6 months after myocardial infarction?
4. What are the factors increasing the risk of postoperative myocardial infarction after noncardiac surgery?

B. Preoperative Evaluation and Preparation

1. Would you discontinue digoxin? Why? What is its half-life?
2. Would you discontinue propranolol? Why? What is its half-life?
3. If the patient who is on propranolol develops hypotension intraoperatively, how would you manage it?
4. What is nifedipine? How does it work?
5. What preoperative tests would you order?
6. How do you evaluate the patient's left ventricular function?
7. What are the three major determinants of myocardial oxygen consumption? How are they measured clinically?
8. What are the rate pressure product (RPP) and the triple index (TI)?
9. What factors determine myocardial oxygen supply?
10. How would you premedicate the patient? Why?

C. Intraoperative Management

C. I. Before Cardiopulmonary Bypass
1. How do you monitor the patient?
2. What is the Allen test?
3. Why do you need both esophageal and rectal temperatures?
4. How do you know that the Swan–Ganz catheter is in the right ventricle (RV) or pulmonary artery (PA)?
5. What is normal pulmonary capillary wedge pressure (PCWP)?
6. Is it necessary to monitor pulmonary artery pressure for coronary artery operations?
7. What are the complications of Swan–Ganz catheterization?
8. How can you detect myocardial ischemia?
9. How would you monitor ECG? Why V_5?
10. If you don't have precordial leads in your ECG machine, how can you monitor the left ventricle?
11. How would you induce anesthesia?
12. How would you maintain anesthesia?
13. What is the better anesthetic agent for this operation—an inhalational or intravenous agent?
14. What are the cardiovascular effects of halothane, enflurane, isoflurane, morphine, and fentanyl?
15. What is the cardiovascular effect of nitrous oxide?
16. What kind of muscle relaxant would you use? Why?
17. If ST–segment depression is seen during surgery, how would you treat it?
18. How would you correct hypertension?
19. How would you treat hypotension?
20. What are the indications for intravenous propranolol during surgery? How much would you give? What are the relative contraindications?
21. How would you correct increased PCWP?
22. During sternal splitting, would you do something?
23. Would you monitor PCWP continuously? Why?

C. II. During Cardiopulmonary Bypass (CPB)
1. What anticoagulant would you give before CPB? How much would you give? What is its mechanism?
2. What is the half-life of heparin? How is it eliminated?
3. How do you monitor heparin dosage? What is the ACT test?
4. What is total cardiopulmonary bypass? What is partial bypass?
5. What is the purpose of putting a left ventricle sump drain through a pulmonary vein?
6. How may types of oxygenators are there? What are the advantages of each type?
7. What kind of priming solution would you use? How much priming solution would you use? Would you prime with blood or not? Why?
8. What are the advantages and disadvantages of hemodilution?

9. What kind of pumps do you use? Are they pulsatile or not?
10. How do you monitor the patient during CPB?
11. How much blood pressure would you keep during CPB? Why?
12. How would you treat hypotension during CPB?
13. How would you treat hypertension (a mean arterial pressure of over 100 torr)?
14. How do you prepare an intravenous infusion of sodium nitroprusside, phentolamine, and nitroglycerin? What are the usual doses? Which do you prefer to use?
15. How much pump flow would you maintain during CPB?
16. How would you adjust the pump flow during hypothermia?
17. How would you adjust the pump flow during hemodilution?
18. What are the advantages of hypothermia?
19. How does blood viscosity change during hypothermia?
20. What are the main causes of death associated with accidential hypothermia?
21. Would you give anesthesia during CPB? Why?
22. Would you give muscle relaxants during CPB? How is the action of muscle relaxant affected during CPB?
23. How do you know the patient is well perfused during CPB?
24. How much gas flow would you use for the oxygenator? What kind of gas would you use? Why?
25. What are the disadvantages of low $PaCO_2$ during CPB?
26. The arterial blood gases and electrolytes during CPB are: pH, 7.36; $PaCO_2$, 42 torr; PaO_2, 449 torr; CO_2 content, 24 mEq/L; Na, 128 mEq/L; K, 5.8 mEq/L; Ht, 20%. The patient's temperature is 27°C. At what temperature are blood gases measured? How would you correct the blood gases according to patient's body temperature? Would you treat the arterial blood gases at 37°C or at patient's body temperature?
27. If the blood level of the oxygenator is low, what would you replace it with? Blood or balanced salt solution?
28. How do you know the fluid balance during CPB?
29. How would you preserve the myocardium during CPB?
30. What is the cardioplegic solution? How much would you use?
31. For how long a period can the aorta be cross clamped?
32. Why does urine become pink after 2 hours of CPB? What is the renal threshold for plasma hemoglobin?
33. At what temperature can the patient be weaned from CPB?
34. Why does it take longer to rewarm than to cool the patient by the pump oxygenator?
35. How would you defibrillate the heart internally during CPB?
36. Why is calcium chloride usually administered right before the patient comes off the pump?
37. If the heart rate is 40/min, what should you do?
38. How does the blood sugar level change during CPB? Why?
39. What are the effects of CPB on platelet and coagulation factors?

C. III. After Cardiopulmonary Bypass

1. How would you reverse heparin? How much protamine would you use?
2. What is the action mechanism of protamine?
3. What are the complications of too much protamine?
4. Why did the patient develop hypotension after administering protamine? How do you treat and prevent this condition?
5. What are the indications for intraaortic balloon pump (IABP)?
6. What are the principles of IABP?
7. What are the complications of IABP?

D. Postoperative Management

1. What are the postoperative complications?
2. Would you reverse the muscle relaxants? Why?
3. When will you wean the patient from the respirator?
4. What criteria would you use in deciding when to wean the patient from the respirator?

A. Medical Disease and Differential Diagnosis

A.1. What is triple vessel coronary artery disease (CAD)? Name the branches of the coronary arteries.

Triple vessel CAD usually involves the following:
- The right coronary artery (RCA)
- The left anterior descending branch (LAD)
- The left circumflex branch (CFX)

The branches of coronary arteries are shown in Figure 7–1. The sinus node is supplied by the RCA in about 55% of human beings and by the left circumflex artery in the remaining 45%. The atrioventricular (A-V) node is provided by the RCA in 90% of human beings and by the left circumflex artery in the remaining 10%. The most common arteries for coronary bypass grafts are left anterior descending, obtuse marginal, and posterior descending arteries.

Braunwald E: Heart Disease, pp 314–338. Philadelphia, WB Saunders, 1980

A.2. What are the indications for coronary artery bypass graft?
- Unstable angina pectoris or episodes of prolonged myocardial ischemia
- Unacceptable angina pectoris, despite optimal medical therapy
- Repeated episodes of myocardial ischemia following myocardial infarction
- Prinzmetal's angina (variant angina) with coronary artery obstruction
- High-grade left main coronary artery obstruction, triple- or double-vessel obstruction, or proximal left anterior descending artery obstruction

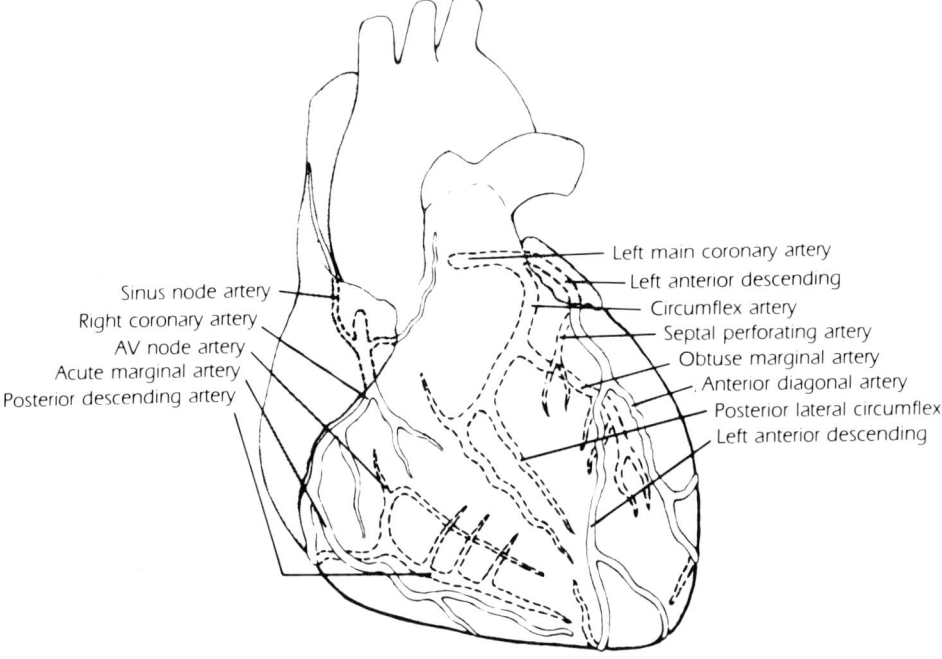

Fig. 7-1. Branches of the coronary arteries

- Acute myocardial infarction, cardiogenic shock, intractable ventricular arrhythmias
- Stable angina pectoris that interferes with desired life style

Braunwald E: Heart Disease, pp 1419–1420. Philadelphia, WB Saunders, 1980

Hurst JW: Coronary Bypass Surgery: Evolution of a point of view. Primary Cardiology Clinics, New York, P.W. Communications, I, No. 4 pp 8–14, 1979

A.3. What is the incidence of perioperative reinfarction for non-cardiac surgery at 0–3 months, 4–6 months, and over 6 months after myocardial infarction?

The incidence of perioperative reinfarction depends on the time interval between myocardial infarction and operation. Topkins and Artusio in 1964 reported a 55% incidence of reinfarction in male patients over 50 years old, undergoing surgery within 6 months of a myocardial infarction. Between 6 months and 2 years, the reinfarction rate was 22% to 25%. After 3 years, the incidence decreased to 1%. The more recent reports are shown in Table 7–1. All reports showed a significant decline in reinfarction rate after 6 months of a myocardial infarction. In 1981, Rao and El–Etr claimed reinfarction rate to be 7.8% and 3.4% in patients who developed infarction 3 and 6 months before surgery. Close hemodynamic monitoring, including systemic and pulmonary arterial pressures, and chest lead V_5 ECG, with immediate and appropriate therapy to control various hemodynamic aberrations has contributed to the lower reinfarction rate. The mortality of reinfarction is about 70% in all reports.

Rao TCK, El–Etr AA: Myocardial reinfarction following anesthesia in patients with recent infarction. Anesth Analg (Cleve) 60:271–272, 1981

Steen P, Tinker JH, Tarhan S: Myocardial reinfarction after anesthesia and surgery. JAMA 239:2566, 1978

Tarhan S, Moffett EA: Myocardial infarction after general anesthesia. JAMA 220:1451, 1972

Topkins MJ, Artusio JF: Myocardial infarction and surgery: A five year study. Anesth Analg (Cleve) 43:716, 1964

Table 7–1. The incidence and mortality of perioperative reinfarction for noncardiac surgery

	TIME INTERVAL			MORTALITY OF REINFARCTION
	0–3 M	4–6 M	OVER 6 M	
Tarhan and Moffett (1972)	37%	16%	5%	66%
Steen and Tarhan (1978)	27%	11%	4.1%	69%
Rao and El–Etr (1981)	7.8%	3.4%	—	67%

A.4. What are the factors increasing the risk of postoperative myocardial infarction after noncardiac surgery?

Goldman and associates found nine factors to have statistically significant independent correlations with cardiac outcome. They are as follows:

- Age over 70 years
- Myocardial infarction in previous 6 months
- S_3 gallop or jugular vein distention
- Important valvular aortic stenosis
- Rhythm other than sinus or premature atrial contractions on preoperative ECG
- Premature ventricular contractions more than 5/min at anytime before surgery
- Poor general medical status:
  PaO_2 less than 60 torr, or $PaCO_2$ more than 50 torr, potassium less than 3.0 or HCO_3 less than 20 mEq/L, BUN more than 50 mg/dl or creatinine more than 3.0 mg/dl, abnormal SGOT or signs of chronic liver disease
- Intraperitoneal, intrathoracic or aortic operation
- Emergency operation

Steen and associates reported the following risk factors associated with significantly increased reinfarction rates:

- Preoperative hypertension
- Intraoperative hypotension
- Non-cardiac thoracic or upper abdominal operations of more than 3 hours duration
- Time interval between previous myocardial infarction and surgery

Generally, the choice of anesthetic agents or site of previous myocardial infarction did not play any role in the occurance of reinfarction.

Goldman L et al: Multifactorial index of cardiac risk in non-cardiac surgical procedures. N Engl J Med 297:845–850, 1977

Steen PA et al: Myocardial reinfarction after anesthesia and surgery. JAMA 239:2566–2570, 1978

B. Preoperative Evaluation and Preparation

B.1. Would you discontinue digoxin? Why? What is its half-life?

In order to prevent digitalis intoxication after cardiopulmonary bypass (CPB), digitalis preparations are usually discontinued one half-life (1.5–1.7 days for digoxin, 5–7 days for digitoxin) before surgery. Digitalis intoxication is quite possible, especially after CPB when acid–base and electrolytes are abnormal. If the patient is in congestive heart failure (CHF) and digitalis-dependent, digitalis is continued until the night before surgery. However, the predisposing factors to digitalis intoxication, especially hypopotassemia, have to be prevented.

Gillman AG, Goodman LS, Gilman A: The Pharmacological Basis of Therapeutics, 6th ed, p 747. New York, MacMillan, 1980

Kaplan J: Cardiac Anesthesia, p 255. New York, Grune & Stratton, 1979

Kebowitz PW: Clinical Anesthesia Procedures of the Massachusetts General Hospital, p 147. Boston, Little, Brown & Co, 1978

B.2. Would you discontinue propranolol? Why? What is its half-life?

Propranolol is generally continued up until the time of surgery. In those patients who have stable angina, propranolol may be gradually tapered during the 48 hours prior to surgery. In those patients who are unstable, however, it should be continued at its full dose. In patients with unstable angina, sudden withdrawal of propranolol may produce an exacerbation of symptoms and may precipitate acute myocardial infarction. The half-life of oral propranolol is 3.4 to 6 hours. Propranolol disappears from the plasma and atria within 24 to 48 hours after discontinuing doses of 30 to 240 mg/day. Shand and Keats have shown that with a 0.5 mg dose of propranolol IV, blood levels as high as 50 ng/ml are obtained, but rapidly drop off to unmeasurable levels within 5 to 10 minutes. There has been no myocardial depression seen with these small intravenous doses.

Kaplan J: Cardiac Anesthesia, p 254. New York, Grune & Stratton, 1979

B.3. If the patient who is on propranolol develops hypotension intraoperatively, how would you manage it?

The specific antagonists for propranolol are not the first choice. The more common causes of intraoperative hypotension such as hypovolemia, deep anesthesia, and surgical manipulation should be corrected first. In rare

Ischemic Heart Disease and Coronary Artery Bypass Graft · 95

instances, it is necessary to administer atropine for bradycardia or isoproterenol, glucagon, calcium, or digitalis to counteract the beta-blockade. Cardiogenic hypotension is usually associated with high pulmonary capillary wedge pressure (PCWP) and low blood pressure.

Kaplan J: Cardiac Anesthesia, p 254. New York, Grune & Stratton, 1979

Schwartz AJ, Wollman H: Anesthetic considerations for patients on chronic drug therapy: L-dopa, MAO inhibitors, tricyclic antidepressants, and propranolol. ASA Refresher Courses in Anesthesiology, 4:108, 1976

B.4. What is nifedipine? How does it work?

Nifedipine is a calcium channel blocker. The commonly used calcium channel blockers in the United States are nifedipine, verapamil, and diltiazem hydrochloride. They inhibit excitation-contraction coupling of myocardial and smooth muscle by blocking calcium influx at cellular membranes. This results in decreased myocardial contractility and in vasodilation. Therefore, myocardial oxygen consumption is decreased. Calcium channel blockers are effective for the treatment of variant angina (Prinzmetal's angina), angina pectoris, and possibly acute myocardial infarction.

Although nitrates and beta adrenergic blockers are effective for angina, the calcium channel blockers are longer acting and may be used in the presence of chronic obstructive pulmonary disease and asthma. Calcium also plays a key role in cardiac electrical activity. The electrical activity of the sinoatrial (S-A) and atrioventricular (A-V) nodal cells are especially dependent on the calcium or "slow current," whereas the rest of the specialized conduction system is more dependent on the sodium or "fast current." Verapamil has a more profound influence on the calcium current of the S-A and A-V nodes. This drug has been most useful in the treatment of supraventricular tachyarrhythmias, which are often caused by reentry through the A-V node. In contrast, nifedripine has less influence on the S-A node and no effect on A-V conduction time. Therefore, nifedipine might be used where further suppression of A-V conduction is undesirable.

Karlsberg RP: Calcium channel blockers for cardiovascular disorders. Arch Intern Med 142:452–455, 1982

B.5. What preoperative tests would you order?

In addition to the routine systemic examinations of all organ systems, special attention should be paid to circulatory functions.

- Renal function—urinalysis, BUN, creatinine
- Hepatic function—bilirubin, albumin/globulin, alkaline phosphatase, SGOT, SGPT
- Pulmonary function—baseline arterial blood gases, spirometry as indicated, chest x-ray
- Hematologic function—complete blood count, PT, PTT, platelets

- Metabolism—electrolytes and blood sugar
- Cardiovascular function—Resting and exercise ECG, catheterization and angiography, left ventricular function, and location and severity of coronary occlusion

B.6. How do you evaluate the patient's left ventricular function?

- By the history of myocardial infarction and angina
- By symptoms and signs of left ventricular failure, dyspnea, nocturnal orthopnea, pitting edema
- Cardiac catheterization and angiography
- Ejection fraction (normal 65%)
- Left ventricular end diastolic pressure (LVEDP) or PCWP (normal 8–12 torr)
- Left ventricular wall motion—akinesia, hypokinesia, or dyskinesia
- Cardiac index (normal 3 L/min/m^2)

Kaplan J: Cardiac Anesthesia, p 247. New York, Grune & Stratton, 1979

B.7. What are the three major determinants of myocardial oxygen consumption? How are they measured clinically?

The three major determinants are myocardial wall tension, contractility, and heart rate.

Myocardial Wall Tension is Measured by:
- Preload—LVEDP, left atrial pressure, or PCWP
- Afterload—systolic ventricular pressure or systolic blood pressure

Contractility is Measured by:
- Invasive technique—maximal velocity of contraction (Vmax) dp/dt (pressure time indices of ventricle)
- Noninvasive technique—Preejection period (PEP)/left ventricular ejection time (LVET)

Heart Rate

Braunwald E: Heart Disease, pp 1280–1283. Philadelphia, WB Saunders, 1980

B.8. What are the rate pressure product (RPP) and the triple index (TI)?

$$RPP = \text{systolic blood pressure (SBP)} \times \text{heart rate (HR)}$$
$$TI = SBP \times HR \times PCWP$$

Both RPP and TI are used to measure myocardial oxygen demand. Angina threshold depends on the severity of coronary artery occlusion. Angina threshold of RPP usually ranges from 15,000 to 20,000 torr/min. A high RPP or TI indicates a potential danger of myocardial ischemia, but a normal or low RPP and TI do not rule out ischemia. Patients with tachycardia and hypotension may have a normal RPP, but both tachycardia (increasing O_2 demand, decreasing O_2 supply) and hypotension (decreasing O_2 supply) may cause myocardial ischemia. Precordial lead V_5 ECG and angina (awake patients) are more important monitors for ischemia. Most important is to keep all three factors (SBP, HR, PCWP) as close as possible to their usual normal values. It is usually recommended to keep RPP below 12,000 and TI below 150,000.

Kaplan J: Cardiac Anesthesia, pp 108–109. New York, Grune & Stratton, 1979

B.9. What factors determine myocardial oxygen supply?

Myocardial oxygen supply = coronary blood flow × arterial oxygen content

$$\text{Coronary blood flow} = \frac{\text{coronary perfusion pressure}}{\text{resistance}}$$

Coronary blood flow depends on the following:
- Aortic diastolic pressure (DP)
- Left ventricular end diastolic pressure (LVEDP)
- Patency of coronary arteries

Arterial O_2 content is determined by the following equation:

$$CaO_2 = 1.34 \times Hb \times O_2 \text{ saturation} + 0.0031 \times PaO_2$$

Braunwald E: Heart Disease, p 1283. Philadelphia, WB Saunders, 1980

B.10. How would you premedicate the patient? Why?

The patient should be well sedated to prevent anxiety which may precipitate angina. We usually give pentobarbital, 2 mg/kg intramuscularly, 1 hour before surgery. Two inches of nitroglycerin paste (Nitropaste) are applied prophylactically to the chest wall.

Even though atropine or scopolamine is not contraindicated, atropine is not given at Cornell Medical Center because of the possibility of tachycardia, which will increase O_2 demand.

C. Intraoperative Management

Before cardiopulmonary bypass

C. I-1. How do you monitor the patient?

- ECG: Simultaneous leads V_5 and II
- Arterial line for BP and arterial blood gases
- Swan–Ganz catheter: PCWP, PAD, hemodynamic study
- CVP line: If the patient has good left ventricular function and no problems are expected
- Urine output
- Temperature: Esophageal and rectal
- Laboratory: ABG, electrolytes, hematocrit, activated coagulation time (ACT), and PvO_2
- Oxygen analyzer for inspired gas mixture

C. I-2. What is the Allen test?

The Allen test is used to detect collateral ulnar circulation. The radial and ulnar arteries are occluded by the examiner's hands. The patient is then asked to make a tight fist to empty blood from the hand. The hand is held above the heart level to help venous drainage. If the patient is under anesthesia, the blood in the hand may be drained by a third person squeezing the hand. Then the hand is opened slowly and put down to the heart level. Only the ulnar compression is released. The flush of the hand is watched.

Normal < 7 seconds
Borderline 7–15 seconds
Abnormal > 15 seconds

A modified Allen test may be done with a Doppler detector or pulsimeter. The Allen test results are abnormal in approximately 3% of young healthy individuals.

Eckenhoff JE: Controversy in Anesthesiology, pp 237–244. Philadelphia, WB Saunders, 1979

Hedley–Whyte J et al: Applied Physiology of Respiratory Care, p 95. Boston, Little, Brown & Co, 1976

C. I-3. Why do you need both esophageal and rectal temperatures?

During cooling and rewarming, there is uneven distribution of body temperature. Esophageal temperature represents core temperature; rectal temperature represents peripheral temperature. During cooling and rewarming, using the pump–oxygenator, esophageal temperature changes rapidly, whereas the rectal temperature changes slowly. During surface cooling or warming, the rectal temperature changes quickly, while the esophageal temperature changes slowly. In order to estimate the average temperature and to achieve even distribution of body temperature, it is necessary to record both esophageal and rectal temperatures.

Galletti PM, Brecher GA: Heart–Lung Bypass, p 294. New York, Grune & Stratton, 1962

Kaplan J: Cardiac Anesthesia, p 413. New York, Grune & Stratton, 1979

C. I-4. How do you know that the Swan–Ganz catheter is in the right ventricle (RV) or pulmonary artery (PA)?

There are two main differences in the pressure tracings.

Diastolic Pressure is Higher in PA than in RV
- PA pressure 20–25/5–10 torr
- RV pressure 20–25/0 torr

Pressure Contour
- PA pressure tracing has dicrotic notch from closure of pulmonary valve.
- RV pressure tracing has plateau and sharp drop in diastole.

In the late diastolic phase, PA pressure is going down while the RV pressure is going up because of ventricular filling.

C. I-5. What is normal PCWP?

- Normal 5–12 torr
- Borderline 13–17 torr
- Heart failure over 18 torr

Braunwald E: Heart Disease, p 1343. Philadelphia, WB Saunders, 1980

C. I-6. Is it necessary to monitor pulmonary artery pressure for coronary artery operations?

The indication to monitor pulmonary artery pressure depends on the left ventricular function. Patients may be divided into two different categories on the basis of left ventricular function. For patients who have good left ventricular function (ejection fractions greater than 0.5 and good ventricular wall motion), the central venous pressure (CVP) correlates well with the pulmonary capillary wedge pressure (PCWP), therefore pulmonary pressure monitoring may not be necessary for this group of patients. On the other hand, for patients with poor left ventricular function (ejection fractions less than 0.4 or ventricular dyssynergy), the CVP does not correlate with the PCWP, therefore pulmonary pressure monitoring is indicated for this group of patients.

Mangano DT: Monitoring pulmonary arterial pressure in coronary–artery disease. Anesthesiology 53:364–369, 1980

Editorial views: To (PA) catheterize or not to (PA) catheterize: That is the question. Anesthesiology 53:361–363, 1980

C. I-7. What are the complications of Swan–Ganz catheterization?

From Venopuncture Sites (as for CVP)
- Common complications:
  - Infection—sepsis
  - Hematoma
  - Air embolism
  - Thrombosis
- Subclavian approach:
  - Pneumothorax
  - Hemothorax
  - Hydrothorax
- Internal jugular approach:
  - Pneumothorax
  - Neck hematoma from puncture of carotid artery
  - Possible vagus nerve injury

The basilar or cephalic vein approach has fewer complications, but the failure rate is higher.

From Swan–Ganz Catheter

Arrhythmias 1.5% to 11%, thromboemboli, pulmonary infarction from continuous wedging, massive hemorrhage from perforation of PA, RA, failure to wedge, hemoptysis, intracardiac knotting, balloon rupture, endocardial thrombi, and tricuspid valve injury.

Hedley–Whyte J et al: Applied Physiology of Respiratory Care, p 107. Boston, Little, Brown & Co, 1976

C. I-8. How can you detect myocardial ischemia?

When the patient is awake, angina pain is the best sign. When the patient is under anesthesia, ST-depression in V_5 ECG is the best sign. We consider 1 mm horizontal or downsloping ST-segment depression from baseline a significant sign of myocardial ischemia (1 mv = 10 mm). Inverted T waves, elevated PCWP, and decreased cardiac contractility may be signs of myocardial ischemia as well.

Kaplan J: Cardiac Anesthesia, p 257. New York, Grune & Stratton, 1979

C. I-9. How would you monitor ECG? Why V_5?

Multiple-lead ECG monitoring provides the best currently available method of detecting perioperative ischemia. It is better to use simultaneous leads II and V_5. If only one channel can be displayed, V_5 should be used. Blackburn showed that 89% of the ST-segment information contained in the conventional 12-lead exercise ECG is found in lead V_5.

Blackburn H et al: Standardization of the exercise electrocardiogram. A systematic comparison of chest lead configurations employed for monitoring during exercise. In Karvamen MJ, Barry AJ: Physical Activity and the Heart, pp 101–133. Springfield, IL, Charles C Thomas, 1967

Kaplan J: Cardiac Anesthesia, p 257. New York, Grune & Stratton, 1979

C. I-10. If you don't have precordial leads in your ECG machine, how can you monitor the left ventricle?

A modified V_5 or CM_5 may be used. Place the right arm (RA) electrode on the middle part of manubrium, the left leg (LL) electrode on the V_5 position, and the left arm electrode on any area of the body for ground, and monitor lead II. Recent claims suggest that the CB_5 lead is simple to apply and provides tracings equivalent to the V_5 when monitoring for ischemia, while allowing easier recognition of P waves. Lead CB_5 is a bipolar lead consisting of a negative (RA) electrode over the center of the right scapula and a positive (LL) electrode over the V_5 position monitoring lead II. The CB_5 lead is useful for thoracic surgery.

Bazaral MG, Norfleet EA: Comparison of CB_5 and V_5 leads for intraoperative electrocardiographic monitoring. Anesth Analg (Cleve) 60:849–853, 1981

C. I-11. How would you induce anesthesia?

A smooth induction is essential to prevent hypotension, hypertension, and tachycardia. Different techniques may be used to achieve a smooth induction. For patients with good left ventricular function, anesthesia is induced with fentanyl, 0.005 mg (0.1 ml)/kg, and thiopental, 2 mg/kg. The patient is ventilated by mask with 100% oxygen or a mixture of 50% nitrous oxide and 50% oxygen. After administration of succinylcholine, 1 mg/kg, and lidocaine, 0.7 mg/kg intravenously, the patient is intubated. Intravenous lidocaine is used to block the tracheal response to intubation. If a potent inhalation agent is to be used for maintenence, anesthesia is induced with thiopental, 4 mg/kg, and deepened with 2.0% enflurane for 3–5 minutes. When adequately anesthetized, the patient is given succinylcholine and intubated. In our experiences, hypertension and tachycardia frequently developed after endotracheal intubation when the same concentrations of isoflurane instead of enflurane were used to deepen anesthesia. For patients with poor left ventricular function, potent inhalation agents such as enflurane, isoflurane, and halothane are avoided during induction and maintenence of anesthesia.

C. I-12. How would you maintain anesthesia?

Again, smooth anesthesia is essential to achieve a balance between myocardial oxygen demand and supply. Different agents and techniques may be used to accomplish the same goal. I personally prefer neuroleptic technique with a moderate dose of fentanyl–droperidol–N_2O–O_2 for maintenence of anesthesia. After the patient is intubated, a mixture of 60% nitrous oxide and 40% oxygen is administered to keep the patient unconscious.

The depth of anesthesia must be titrated to meet the requirements of the varying intensities of surgical stimulation. Skin incision and sternal splitting are very painful. But the strongest stimulation is usually from sternal retraction with the self-retaining retractor. Droperidol, 0.1 ml (0.25 mg)/kg, and fentanyl, 0.1 ml/kg, are given right before skin incision and are usually strong enough to block the cardiovascular response from sternal splitting and retraction. Very high doses of fentanyl, with or without droperidol, and oxygen without nitrous oxide have been successfully used for cardiac anesthesia. Since we can maintain very smooth anesthesia with much lower doses, (usually $1/10$–$2/10$ of the reported doses), we do not want to waste the expensive drugs. Meanwhile, we believe mild cardiac depression from nitrous oxide may decrease the cardiac oxygen demand similar to the effect of propranolol. The possibility of oxygen toxicity from the use of 100% oxygen should also be kept in mind.

Stanley TH, Philbin DM, Coggins CH: Fentanyl–oxygen anesthesia for coronary artery surgery: Cardiovascular and antidiuretic hormone responses. Can Anaesth Soc J 26:168–172, 1979

Quintin L et al: Oxygen–high dose fentanyl–droperidol anesthesia for aortocoronary bypass surgery. Anesth Analg (Cleve) 60:412–416, 1981

C. I-13. What is the better anesthetic agent for this operation–an inhalational or intravenous agent?

The choice of anesthetic agents is still debatable. Both inhalational and intravenous agents have been used successfully. They both have advantages and disadvantages. Understanding the cardiovascular effects of each anesthetic agent and careful titration of each drug will improve the balance between myocardial oxygen demand and supply. Early detection and appropriate control of the major determinants of myocardial oxygen consumption (BP, HR, PCWP) are mandatory if myocardial ischemia is to be avoided.

Merin et al concluded that neither fentanyl nor halothane protected against ischemia produced by a 60% decrease in left anterior descending coronary artery blood flow for 30 minutes in swine. No advantage was seen for either anesthetic regimen in the acute ischemic, non-failing heart.

Eckenhoff JE: Controversy in Anesthesiology, p 2. Philadelphia, WB Saunders, 1979

Lowenstein E: Anesthetic considerations in coronary–artery disease. ASA Refresher Courses in Anesthesiology 4:51–64, 1976

Merin RG et al: Myocardial Functional and metabolic responses to ischemia in swine during halothane and fentanyl anesthesia. Anesthesiology 56:84–92, 1982

C. I-14. What are the cardiovascular effects of halothane, enflurane, isoflurane, morphine, and fentanyl?

In general, halothane, enflurane, and isoflurane produce a dose-related depression in ventricular function and vascular tonus. Halothane sensitizes the heart to catecholamine more than enflurane and isoflurane. Narcotics such as morphine and fentanyl at their clinical dosage have minimal cardiovascular effects. Both may cause bradycardia. Neither sensitize the heart to catecholamine or depress myocardial function. The cardiovascular effects of morphine depend on the dosage used. Large doses of morphine sulfate have reportedly caused myocardial lactate production and reduction in coronary blood flow in animals. Sethna found that morphine sulfate, 0.25 mg/kg IV, did not produce a global myocardial ischemia in patients with coronary artery disease. High doses of morphine, 1 mg/kg, produce a significant decrease in arterial blood pressure and systemic vascular resistance accompanied by an average 750% increase in plasma histamine. On the other hand, high doses of fentanyl, 0.050 mg/kg, do not produce any significant changes in blood pressure, vascular resistance and plasma histamine levels.

Kaplan J (ed): Cardiac Anesthesia, pp 7–24. New York, Grune & Stratton, 1979

Rosow CE et al: Histamine release during morphine and fentanyl anesthesia. Anesthesiology 56:93–96, 1982

Sethna DH et al: Cardiovascular effects of morphine in patients with coronary arterial disease. Anesth Analg (Cleve) 61:109–114, 1982

C. I-15. What is the cardiovascular effect of nitrous oxide?

Nitrous oxide is a weak central nervous system depressant. It has been generally considered to have minimal effects on other organ systems. Recent studies, however, have shown that 40% of N_2O can produce a small

Ischemic Heart Disease and Coronary Artery Bypass Graft · 103

but significant depression of ventricular function in man. In addition, N_2O added to narcotic agents results in more marked ventricular depression. When added to other inhalational anesthetics, N_2O increases arterial pressure and systemic vascular resistance, suggesting that it has a vasoconstrictor action.

Brown BR Jr: Anesthesia and the Patient with Heart Disease, p 9. Philadelphia, F.A. Davis, 1980

Merin RG: The function of the heart: Effects of anesthetics and adjuvant drugs. ASA Refresher Courses in Anesthesiology 6:81–95, 1978

C. I-16. What kind of muscle relaxant would you use? Why?

We usually use d-tubocurarine. When full paralyzing doses are given in a bolus, d-tubocurarine tends to produce bradycardia and hypotension from ganglionic blockade and histamine release, whereas pancuronium and gallamine generally cause tachycardia and hypertension from vagolytic effect and norepinephrine released from cardiac sympathetic nerves. We give d-tubocurarine in increments of 6 mg dose every 5 to 10 minutes until patients are fully paralyzed (0.3 mg/kg). Blood pressure and heart rate are usually not changed by this small dose and slow injection rate. Pancuronium is a better choice if hypotension (BP < 80 torr systolically) and bradycardia (HR < 50/m) are present. Otherwise, pancuronium may increase myocardial O_2 consumption due to tachycardia and hypertension.

Gillman AG, Goodman LS, Gilman A: The Pharmacological Basis of Therapeutics, 6th ed, p 229. New York, MacMillan, 1980

C. I-17. If ST–segment depression is seen during surgery, how would you treat it?

ST–segment depression indicates myocardial ischemia, either from increased O_2 demand or decreased O_2 supply. The treatment includes the following:

- Increase O_2 supply: correct hypotension and hypoxemia
- Decrease O_2 demand: correct hypertension, tachycardia, increased PCWP or CVP by deepening anesthesia or the use of vasodilators and propranolol. All the major determinants have to be considered and corrected to their usual normal levels.

Gerson and associates (in experimental dogs) found that elevation of ST segments induced by occlusion of the coronary artery was more limited with halothane than with a combination of nitroprusside and propranolol. The more favorable effect of halothane was explained by its effects on coronary vascular reserve and the known effect of nitroprusside to reduce myocardial blood flow to ischemic myocardium.

If there are no obvious changes in blood pressure, heart rate, and pulmonary wedge pressure, nitroglycerin is indicated for coronary spasm.

Nitroglycerin may be given by intravenous drip or bolus nasal administration of 0.8 mg in 1 ml of normal saline.

Gerson JI et al: Treatment of myocardial ischemia with halothane or nitroprusside-propranolol. Anesth Analg (Cleve) 61:10–14, 1982

Hill AB et al: Intranasal administration of nitroglycerin. Anesthesiology 54:346–348, 1981

C. I-18. How would you correct hypertension?

Blood pressure = blood flow × resistance

Hypertension is usually due to inadequate depth of anesthesia. Occasionally it is due to fluid overloading. The treatment of hypertension includes the following:

- Deepen the anesthesia. Inhalational agents such as halothane, enflurane, and isoflurane are more effective than narcotics because of their vasodilator effect.
- Vasodilators—when inhalational agents are not used.
  - Sodium nitroprusside produces more arteriolar dilation than venodilation.
    Dose: 10–100 µg/min IV drip titration
  - Nitroglycerin produces more venodilation than arteriolar dilation.
    Dose: 20–200 µg/min IV drip titration

Gerson JI et al: Arterial and venous dilation by nitroprusside and nitroglycerin—is there a difference? Anesth Analg 61:256–260, 1982

Kaplan J: Cardiac Anesthesia, p 264. New York, Grune & Stratton, 1979

C. I-19. How would you treat hypotension?

Hypotension is usually due to hypovolemia, deep anesthesia, bradycardia, or congestive heart failure (CHF). The treatments are as follows:

- Increase fluid infusion and put the patient in head-down position when CVP or PCWP is low
- Lighten the level of anesthesia or use a vasoconstrictor—phenylephrine, 0.1 mg IV increments to correct vasodilation produced by anesthesia
- Atropine, 0.2 to 2.0 mg, for bradycardia or isoproterenol, 1 mg/100 ml D_5W IV drip titration
- Treat CHF when PCWP is high:
  - Lighten the level of anesthesia
  - Restrict fluids
  - Diuretics: furosemide (Lasix) 20 to 40 mg, IV
  - Inotropes: $CaCl_2$ (0.5–1.0 gm)
    Dopamine, 5 to 20 µg/kg/min, IV drip
    Dopride (dopamine and nitroprusside)
    Norepinephrine
  - IABP (Intra-aortic balloon pump)

Kaplan J: Cardiac Anesthesia, p 435. New York, Grune & Stratton, 1979

Ischemic Heart Disease and Coronary Artery Bypass Graft · 105

C. I-20. What are the indications for intravenous propranolol during surgery? How much would you give? What are the relative contraindications?

Indications
- ST-segment depression associated with tachycardia; no response to deepening the level of anesthesia
- Supraventricular tachycardia over 120/m
- Recurrent ventricular arrhythmias

Contraindications
- Congestive heart failure
- Asthma, chronic obstructive pulmonary disease

Dosage: 0.25 mg increments every 1–2 minutes—total dose 2–3 mg.

Kaplan J: Cardiac Anesthesia, p 265. New York, Grune & Stratton, 1979

C. I-21. How would you correct increased PCWP?

It is important to treat the patient as a whole. All monitors have to be considered together not only one single parameter. Increased PCWP is usually due to a light level of anesthesia or congestive heart failure (CHF). Combining the readings of PCWP and blood pressure will make differential diagnosis.

Inadequate anesthesia—increased PCWP with hypertension
℞:
- Deepen the level of anesthesia with inhalational agents such as halothane or enflurane, which also have a vasodilator effect.
- Give a vasodilator. Nitroglycerin is a better venodilator than nitroprusside.

CHF—increased PCWP with hypotension
℞:
- Lighten the level of anesthesia
- Restrict fluids
- Use vasodilators
- Give diuretics
- Use inotropes

Kaplan J: Cardiac Anesthesia, p 264. New York, Grune & Stratton, 1979

C. I-22. During sternal splitting, would you do something?

Stop ventilation and deflate the lungs to prevent lung injury from the electric saw.

C. I-23. Would you monitor PCWP continuously? Why?

No, If the Swan–Ganz catheter balloon is inflated continuously, pulmonary infarction distal to the occlusion may ensue. Usually PADP is monitored continuously because PADP is very close to PCWP.

Miller RD: Anesthesia, p 191. New York, Churchill Livingstone, 1981

106 · Anesthesiology

During cardiopulmonary bypass (CPB)

C. II-1. What anticoagulant would you give before CPB? How much would you give? What is its mechanism?

Heparin has been used conventionally in doses of 3 mgs or 300 units/kg of body weight, assuming an initial concentration of at least 2 to 4 units/ml of whole blood. Empirically, after 2 hrs of the initial dose, subsequent doses of 1 mg/kg are given for each additional hour of bypass. Because there is marked individual variation, heparin doses are best monitored by the celite activated coagulation time test.

Heparin acts indirectly by means of a plasma cofactor. The heparin cofactor, or antithrombin III, is an $\alpha 2$-globulin and a protease inhibitor that neutralizes several activated clotting factors, XIIa, kallikrein, XIa, IXa, Xa, IIa, and XIIIa. Antithrombin III forms irreversible complexes with thrombin (IIa) and, as a result, both proteins are inactivated. Heparin markedly accelerates the velocity, but not the extent of the reactions of antithrombin III.

Gillman AG, Goodman LS, Gilman A: The Pharmacological Basis of Therapeutics, 6th ed, p 1349. New York, MacMillan, 1980

Kaplan J: Cardiac Anesthesia, p 427. New York, Grune & Stratton, 1979

C. II-2. What is the half-life of heparin. How is it eliminated?

The biological half-life of heparin varies with dosages and temperature. It has a remarkable individual variation. The average half-life is approximately 100 minutes in normothermic man for the initial doses of 3 mg/kg, increasing with higher dosage and decreasing temperature. When 1, 4, or 8 mg/kg of heparin is given intravenously, the approximate half-life is 1, 2, and 3 hours respectively.

Heparin is metabolized in the liver by an enzyme termed heparinase, and the inactive metabolic products are excreted in the urine. In patients with renal failure or liver cirrhosis, the half-life of heparin is significantly longer than in normal subjects.

Gillman AG, Goodman LS, Gilman A: The Pharmacological Basis of Therapeutics, 6th ed, p 1350. New York, MacMillan, 1980

Kaplan J: Cardiac Anesthesia, p 427. New York, Grune & Stratton, 1979

C. II-3. How do you monitor heparin dosage? What is the ACT test?

Heparin therapy can be assessed by the PTT, heparin assay, heparin–protamine titration, and the ACT test. The most convenient and practical method used to monitor heparin therapy in the operating room is the celite activated coagulation time (ACT) test. There is a very good correlation between the ACT, plasma heparin units, and thrombin time. Two ml of blood are put into a test tube containing celite to activate coagulation. Then the tube is kept at 37°C and clot formation is watched for ACT. The normal control value of ACT is 120 to 150 seconds. A baseline value is determined before the administration of heparin, and the test is repeated 20 minutes after heparin is given and at intervals of 60 minutes thereafter. With the dose of heparin in milligrams per kilogram on the vertical axis and ACT in seconds on the horizontal axis, a dose response curve can be plotted. ACT values are maintained at at least twice control value and not less than 350 seconds. At Cornell Medical Center, we keep the ACT above 480 seconds.

Bull MH, Huse WM, Bull BS: Evaluation of tests used to monitor heparin therapy during extracorporeal circulation. Anesthesiology 43:346–353, 1975

Kaplan J: Cardiac Anesthesia, p 427. New York, Grune & Stratton, 1979

C. II-4. What is total cardiopulmonary bypass? What is partial bypass?

Total bypass indicates that all the venous return from superior and inferior venae cavae and coronary sinus is drained to the oxygenator and no blood is pumped by the right ventricle to the lungs. The pulmonary artery tracing becomes nonpulsatile. Partial bypass means that some of the blood return is still pumped by both right and left ventricles. Some venous blood is drained to the oxygenator and pumped back to the arterial side. Femoral–femoral bypass is one example.

Arens JF: Extracorporeal circulation: Practical considerations in the use of the heart pump. ASA Refresher Courses in Anesthesiology, 4:13–24, 1976

C. II-5. What is the purpose of putting a left ventricle sump drain through a pulmonary vein?

Even though all the venous return is bypassed from the right ventricle, 2% to 5% of cardiac output is draining to the left ventricle. This is the physiological shunt from the bronchial, thebesian, and pleural veins. The left ventricular sump drain prevents overdistension of the left ventricle, which may cause postpump heart failure. A suction needle inserted proximal to the aortic cross-clamp may serve the same purpose.

Arens JF: Extracorporeal circulation: Practical considerations in the use of the heart pump. ASA Refresher Courses in Anesthesiology, 4:13–24, 1976

C. II-6. How many types of oxygenators are there? What are the advantages of each type?

There are two basic types of oxygenators in terms of their interface with blood.

Direct Gas Interface
- Disc
- Vertical screen
- Bubble

Without Gas Interface

- Membrane: solid or microporous
- Fluid-fluid using flurocarbon liquid

The disc and screen oxygenators are not disposable and have proven to be somewhat difficult to clean, prepare, and resterilize.

The bubble oxygenator has the advantages of simplicity, disposability, and relatively low cost. It is the most popular oxygenator used at the present time.

The disadvantages of gas interface oxygenators include the following:

- Protein denaturation
- Increased fragility of cells
- Susceptibility to hemolysis
- Denaturation of platelet membrane materials resulting in platelet aggregation, clumping
- Formation of air embolism
- Large priming volume
- Variable reservoir level resulting in potential shifts of blood volume between intracorporeal and extracorporeal circuit

The membrane oxygenator has become more economical and efficient and less traumatic to blood. Its advantages include eliminating blood-gas interface effects, promoting constant blood volume, and affording ease of operation. The disadvantages of membrane oxygenators include the following:

- Expense
- Potential difficulty in eliminating all bubbles during priming
- Moderately large priming volume

The major differences in changes of clotting factors between the bubble and membrane oxygenators become apparent after 4 to 6 hours of extracorporeal circulation (ECC).

Ionescu MI, Wooler GH: Current Techniques in Extracorporeal Circulation, pp 13–24. London, Butterworth & Co, 1976

Kaplan J: Cardiac Anesthesia, pp 401–410. New York, Grune & Stratton, 1979

C. II-7. What kind of priming solution would you use? How much priming solution would you use? Would you prime with blood or not? Why?

The usual priming solution for adults at Cornell Medical Center includes 2000 ml of balanced salt solution (normosol) and 200 ml of 20% mannitol. The priming volumes vary with the size of the oxygenators used and the tubing volume; most oxygenators for adult patients have priming volumes of 500 to 1000 ml. In general, blood is added to the oxygenator if the patient is markedly anemic (pre-pump hematocrit below 30%) or if the priming volume is large in relation to the patient's blood volume, such as in pediatric patients. In order to maintain oxygen carrying capacity, we try to keep hematocrit levels above 20%. Mannitol has long been used as an osmotic diuretic in situations where hemolysis or diminished renal function is expected. Mannitol has been found to decrease the incidence of renal failure during hypotension by promoting osmotic diuresis and increasing renal blood flow by decreasing renal vascular resistance.

Ionescu MI, Wooler GH: Current Techniques in Extracorporeal Circulation, pp 117–122. London, Butterworth & Co, 1976

Kaplan J: Cardiac Anesthesia, pp 410–411. New York, Grune & Stratton, 1979

C. II-8. What are the advantages and disadvantages of hemodilution?

Advantages of Hemodilution
- An increase in microcirculation due to a decreasing blood viscosity
- Decreased metabolic acidosis
- Increased urine output
- Reduced blood demands
- Reduced incidence of hepatitis or reactions from blood transfusions
- Reduced postoperative blood loss

Disadvantages of Hemodilution
- Decreased oxygen carrying capacity
- Postoperative extracellular fluid overload
- Possible pulmonary edema
- Hypotension from decreased viscosity and peripheral resistance
- Decreased concentration of calcium, magnesium, phosphate, and zinc

Cooper JD et al: Lung water accumulation with acute hemodilution in dogs. Thorac Cardiovasc Surg 69:957–965, 1975

Ionescu MI, Wooler GH: Current Techniques in Extracorporeal Circulation, pp 129–134. London, Butterworth & Co, 1976

Kaplan J: Cardiac Anesthesia, pp 411–412. New York, Grune & Stratton, 1979

Lawson NW et al: Use of hemodilution and fresh autologous blood in openheart surgery. Anesth Analg (Cleve) 53:672–683, 1974

Verska JJ et al: A comparative study of cardiopulmonary bypass with nonblood and blood prime. Ann Thorac Surg 18:72–80, 1974

C. II-9. What kind of pumps do you use? Are they pulsatile or not?

The most commonly used pumps are modified DeBakey type roller pumps. They are nonpulsatile. Use of the intraaortic balloon pump can make the perfusion pulsatile. Some studies indicate that with prolonged perfusion, pulsatile flow appears to be superior for organ function; however, scientists are less certain that it is an important factor during short-term bypass.

Ionescu MI, Wooler GH: Current Techniques in Extracorporeal Circulation, pp 7–8. London, Butterworth & Co, 1976

Kaplan J: Cardiac Anesthesia, pp 393–395. New York, Grune & Stratton, 1979

C. II-10. How do you monitor the patient during CPB?

Clinical Monitoring

- Mean arterial blood pressure should be kept between 50 and 100 torr to maintain tissue perfusion.
- Pulmonary artery pressure should be low or zero to prevent over distention of the left ventricle.
- Central venous pressure should be low or zero to make sure there is no obstruction to venous return from the head.
- Pump flow rate should be adequate for tissue perfusion and oxygenation.
- Urine output should be maintained above 1 ml/kg/hr by adequate perfusion.
- ECG
- EEG is used in patients in whom cerebral problems may occur.
- Both rectal and esophageal temperatures are recorded.
- The level of anesthesia should be maintained.
- Pupillary size should remain normal and equal.

Laboratory Monitoring at Least Once Every Hour
- Arterial blood gases—kept at normal range
- Venous PO_2 should be 40 to 45 torr
- Hematocrit maintained between 20% and 30%
- Electrolytes $Na+$, $K+$
- ACT measured each hour and maintained above 400 to 480 seconds.
- If urine sugar is negative or more than 3+ in a diabetic patient, blood sugar measurement is necessary.

Arens JF: Extracorporeal circulation: Practical considerations in the use of the heart pump. ASA Refresher Courses in Anesthesiology, 4:13–24, 1976

Kaplan J: Cardiac Anesthesia, pp 420–422. New York, Grune & Stratton, 1979

C. II-11. *How much blood pressure would you keep during CPB? Why?*

The mean arterial pressure is usually maintained at approximately 50 to 100 torr to assure adequate tissue perfusion. Blood pressure depends on cardiac output (pump flow) and total peripheral resistance. We believe that adequate cardiac output (pump flow) is more important for tissue perfusion than blood pressure.

Arens JF: Extracorporeal circulation: Practical considerations in the use of the heart pump. ASA Refresher Courses in Anesthesiology, 4:13–24, 1976

C. II-12. *How would you treat hypotension during CPB?*

$$\text{Mean arterial pressure (MAP)} = \text{cardiac output (CO)} \times \text{total peripheral resistance (TPR)}$$

Hypotension may be caused by low cardiac output or low peripheral resistance. First, cardiac output should be corrected by increasing the pump flow rate. Then, if the cardiac output is adequate, peripheral resistance can be raised by giving vasopressors. We use the primarily alpha-adrenergic vasopressor, phenylephrine in increments of 0.5 mg to raise the MAP to 50 torr. According to Poiseuille's law, low TPR usually is due to decreased viscosity or increased vascular diameter (vasodilation). During CPB using blood-free priming solutions, total viscosity is reduced by hemodilution even though plasma viscosity is increased by hypothermia. A short period of hypotension with a MAP of approximately 30 to 40 torr is usually seen in the first 5 to 10 minutes of bypass. It is due to the following causes:

- Inadequate pump flow at the beginning of bypass
- Hypoxic vasodilation from initial perfusion with blood-free primes carrying no oxygen
- Vasodilation from vasoactive materials released because of the initial reaction of the serum proteins, blood cells and platelets with the foreign surfaces of the heart–lung machine
- Decreased plasma levels of catecholamines by hemodilution

Kaplan J: Cardiac Anesthesia, pp 421–423. New York, Grune & Stratton, 1979

Pratilas V et al: Hypotension and plasma catecholamines during extracorporeal circulation. Anesthesiology Review, VIII, No. 11:9–12, 1981

C. II-13. *How would you treat hypertension (a MAP of over 100 torr)?*

Hypertension during bypass is usually the result of inadequate depth of anesthesia, which causes increased catecholamine output and increased vascular resistance. Pump flow rate should not be reduced to lower the pressure. Low pump flow may cause tissue hypoxia even though blood pressure is high. The most effective treatment involves administering an inhalation agent such as halothane, enflurane, or isoflurane through the vaporizer in the heart–lung machine. Intravenous agents such as sodium pentothal, diazepam, and large doses of narcotics may be used, but they are frequently not effective and have to be supplemented with vasodilator drugs. One may use nitroprusside, nitroglycerin, phentolamine, or chlorpromazine.

Kaplan J: Cardiac Anesthesia, p 423. New York, Grune & Stratton, 1979

Stanely TH et al: Plasma catecholamine and cortisol responses to fentanyl–oxygen anesthesia for coronary–artery operations. Anesthesiology 53:250–253, 1980

C. II-14. *How do you prepare an intravenous infusion of sodium nitroprusside, phentolamine, and nitroglycerin? What are the usual doses? Which do you prefer to use?*

Intravenous solutions may be prepared by adding 10 to 20 mg of the above vasodilators to 100 ml of 5% dextrose in water to make a concentration of 100-200 μg/ml. The usual doses are 1-10 μg/kg/min determined by careful titration. We prefer nitroglycerin infusion. Sodium nitroprusside dilates both arterial and venous smooth muscle. It is very effective in reducing both preload and afterload. It may cause cyanide and thiocyanate toxicity. Because arteriolar vasodilation occurs, intracoronary steal may happen.

The solution has to be covered with aluminum foil to prevent decomposition from exposure to light. In addition to alpha-adrenergic blockade, phentolamine has a vasodilating action on vascular smooth muscle not mediated by adrenergic receptors. It also has beta stimulation and may cause arrhythmias. Nitroglycerin primarily causes venodilation, resulting in reduction of preload and myocardial oxygen consumption. At larger doses and by the intravenous route, it has mild arteriolar dilation and reduces afterload. It has no known toxicity and does not produce intracoronary steal. It may redistribute blood flow to the subendocardium and increase collateral circulation through the myocardium. The nitroglycerin infusion can be prepared by the hospital pharmacy. Twelve or 24 mgs of nitroglycerin (20 or 40 tablets of 0.6 mgs each) are dissolved in 20 ml of a 0.9 percent solution of sodium chloride. It is then sterilized by passing through a millipore filter. This solution is added to 220 ml of dextrose in water to provide a final nitroglycerin concentration of 50 or 100 μg/ml. The intravenous nitroglycerin is commercially available now.

Kaplan J: Cardiac Anesthesia, pp 47–52. New York, Grune & Stratton, 1979

C. II-15. *How much pump flow would you maintain during CPB?*

The pump blood flow is equivalent to cardiac output and to supply tissue oxygenation. The normal average cardiac output for adults is 70 ml/kg/min or 3.1 liters/min/m². Because of higher metabolism, pediatric patients need higher flow rates for each unit of body weight. Usually 70% of normal cardiac output is enough to maintain tissue oxygenation. When body surface is used, both pediatric and adult patients require about the same pump flow, 2.2 to 3.1 liters/min/m². In summary, at normothermia and normal hemoglobin levels, the pump flow is as follows:

Adults	50–70 ml/kg/min
	or
	2.2–3.1 liters/min/m²
Children	100–150 ml/kg/min
	or
	2.2–3.1 liters/min/m²

Clinically, hypothermia and hemodilution are used. Therefore, pump blood flow should be adjusted accordingly to match the oxygen supply with demand.

Pierce C II: Extracorporeal Circulation for Open-Heart Surgery, pp 6–8. Springfield, Charles C Thomas, 1969

C. II-16. *How would you adjust the pump flow during hypothermia?*

Hypothermia decreases oxygen consumption. Therefore, the pump flow may be decreased proportionally if the blood oxygen content does not change. The oxygen consumptions at different body temperatures are listed below.

Temperature	°C	37	32	30	28	25	20	10
Oxygen consumption	%	100	60	50	40	25–30	20	10

The pump flow at 30°C is 50% of the flow at 37°C (50–70 ml/kg/min). Therefore, a pump flow of 25 to 35 ml/kg/min is adequate for adults at 30°C without hemodilution. During profound hypothermia, (10°–20°C) the patients usually can tolerate total circulatory arrest without pump support for about 60 to 90 minutes. The decrease in metabolism during hypothermia is not a linear process. From 37°C to 30°C, the metabolism decreases about 7% by each degree centigrade. Below 30°C decrease in metabolism slows down.

Blair E: Clinical Hypothermia, p 88. New York, McGraw–Hill, 1964

C. II-17. How would you adjust the pump flow during hemodilution?

Oxygen delivery = cardiac output × arterial oxygen content
Arterial oxygen content = $1.34 \times Hb \times O_2$ saturation + $0.003 \times PaO_2$

Hemodilution reduces hemoglobin concentration and hence decreases oxygen content. In order to deliver the same amount of oxygen, the pump flow has to be increased accordingly during hemodilution. For example, if the hematocrit is diluted from 40% to 20% during CPB, the pump flow has to be increased by the factor 40/20. Clinically, both hypothermia and hemodilution are applied simultaneously, so that the adjustment has to be done at the same time. For example, the pump flow for adults at a temperature of 30°C and a hematocrit of 25% will be as follows:

50 to 70 ml/kg/min × 50% × 40/25 = 40 to 56 ml/kg/min

Kaplan J: Cardiac Anesthesia, p 410 New York, Grune & Stratton, 1979

C. II-18. What are the advantages of hypothermia?

Hypothermia decreases oxygen consumption and helps to preserve tissue function during hypoxic or ischemic insult. Pump flow may be decreased during CPB with hypothermia.

Galletti PM, Brecher GA: Heart–Lung Bypass, p 287. New York, Grune & Stratton, 1962

C. II-19. How does blood viscosity change during hypothermia?

Blood viscosity varies inversely with temperature; a 2% increase occurs for every 1°C decrease in temperature. Hemodilution with balanced salt solution will decrease blood viscosity. It has been recommended that the hematocrit be adjusted to the same numerical value as the core body temperature in °C.

Hedley–Whyte J et al: Applied Physiology of Respiratory Care, p 358. Boston, Little, Brown & Co, 1976

C. II-20. What are the main causes of death associated with accidental hypothermia?

Ventricular fibrillation and asystole are the major rhythm disturbances leading to cardiac arrest in hypothermia. In humans externally cooled for cardiac surgery, ventricular fibrillation generally occurs at 23°C and asystole at 20°C. However, asystole and ventricular fibrillation have been reported at 21° to 28°C. Respiratory arrest usually accompanies cardiac arrest during accidental hypothermia.

Southwick FS, Dalglish PH: Recovery after prolonged asystolic cardiac arrest in profound hypothermia. JAMA 243: 1250–1253, 1980

C. II-21. Would you give anesthesia during CPB? Why?

Yes. Anesthesia is maintained with intermittent administration of intravenous barbiturate, narcotic, or inhalation agents to achieve analgesia, control blood pressure, and prevent shivering. Intravenous agents are diluted by the priming solution during CPB. Meanwhile, hypothermia itself produces anesthesia and prolongs the action duration of intravenous agents by decreasing hepatic metabolism and urinary excretion.

Lebowitz PW: Clinical Anesthesia Procedures of the Massachusetts General Hospital, p 154. Boston, Little, Brown & Co, 1978

C. II-22. Would you give muscle relaxants during CPB? How is the action of muscle relaxant affected during CPB?

Yes. Muscle relaxants are given to prevent diaphragmatic movement that interferes with surgery and to prevent shivering during hypothermia. Shivering may increase oxygen consumption to as high as 486% of normal. The effect of a muscle relaxant is altered by both hypothermia and hemodilution. The plasma concentration of muscle relaxants is diluted by the priming solution. Therefore, more relaxant is required to maintain the same degree of relaxation. Hypothermia was originally reported to decrease the effect of nondepolarizing relaxants, because decreased cholinesterase enzyme activity during hypothermia resulted in more acetylcholine accumulation to compete with the nondepolarizing relaxant. The best way to monitor muscle relaxation is by using a peripheral nerve stimulator. Contrary to the earlier reports, it is now established that less d-tubocurarine or pancuronium is needed to maintain muscle relaxation during hypothermia because hypothermia reduces renal and biliary excretions of both d-tubocurarine and pancuronium. Ham et al reported that hypothermia in man does not affect d-tubocurarine pharmacokinetics or the sensitivity of the neuromuscular junction to d-tubocurarine. Hypothermia does prolong the onset of paralysis.

Ham J et al: Pharmacokinetics and dynamics of d-tubocurarine during hypothermia in humans. Anesthesiology 55:631–635, 1981

Lebowitz PW: Clinical Anesthesia Procedures of the Massachusetts General Hospital, p 152. Boston, Little, Brown & Co, 1978

C. II-23. How do you know the patient is well perfused during CPB?

If the perfusion pressure is maintained between 50 and 100 torr, and the pump flow rate is adequately maintained according to the degree of hypothermia and hemodilution, there should be adequate urine output, more than 1 ml/kg/hr, no metabolic acidosis, and normal mixed venous oxygen tension of 40 to 45 torr.

Kaplan J: Cardiac Anesthesia, pp 420–421. New York, Grune & Stratton, 1979

C. II-24. How much gas flow would you use for the oxygenator? What kind of gas would you use? Why?

Normal alveolar ventilation is 4 liters per minute and pulmonary circulation is 5 liters per minute. The V:Q ratio is 0.8. The oxygenator is not as efficient as human lungs. We usually start with 2 liters of gas for each liter of pump flow rate, and then adjust the gas flow rate according to blood $PaCO_2$ and PaO_2. The gas flow may be decreased if the $PaCO_2$ is low and the PaO_2 is too high. The gas:blood-flow ratio may be increased if the $PaCO_2$ is over 40 torr or the PaO_2 under 100 torr. We use a mixture of 99% oxygen and 1% carbon dioxide for the oxygenator. Because of low CO_2 production during hypothermia, high CO_2 elimination from high gas flow and high CO_2 diffusion capacity, the $PaCO_2$ may be very low. Therefore, 1% to 5% CO_2 is added to oxygen to increase $PaCO_2$.

Ionescu MI, Wooler GH: Current Techniques in Extracorporeal Circulation, p 95. London, Butterworth & Co, 1976

Lebowitz PW: Clinical Anesthesia Procedures of the Massachusetts General Hospital, p 153. Boston, Little, Brown & Co, 1978

C. II-25. What are the disadvantages of low $PaCO_2$ during CPB?

- Cerebral blood flow decreases about 2% for each torr decrease in $PaCO_2$ when $PaCO_2$ is in the range of 20 to 60 torr due to cerebral vasoconstriction.
- Respiratory alkalosis shifts the oxygen dissociation curve to the left which increases the O_2 affinity to hemoglobin and decreases oxygen release to the tissues.
- Hypokalemia occurs because of the intracellular shift of potassium during alkalosis.

Smith AL, Wollman H: Cerebral blood flow and metabolism: Effects of anesthetic drugs and techniques. Anesthesiology 36:378–400, 1972

C. II-26. The arterial blood gases and electrolytes during CPB are: pH 7.36, $PaCO_2$ 42 torr, PaO_2 449 torr, CO_2 content 24 mEq/liter, Na 128 mEq/L, K 5.8

mEq/L, Ht 20%. *The patient's temperature is 27°C. At what temperature are blood gases measured? How would you correct the blood gases according to patients body temperature? Would you treat the arterial blood gases at 37°C or at patient's body temperature?*

Blood gases are measured at a constant temperature of 37°C. They may be corrected according to body temperature. Each degree centigrade below 37°C increases blood pH by 0.015. If pH is 7.40 at 37°C *in vitro, in vivo* pH will be 7.55 at 27°C body temperature (7.40 + 0.015 × (37 − 27) = 7.55). The pH increases at lower temperatures, because of increased Pka and decreased CO_2 tension from increased CO_2 blood solubility during hypothermia. *In vivo*, PaO_2 is decreased because of increased oxygen solubility during hypothermia. At Cornell Medical Center, we measure blood gases at 37°C and interpret at 37°C without correcting them to body temperature. The normal values of blood gases at 37°C are: pH 7.40 ± 0.05. $PaCO_2$ 40 ± 5. PaO_2 95 ± 5; we should compare the blood gases at 37°C. During hypothermia, the normal values of blood gases are not the same as those at 37°C. The same blood specimen has different PO_2 values when measured at different temperatures. Yet, the oxygen content remains unchanged. It is easier to calculate the oxygen content at 37°C than at other temperatures where oxygen dissociation curves are shifted. We agree with Ream et al, when they considered temperature correction of blood gases as an example of the emperor's new clothes. We can conclude, therefore that the use of the uncorrected value of pH in managing the hypothermic patient appears to be preferable, because the desired value does not change with temperature. For the management of acid–base status, the uncorrected PCO_2 should be used.

Ream AK et al: Temperature correction of PCO_2 and pH in estimating acid–base status: An example of the emperor's new clothes. Anesthesiology 56:41–44, 1982

C. II-27. *If the blood level of the oxygenator is low, what would you replace it with? Blood or balanced salt solution?*

We try to maintain a hematocrit of at least 20%, during hemodilution. If the hematocrit is below 20%, blood is given to the oxygenator. If the hematocrit is above 20%, normosol is given to the oxygenator.

Lebowitz PW: Clinical Anesthesia Procedures of the Massachusetts General Hospital, p 154. Boston, Little, Brown & Co, 1978

C. II-28. *How do you know the fluid balance during CPB?*

During CPB, all intravenous lines are shut off. The intake includes cardioplegic solution, fluid or blood added to the oxygenator during CPB, and the decreased blood level in the oxygenator. The output includes urine and the increased blood level in the oxygenator.

C. II-29. How would you preserve the myocardium during CPB?

The most popular method of protecting the myocardium is to reduce myocardial oxygen demand by hypothermia and cardioplegia. Hypothermia is induced by a combination of systemic blood cooling by heat exchangers in the oxygenator, local application of cold saline solution to the external surface and chambers of the heart (if the heart is open), and infusion of cold cardioplegic solution through the aortic root or coronary ostium to the coronary arterial tree. The myocardial temperature may be decreased to 10° to 15°C.

Jynge P, Hearse DJ, Brainbridge MV: Myocardial protection during ischemic cardiac arrest. J Thorac Cardiovasc Surg 73:848, 1977

C. II-30. What is the cardioplegic solution? How much would you use?

Cardioplegic solution contains mainly high concentrations of potassium (10–30 mEq/L) or magnesium (160 mEq/L) to relax the heart. Flaccid cardioplegia itself reduces myocardial oxygen consumption and provides optimal conditions for surgery. Bicarbonate or THAM is usually added to raise the pH to levels between 7.4 and 7.80 to increase the intracellular shift of potassium and to decrease the metabolic acidosis from ischemia. Steroids, calcium, and procaine may be added to stabilize lysosomal and cell membranes. Glucose and insulin are added to provide energy and improve the intracellular shift of potassium. At Cornell Medical Center, we put 20 mEq of potassium chloride and 10 mEq of sodium bicarbonate to 1000 ml of 5% glucose in 0.25% salt solution, resulting in a final pH of 7.83, potassium of 20 mEq/L and osmolarity of 380 mOsm/L.

Intermittent, continuous or single infusion of cardioplegic solution have been used. Usually 300 to 600 ml of cold cardioplegic solution are needed to paralize the myocardium and cool the myocardium to 10° to 20°C.

Jynge P, Hearse DJ, Brainbridge MV: Myocardial protection during ischemic cardiac arrest. J Thorac Cardiovasc Surg 73:848, 1977

C. II-31. For how long a period can the aorta be cross clamped?

With myocardial hypothermia at 10° to 20°C and cardioplegia, the aorta may be cross clamped for 60 to 90 minutes without coronary perfusion. The shorter the cross clamping time is, the better the myocardial function will be. If the cross clamp time is expected to be prolonged, myocardial hypothermia should be maintained and coronary perfusion through a separate pump should be considered.

Follette D et al: Prolonged safe aortic clamping by combining stabilization, multi-dose cardioplegia, appropriate pH, reperfusion. J Thorac Cardiovasc Surg 74:682, 1977

C. II-32. Why does urine become pink after 2 hours of CPB? What is the renal threshold for plasma hemoglobin?

Pink urine is a sign of massive hemolysis. Hemolysis is mainly associated with the frothing, violent turbulence, acceleration, and sheer forces of negative pressures generated by the suction apparatus and is associated only to a lesser degree with the action of the pumps or with the gas–blood interface effects in the oxygenator. The renal threshold for hemoglobin is 100 to 150 mg/100 ml. It is advisable to maintain a high output of alkaline urine to prevent possible tubular damage from acid hematin crystals which are converted from hemoglobin.

Kaplan J: Cardiac Anesthesia, pp 415–416. New York, Grune & Stratton, 1979

C. II-33. At what temperature can the patient be weaned from CPB?

An esophageal temperature of 37°C and a rectal temperature at least 33°C must be reached before the patient can come off the pump. After discontinuation of the pump, surface warming should be continued to prevent hypothermia due to redistribution of heat in the body. Usually, esophageal temperature will decrease and rectal temperature will increase during heat redistribution.

Lebowitz PW: Clinical Anesthesia Procedures of the Massachusetts General Hospital, pp 144–157. Boston, Little, Brown & Co, 1978

C. II-34. Why does it take longer to rewarm than to cool the patient by the pump oxygenator?

It usually takes 5 to 10 minutes to cool the patient from 37°C to 25°C of average body temperature. It takes 20 to 40 minutes to rewarm the patient from 28°C to 35°C. The speed of heat exchange by the blood stream depends on the temperature gradient between venous blood and water in the heat exchanger, the pump blood flow rate, and the water flow rate of the heat exchanger. The initial venous blood temperature is 37°C and the water temperature of the heat exchanger is 0° to 4°C. The temperature gradient is 34° to 37°C. During rewarming, the water temperature is limited to 42°C or less to prevent denaturation and destruction of blood. The temperature gradient is limited to 10°C or less to prevent gas embolism due to too much of a decrease in gas solubility in the blood with a sharp increase in temperature. The heat exchanger water flow does not differ much during cooling and rewarming. However, the pump blood flow is usually maintained at a very high level during the initial cooling because of low blood pressure in the beginning of cooling. During rewarming the pump blood flow is frequently maintained at a low level because the blood pressure is usually high and the body temperature is still low. Rewarming may be speeded up by administering inhalation anesthetics or employing vasodilators to decrease vascular resistance and thereby increasing pump flow to maintain the same blood pressure. Because the increased vascular resistance is usually due to inadequate anesthesia during rewarming, we prefer inhalation anesthetics to vasodilators.

Kaplan J: Cardiac Anesthesia, pp 398–399. New York, Grune & Stratton, 1979

Stanely TH et al: Plasma catecholamine and cortisol responses to Fentanyl-oxygen anesthesia for coronary–artery operations. Anesthesiology 53:250–253, 1980

C. II-35. How would you defibrillate the heart internally during CPB?

The heart is defibrillated internally by a DC defibrillator, usually 10 to 20 watt second. If the heart remains in ventricular fibrillation, blood gases, electrolytes, and temperature are rechecked and lidocaine 1 to 2 mg/kg is administered before DC defibrillation. Rarely, propranolol and bretylium are added to treat intractable ventricular fibrillation or tachycardia.

Kaplan J: Cardiac Anesthesia, p 430. New York, Grune & Stratton, 1979

C. II-36. Why is calcium chloride usually administered right before the patient comes off the pump?

With hemodilution, the ionized calcium frequently falls to about 1.5 mEq/l (normal 1.9–2.2 mEq/L). Calcium chloride, 0.5 to 1.0 gm, is usually given to increase myocardial contractility and reverse potassium cardioplegia.

Kaplan J: Cardiac Anesthesia, p 431. New York, Grune & Stratton, 1979

C. II-37. If the heart rate is 40/min, what should you do?

Atropine may be administered to treat sinus or nodal bradycardia. Frequently, temporary AV block is found at the end of bypass because of potassium cardioplegia and ischemic insult during aortic cross clamping. A temporary epicardial pacemaker may be needed if atropine is not effective. Atrial pacing is preferred because of better cardiac output with atrial kick. Ventricular pacing is necessary if there is complete AV block. AV sequential pacing is indicated when ventricular pacing does not provide adequate cardiac output.

Kaplan J: Cardiac Anesthesia, p 431. New York, Grune & Stratton, 1979

C. II-38. How does the blood sugar level change during CPB? Why?

Blood sugar levels are elevated during perfusion, possibly indicating a defect in glucose utilization due to catecholamine inhibition of insulin secretion, or to the direct effect of catecholamine on the catabolism of glycogen to blood glucose. Catecholamines are markedly elevated during bypass.

Ionescu MI, Wooler GH: Current Techniques in Extracorporeal Circulation, p 113. London, Butterworth & Co, 1976

Stanley TH et al: Plasma catecholamine and cortisol responses to Fentanyl–oxygen anesthesia for coronary–artery operations. Anesthesiology 53:250–253, 1980

C. II-39. What are the effects of CPB on platelet and coagulation factors?

Platelet counts fall more with the bubble type oxygenator than with the membrane type oxygenator, but rarely below the levels clinically required for hemostasis. Thrombocytopenia is mainly caused by hemodilution, aggregation, adhesion, and the ADP–release reaction induced by the foreign surfaces and the blood–gas interface. Heparin may potentiate platelet aggregation and adhesions. The level of coagulation factors decreases at the beginning of bypass because of hemodilution, surface absorption by the plastic, glass, and metal, and protein denaturation induced by blood-gas interface. At the same time, the synthesis of clotting factors by the liver increases so that the concentration of clotting factors returns to normal within a period of hours. Membrane oxygenators cause few changes in clotting factors.

Ionescu MI, Wooler GH: Current Techniques in Extracorporeal Circulation, pp 16–22. London Butterworth & Co, 1976

Kaplan J: Cardiac Anesthesia, pp 16–22. New York, Grune & Stratton, 1979

After Cardiopulmonary Bypass

C. III-1. How would you reverse heparin? How much protamine would you use?

It has been recommended that 1.1 to 1.3 mg of protamine sulfate are needed to reverse each 100 units of remaining heparin calculated by ACT dose–response curve or protamine titration test. At Cornell Medical Center, we give 1.0 mg of protamine to reverse each 100 units or 1 mg of heparin initially administered. Only the initial dose of heparin is counted. The subsequently added dose of heparin, to keep the ACT level above 480 seconds, is not considered because of its metabolism and elimination. The ACT test is repeated 20 minutes after the administration of protamine. ACT usually returns to its control level. If the ACT is still prolonged, additional protamine is given according to the ACT dose response curve.

Bull MH, Huse WM, Bull BS: Evaluation of tests used to monitor heparin therapy during extracorporeal circulation. Anesthesiology 43:346–353, 1975

C. III-2. What is the action mechanism of protamine?

Heparin is a strong organic acid. Protamine is a strong organic base. They combine ionically to form a stable salt and lose their own anticoagulant activity.

Gillman AG, Goodman LS, Gilman A: The Pharmacological Basis of Therapeutics, 6th ed, p 1352. New York, MacMillan, 1980

C. III-3. What are the complications of too much protamine?

Protamine itself is an anticoagulant. Too much protamine will cause postoperative hemorrhage.

Gillman AG, Goodman LS, Gilman A: The Pharmacological Basis of Therapeutics, 6th ed, p 1352. New York, MacMillan, 1980

C. III-4. Why did the patient develop hypotension after administering protamine? How do you treat and prevent this condition?

The precise mechanisms of the hypotensive effects of protamine are not entirely clear. The possible causes are vasodilation and myocardial depression from bolus administration of large doses of protamine sulfate. The treatments are as follows:

- Stop protamine administration temporarily
- Lighten the anesthesia
- Increase blood volume or give small doses of phenylephrine, 0.1 mg increments, if PCWP is low
- Give diuretics and inotropes if PCWP is high
- Go back on bypass temporarily

Conahan reported that in 15 adult patients there were no statistically significant changes in mean arterial pressure, cardiac output, and central venous pressure after administration of protamine sulfate (3 mg/kg over 5 min), even though some patients had a 40 torr drop in blood pressure. Our clinical observation has indicated that 3.0 mg/kg of protamine given in 3 to 5 minutes occasionally can precipitate severe hypotension.

Conahan TJ et al: Cardiovascular effects of protamine sulfate in man. Anesth Analg 60:33–36, 1981

C. III-5. What are the indications for intraaortic balloon pump (IABP)?

IABP is primarily used for cardiogenic shock not responsive to maximal pharmacological support. The indications include the following:

Ischemic Heart Disease
- Cardiogenic shock
- Acute myocardial infarction complicated by
  - mechanical defects—ventricular or septal rupture, acute mitral insufficiency, or ventricular aneurysm
  - Continued ischemic pain and extension of infarction
  - Refractory ventricular arrhythmias
- During cardiac catheterization
- Undergoing noncardiac surgery

Cardiac Surgery
- Before CPB and postoperatively
- After CPB—low output syndrome

Pulsatile CPB—rare

Pediatric Congenital Heart Disease—rare

Neurosurgery—temporarily increase total cerebral blood flow in specific circumstances

Ionescu MI, Wooler GH: Current Techniques in Extracorporeal Circulation, p 496. London, Butterworth & Co, 1976

Kaplan J: Cardiac Anesthesia, pp 450–460. New York, Grune & Stratton, 1979

C. III-6. What are the principles of IABP?

IABP counterpulsation is designed to increase the myocardial oxygen supply during diastole and to decrease myocardial oxygen demand during systole. The balloon is inflated during diastole to increase the diastolic aortic pressure, resulting in increased coronary blood flow. The balloon is deflated just prior to the next systole to decrease the intraaortic pressure and afterload, resulting in decreased myocardial oxygen consumption. The cardiac output is increased because of increased coronary perfusion and decreased resistance.

Ionescu MI, Wooler GH: Current Techniques in Extracorporeal Circulation, p 155. London, Butterworth & Co, 1976

C. III-7. What are the complications of IABP?

- Ischemia of the leg
- Dissection of the aorta
- Thrombus formation and embolization
- Thrombocytopenia
- Infection
- Gas embolization
- Inability to place the IABP

Kaplan J: Cardiac Anesthesia, p 463. New York, Grune & Stratton, 1979

D. Postoperative Management

D.1. What are the postoperative complications?

Cardiovascular—congestive heart failure, arrhythmias, low output syndrome, myocardial ischemia or infarction due to surgical manipulation, prolonged CPB and aortic cross-clamp (coronary ischemia), use of cardioplegic solution, and occlusion or kinking of grafts

Pulmonary—pump lung or adult respiratory distress syndrome due to the following:

- Decreased blood flow to the lung during total CPB
- Deflated alveoli during CPB, resulting in decreased surfactant and decreased distensibility
- Fluid overloading
- Hyperoxia during CPB

- Left ventricular failure
- Microemboli

Renal
- Polyuria from hemodilution and diuretics
- Oliguria from hypoperfusion

Hemorrhage
- Too much or too little protamine to reverse heparin
- Thrombocytopenia and decreased coagulation factors
- Disseminated intravascular coagulopathy
- Poor surgical hemostasis

Embolism—due to air, destroyed or aggregated formed blood elements, fat, endogenous and exogenous debris
Neurological—functional changes in behavior, personality, or other brain functions; cerebral embolism
Hyperglycemia—due to increased catecholamine levels
Hypopotassemia—due to hemodilution and diuretics

Arens JF: Extracorporeal circulation: Practical considerations in the use of the heart pump. ASA Refresher Courses in Anesthesiology 4:13–24, 1976

D.2. Would you reverse the muscle relaxants? Why?

No. We usually keep the patient on the respirator over night to prevent postoperative respiratory failure. Moreover, atropine and neostigmine may cause severe tachycardia or bradycardia in ischemic cardiac patients.

Arens JF: Extracorporeal circulation: Practical considerations in the use of the heart pump. ASA Refresher Courses in Anesthesiology 4:13–24, 1976

D.3. When will you wean the patient from the respirator?

Generally, the patient is weaned from the respirator the following morning after surgery. If the operative course is very smooth and if the patient has good ventricular function, the patient may be weaned from the respirator early, usually 2 to 6 hours after surgery.

Kaplan J: Cardiac Anesthesia, p 478. New York, Grune & Stratton, 1979

D.4. What criteria would you use in deciding when to wean the patient from the respirator?

- Consciousness—awake and alert
- Stable vital signs
- Acceptable arterial blood gases—pH, 7.35–7.45; PO_2, over 80 torr with F_IO_2 0.4; PCO_2, 35–45 torr
- Acceptable respiratory mechanics
  - Vital capacity greater than 10–15 ml/kg
  - Maximal inspiratory force—greater than 20–25 cm H_2O

- Hemostasis—less than 200 ml/hr of chest tube drainage
- Stable metabolic state—normal temperature and electrolytes

When the patient can satisfy the above criteria, the patient is put on T-piece with 50% oxygen. If the patient tolerates the T-piece well for 30 minutes and arterial blood gases are acceptable, the patient is extubated.

Kaplan J: Cardiac Anesthesia, p 478. New York, Grune & Stratton, 1979

8 Valvular Heart Disease

Marjorie J. Topkins

A 55-year-old man was admitted with a three day history of palpitation, coughing, orthopnea, wheezing, shortness of breath while climbing one flight of stairs, and substernal pain relieved by sitting up. All symptoms were worse at night. (Three years ago, a murmur was heard by his physician and echocardiography was performed.) On this admission the following was noted: ABG pH 7.46, P_{CO_2} 29, P_{O_2} 51, CO_2 21, oxygen saturation 85.5%, WBC 12,000, bp 120/80, pulse 110, respiration 26, temperature 38.3°C. A holosystolic murmur was heard throughout, but it was greatest at the apex. Point of maximal impulse—6th interspace. ECG—apical myocardial infarction or ischemia, left ventricular hypertrophy with strain, and digitalis effect.

A. Medical Disease and Differential Diagnosis

1. What is the presumptive diagnosis? Differential diagnosis?
2. What are some of the causes of mitral insufficiency?
3. What is floppy valve syndrome?
4. What are the complications of mitral regurgitation?
5. What is the natural history of the disease?
6. Describe the murmur of the following: mitral insufficiency, mitral stenosis, aortic insufficiency, aortic stenosis, and floppy valve syndrome.
7. What is the New York Heart Association classification of heart disease?
8. What are the differences between acute and chronic mitral regurgitation (MR)?

B. Preoperative Evaluation and Preparation

1. What diagnostic tests are available to evaluate the disease or to confirm the presumptive diagnosis?

2. How will you treat pulmonary edema in this patient? Is there a role for the following:
   - Beta-blockade
   - Digitalis preparations
   - Diuretics
   - Nitroprusside
3. What are the electrocardiographic findings in mitral regurgitation? Which ones would you treat?
4. Discuss myocardial oxygen consumption (MVO_2) in the patient with mitral regurgitation versus aortic regurgitation.
5. How is the mitral valve area measured? How is the aortic valve area measured?
6. Discuss the rationale for premedicating this patient.

C. Intraoperative Management

1. What monitoring will be used? What information will you obtain from each?
2. What anesthetic management will you employ and why?
3. Discuss the use of nitroprusside and nitroglycerine in mitral regurgitation (MR).
4. Which muscle relaxant will you use and why?

D. Postoperative Management

1. Discuss the use of the intraaortic balloon pump (IABP) in this patient after bypass.
2. What parameters will you monitor postoperatively?
3. Discuss postoperative ventilation.

A. Medical Disease and Differential Diagnosis

A.1. What is the presumptive diagnosis? Differential diagnosis?

The presumptive diagnosis is valvular heart disease, specifically mitral valvular disease. The history of recent onset of palpitations, dyspnea, cough, orthopnea, shortness of breath, substernal pain, all worse at night, and the holosystolic murmur suggest acute mitral insufficiency. The nocturnal increase in symptoms suggests pulmonary overload in the supine position. Left ventricular hypertrophy is a component of acute mitral insufficiency. The ECG evidence of myocardial infarction or ischemia suggests a possible cause for the acute rupture. The differential diagnosis includes the following:

- Hypertrophic cardiomyopathy—both have pansystolic murmurs, prominent left ventricles, and third heart sound

- Ventricular septal defect (VSD) has pansystolic murmur, overactive left ventricle, and third heart sound.
- Endocardial cushion defects with ostium primum atrial defect and mitral incompetence
- Acquired VSD secondary to rupture of septum

Sokolow M, McIlroy MB: Clinical Cardiology, p 383. Los Altos, CA, Lange Medical Publications, 1977

A.2. What are some of the causes of mitral insufficiency?

Mitral insufficiency is either acute or chronic. The following are some of the causes:

- Rheumatic fever with subsequent rheumatic endocarditis is responsible for 50% of cases of mitral insufficiency.
- Degenerative changes with stretching and tearing of chordae tendineae
- Infective endocarditis
- Ischemic heart disease especially posterior inferior myocardial infarction with subsequent ischemia or rupture of the papillary muscle
- Congenital heart disease. Clefts of the mitral valve, Marfan's syndrome, and osteogenesis imperfecta are associated with isolated mitral insufficiency.
- Mitral valve ring calcification
- Traumatic heart disease; i.e., steering wheel injury

Sokolow M, McIlroy MB: Clinical Cardiology, p 375. Los Altos, CA, Lange Medical Publications, 1977

A.3. What is floppy valve syndrome?

Floppy valve syndrome or click murmur syndrome or mitral valve prolapse was first described by Barlow and is usually considered a hemodynamically insignificant lesion. However, it may cause acute mitral insufficiency. The incidence is 4% to 6% in young women and over 90% in Marfan's syndrome, usually in the third to fifth decade.

Sokolow M, McIlroy MB: Clinical Cardiology, p 377. Los Altos, CA, Lange Medical Publications, 1977

A.4. What are the complications of mitral regurgitation (MR)?

- Systemic emboli, frequently due to infective endocarditis, occur in 20% of cases
- Infective endocarditis—20%
- Rheumatic myocarditis
- Coronary artery disease, hypertension, and atherosclerosis are almost invariably present in elderly patients with MR.
- Ventricular arrhythmias and sudden death especially in the click murmur syndrome

Sokolow M, McIlroy MB: Clinical Cardiology, pp 383–384. Los Altos, CA, Lange Medical Publications, 1977

A.5. What is the natural history of the disease?

The symptoms of dyspnea on exertion and fatigability may persist for many years. However, once severe congestive failure ensues, the disease progresses rapidly. Fifty percent of patients in NYHA Class III are dead in 6 years, and 50% of patients in Class IV are dead in 2 years. If mitral regurgitation is due to cardiomyopathy or disease, the prognosis is poor.

Thomas SJ, Lowenstein E: Anesthetic management of valvular heart disease. International Anesthesiology Clinics, 17:87, 1979

A.6. Describe the murmur of the following: mitral insufficiency, mitral stenosis, aortic insufficiency, aortic stenosis, and floppy valve syndrome?

Mitral insufficiency produces a pansystolic murmur. Mitral stenosis produces a presystolic murmur. Aortic insufficiency produces immediate diastolic murmur. Aortic stenosis produces a systolic ejection murmur. Floppy valve syndrome produces a late systolic murmur.

Sokolow M, McIlroy MB: Clinical Cardiology, pp 55–57. Los Altos, CA, Lange Medical Publications, 1977

A.7. What is the New York Heart Association classification of heart disease?

The New York Heart Association classification of heart disease evaluates both functional and therapeutic status of the patient. The functional status of the patient is divided into four classes.

Class I—No limitation of physical activity

Class II—Slight limitation of physical activity. The patient is comfortable at rest, but ordinary activity produces fatigue, palpitations, dyspnea or angina.

Class III—Marked limitation of physical activity. The patient is comfortable at rest, but less than ordinary activity produces fatigue, palpitation, dyspnea or angina.

Class IV—Unable to carry on any physical activity without discomfort. Symptoms of cardiac insufficiency or angina may be present at rest.

Class II is occasionally divided into two parts.

II-a—Climbing stairs may produce symptoms while ordinary walking does not.

II-b—Some limitation on any physical activity

The therapeutic classification is divided into 5 classes.

Class A—Physical activity is not restricted.

Class B—Ordinary activity need not be restricted. Competitive efforts are avoided.

Class C—Ordinary activity should be moderately restricted. All strenuous activity must be discontinued.

Class D—Ordinary activity should be markedly restricted.

Class E—Patient should be at complete rest.

> Criteria Committee of the New York Heart Association, Inc: Diseases of the Heart and Blood Vessels (Nomenclature and Criteria for Diagnosis), 6th ed. Boston, Little, Brown & Co, 1964
>
> Sokolow M, McIlroy MB: Clinical Cardiology, p 37. Los Altos, CA, Lange Medical Publications, 1977

A.8. What are the differences between acute and chronic mitral regurgitation (MR)?

Etiology

Acute MR is most commonly caused by rupture of chordae tendineae secondary to endocarditis, papillary muscle dysfunction secondary to myocardial ischemia, and papillary muscle rupture secondary to acute myocardial infarction. Chronic MR results from many causes, most commonly rheumatic valvular disease that is almost always associated with some mitral stenosis. Other causes include papillary muscle dysfunction, floppy valve syndrome, rupture of chordae tendineae, bacterial endocarditis, and cardiomyopathy.

Hemodynamics

In acute MR, the smaller and less distensible atrium does not absorb the regurgitant flow as in chronic MR. Therefore, left ventricular end-diastolic pressure (LVEDP), left atrial V-wave pressure, and pulmonary venous and arterial pressures are higher in acute MR than in chronic MR.

In chronic MR, the left atrium is enlarged and more distensible; therefore, little pressure is reflected in the pulmonary circulation. The left ventricle is dilated and hypertrophic in chronic MR; this condition results in higher left ventricular end-systolic and end-diastolic volumes.

Rhythm

In chronic MR, atrial fibrillation is the most common rhythm. The presence of normal sinus rhythm suggests acute MR rather than chronic MR.

> Kaplan JA: Cardiac Anesthesia, pp 213–219. New York, Grune & Stratton, 1979

B. Preoperative Evaluation and Preparation

B.1. What diagnostic tests are available to evaluate the disease or to confirm the presumptive diagnosis?

In addition to the history, physical, and routine laboratory studies, there are both invasive and noninvasive procedures that aid the physician in evaluating the patient and his disease. Noninvasive procedures include PA lateral and oblique chest x-rays, and may include a barium swallow to outline the atrium as well. Left ventricular and atrial enlargement are seen in chronic regurgitation. In acute regurgitation, the heart may be normal in size, and pulmonary congestion and edema may be the only findings. Within a week or two, chamber enlargement begins and the chamber may approach the size seen in chronic regurgitation in a year if the patient survives.

Calcification of the mitral ring can be visualized in fluoroscopy. Echocardiography is used to visualize the mitral valve leaflets, their movement, and their competence. Echocardiography is a sensitive means of detecting minor degrees of mitral valve prolapse. Chamber size (left atrium and ventricle) can be approximated by echocardiography as well. Radionuclide imaging can yield information concerning ventricular wall motion and can be used to calculate the ejection fraction. Invasive techniques include right and left heart catheterization and angiography. In acute mitral regurgitation, a wide pulse pressure in the wedge or left atrial pressure is significant. Giant-v-waves as high as 80 torr and averaging 50 torr are characteristic. V-waves are also seen in the pulmonary artery pressure tracing. In chronic mitral regurgitation, left atrial pressure is only moderately elevated with v-waves up to 30 torr. If the left atrium is large, the pressures are not usually impressive. Left ventricular end-diastolic pressure (LVEDP) is important. If elevated, hypertension, rheumatic myocarditis, or coronary artery disease should be suspected.

Angiography done on the same occasion will determine the magnitude of the regurgitant fraction. Coronary arteriography will evaluate the coronary arteries so that their contribution to the pathophysiology can be assessed.

Sokolow M, McIlroy MB: Clinical Cardiology, pp 381–383. Los Altos, CA, Lange Medical Publications, 1977

B.2. How will you treat pulmonary edema in this patient? Is there a role for the following:

- Beta-blockade
- Digitalis preparations
- Diuretics
- Nitroprusside

Beta-blockade given with norepinephrine in mitral regurgitation produces an increase in mean arterial pressure, an increase in LAP and even greater rise in regurgitant flow and a fall in forward flow. When norepinephrine is given without beta-blockade, mean left atrial pressure rises, but there is no decrease in forward flow and no increase in regurgitant flow. Beta-adrenergic effects are necessary to overcome the adrenergic effects on arterial impedance. Therefore, beta-blockade would appear to have a negative effect on pulmonary edema.

Digitalis preparations will decrease the size of the left ventricle and the regurgitant fraction, thereby improving the pulmonary edema.

Diuretics decrease the afterload and, to some extent, preload. Therefore, diuretics should improve the pulmonary edema. Care must be taken, however, to avoid hypokalemia.

Nitroprusside by decreasing the afterload, will increase forward flow, decrease the heart size, and decrease the regurgitant fraction. The pulmonary edema should improve.

Kaplan J: Cardiac Anesthesia, pp 217–219. New York, Grune & Stratton, 1979

Thomas SJ, Lowenstein E: Anesthetic Management of the patient with valvular heart disease. Int Anesthesiol Clin 17:67–96, 1979

B.3. What are the electrocardiographic findings in mitral regurgitation? Which ones would you treat?

Left ventricular hypertrophy is greater in acute regurgitation. An incomplete right-bundle-branch block (rsR′ in V_1) is seen in 5% of patients. Left bundle branch block is less common and indicates ventricular disease. Atrial arrhythmias develop with time. Atrial fibrillation is more common than atrial premature contractions, atrial tachycardia, or atrial flutter. The absence of atrial fibrillation in a symptomatic patient suggests acute incompetence. P Mitrale may be seen in click murmur syndrome. Atrial and ventricular premature beats are often seen. Rapid ventricular response in atrial fibrillation and multiple premature contractions should be treated, especially if hemodynamically significant.

Sokolow M, McIlroy MB: Clinical Cardiology, pp 379–381. Los Altos, CA, Lange Medical Publications, 1977

B.4. Discuss myocardial oxygen consumption (MVO_2) in the patient with mitral regurgitation versus aortic regurgitation (AR).

Doubling pressure work involves large increases in wall tension, a major determinant of myocardial oxygen consumption. Doubling volume work, which may occur in mitral and aortic regurgitation, results in a small increase in myocardial oxygen consumption (MVO_2). Pressure developed in the hypertrophied left ventricle is rapidly absorbed by the dilated left atrium into which the left ventricle empties in part through the regurgitant mitral valve. In aortic regurgitation, pressure developed in the left ventricle is opposed by the aortic pressure which offers greater impedance to left ventricular ejection than the lower pressured left atrium does in mitral regurgitation. The left ventricle in AR dilates and hypertrophies more to effect forward flow. Therefore, MVO_2 increases in AR. In addition, the lower diastolic pressure of AR decreases myocardial perfusion and angina may result.

Kaplan JA: Cardiac Anesthesia, p 202. New York, Grune & Stratton, 1979

Thomas SJ, Lowenstein E: Anesthetic management of patients with valvular heart disease. Int Anesthesiol Clin 17:73, 1979

B.5. How is the mitral valve area measured? How is the aortic valve area measured?

As a valve becomes stenotic, flow becomes turbulent and proportional to the square root of the pressure gradient. A 50% decrease in valve size is necessary before a significant transvalvular pressure gradient can be detected at catheterization. As stenosis increases, greater increases in pressure gradient are needed to produce the same flow.

The valve area is expressed in centimeters squared and relates flow across the valve and the square root pressure gradient across that valve.

$$\text{Mitral valve area (cm}^2) = \frac{\text{Mitral valve flow}}{31 \sqrt{\text{mean mitral valve gradient}}}$$

$$\text{Where mitral valve flow} = \frac{\text{Cardiac output in ml/min}}{\text{diastolic filling period in sec/min}}$$

$$\text{Aortic valve area (cm}^2) = \frac{\text{Aortic valve flow}}{44.5 \sqrt{\text{mean aortic valve gradient}}}$$

$$\text{Where aortic valve flow} = \frac{\text{cardiac output in ml/min}}{\text{systolic ejection period in sec/min}}$$

Kaplan JA: Cardiac Anesthesia, pp 202–203. New York, Grune & Stratton, 1979

B.6. Discuss the rationale for premedicating this patient.

Patients with mitral regurgitation require a normal or slightly elevated heart rate except when significant mitral stenosis is associated with the regurgitation. Scopolamine and a narcotic provide good sedation with little effect on the heart rate. Atropine in usual doses has little effect on heart rate; however, atropine could be useful in pure mitral regurgitation to maintain heart rate and thereby augment forward flow. If an antisialagogue is required or desired, scopolamine is superior to atropine and has a central depressant effect as well. Light premedication is satisfactory in these cases as compared with patients undergoing coronary artery bypass surgery in whom anginal attacks might be precipitated by anxiety.

Kaplan JA: Cardiac Anesthesia, p 53. New York, Grune & Stratton, 1979

Thomas SJ, Lowenstein E: Anesthetic management of patients with valvular heart disease. Int Anesthesiol Clin, 17:89–90, 1979

C. Intraoperative Management

C.1. What monitoring will be used? What information will you obtain from each?

- ECG for rate, rhythm, and evidence of myocardial ischemia manifested by depression of S-T segment or inversion of T-waves
- Arterial line for blood gases as well as pressure
- Pulmonary artery catheter to measure central venous pressure, pulmon-

ary artery pressure, pulmonary capillary wedge pressure, and cardiac output. The wedge pressure is an indirect measurement of left atrial pressure and therefore left ventricular filling pressure. It is useful when determining optimal preload postoperatively. Wedge pressure is an essential guide when using vasodilators for afterload reduction.
- Temperature—Esophageal and rectal
- Urinary output

Kaplan JA: Cardiac Anesthesia, pp 219–220. New York, Grune & Stratton, 1977

Lappas DG, Gayes JM: Intraoperative monitoring. Int Anesthesiol Clin 17:157–173, 1979

Thomas SJ, Lowenstein E: Anesthetic management of patients with valvular heart disease. Int Anesthesiol Clin 17:89, 1979

C.2. *What anesthetic management will you employ and why?*

All commonly used inhalation anesthetics cause myocardial depression which is dose related. In addition, they alter peripheral resistance and heart rate in various ways.

- Enflurane has little or no effect on peripheral resistance and heart rate. Cardiac output is decreased.
- Halothane decreases peripheral resistance with no change in heart rate. Cardiac output is decreased.
- Nitrous oxide increases peripheral resistance with little change in heart rate. Cardiac output is decreased.
- Isoflurane decreases peripheral resistance and increases heart rate and is only a mild myocardial depressant. Cardiac output is maintained.
- Morphine produces little myocardial depression. Cardiac output is increased and peripheral resistance decreased. MVO_2 is decreased in patients with valvular heart disease.
- Innovar in anesthetic doses increases cardiac output and maximum acceleration of left ventricular ejection with a slight decrease in tension–time index with minimal effects on MVO_2.
- Isoflurane, halothane, enflurane, in that order, would appear to be better for patients with mitral regurgitation. Morphine anesthesia would appear to be the preferred intravenous anesthetic.

Philbin DM, Bland JHL: Cardiovascular effects of anesthetics: An introduction. Int Anesthesiol Clin 17:1–9, 1979

Stevens WC: Anesthetic Management. Anesth Analg (Cleve) 55:622, 1976

Thomas SJ, Lowenstein E: Anesthetic management of patients with valvular heart disease. Int Anesthesiol Clin 17:92, 1979

C.3. *Discuss the use of nitroprusside and nitroglycerine in mitral regurgitation (MR).*

Nitroprusside and nitroglycerine will decrease systemic vascular resistance (SVR) and promote forward flow. Nitroglycerine may be of greater benefit in patients in whom MR is secondary to ischemic heart disease with secondary papillary muscle dysfunction. The mechanism of action is increased venous pooling and decreased preload and afterload, with resultant decrease in myocardial oxygen demand and possible redistribution of coronary blood flow causing an increase in myocardial oxygen supply.

Kaplan JA (ed): Cardiac Anesthesia, p 210. New York, Grune & Stratton, 1979

Kaplan JA (ed): Cardiac Anesthesia, pp 49–51. New York, Grune & Stratton, 1979

C.4. Which muscle relaxant will you use and why?

A muscle relaxant that maintains or increases the heart rate and decreases peripheral resistance, thereby promoting forward flow, is the relaxant of choice in mitral regurgitation. Pancuronium or gallamine would be the preferred agents. However, if significant stenosis is associated with the regurgitation, the tachycardia produced by pancuronium or gallamine might decrease significantly the diastolic filling time of the left ventricle.

Savarese JJ, Philbin DM: Cardiovascular effects of neuromuscular blocking drugs, Int Anesthesiol Clin 17:13–54, 1979

D. Postoperative Management

D.1. Discuss the use of the intraaortic balloon pump (IABP) in this patient after bypass.

The indications for IABP postbypass are low output syndrome and intraoperative myocardial infarction. The use of IABP has decreased over the last few years as better techniques at myocardial preservation have been devised and procedures are accomplished with shorter pump times. There is greater use of inotropic agents and vasodilatation when coming off the pump. There are, however, a few patients who require IABP. If this patient fails to respond to the usual measures, the balloon can be inserted percutaneously into the femoral artery and advanced up the aorta to lie just caudad to the left subclavian artery. When ballooning commences, it is timed with the arterial pulse wave. In essence, the balloon decreases the work of the heart by lowering systolic pressure and decreasing impedance to ventricular outflow and slowing the rate. At the same time it augments the diastolic aortic pressure above the level of the systolic pressure, thereby improving myocardial perfusion. The results are increased cardiac output, ejection fraction, and cerebral and renal blood flow.

Kaplan JA: Cardiac Anesthesia, p 442. New York, Grune & Stratton, 1979

D.2. What parameters will you monitor postoperatively?

- Systemic blood pressure, pulmonary artery diastolic and wedge pressures, and central venous pressure. High systemic pressures must be avoided to prevent excessive afterload and increased myocardial work (pressure work) and to prevent bleeding from the cannula site in the aorta or from a suture line if the aorta was incised. Hypotension must be diagnosed as to cause. The pulmonary artery wedge pressure is monitored as an indirect measurement of left ventricular filling pressure. High pulmonary wedge pressures with a low systemic pressure may indicate a failing myocardium. Low wedge pressures with low systemic pressures indicate inadequate volume. Low wedge pressure and high systemic pressure may indicate increased peripheral vascular resistance with a low volume. Finally, a high wedge and a high systemic pressure may indicate fluid overload or peripheral vasoconstriction. Each must be treated differently, with an inotropic agent, volume and peripheral dilator such as nitroprusside or peripheral dilator alone.

- ECG for arrhythmia, rate, and evidence of ischemia
- Blood gases and chemistries. These are monitored to ensure the adequacy of ventilation and the adequacy of oxygen delivery to the tissues. Metabolic acidosis suggests inadequate perfusion. Respiratory acidosis indicates inadequate ventilation. Respiratory alkalosis means excessive ventilation. Respiratory alkalosis results in a shift of the oxygen dissociation curve to the left, decreasing the P_{50}. Coronary blood flow is decreased 30% when P_aCO_2 is decreased to 20 torr. Respiratory alkalosis and hypocarbia can cause a rapid shift of potassium from the blood into the cells. The resultant hypokalemia may precipitate arrhythmias. Mild acidosis facilitates oxygen delivery. Electrolytes must be monitored as well as glucose, BUN, and cardiac enzymes.
- Temperature. Hypothermia can shift the oxygen dissociation curve to the left; it can be a cause for arrhythmias and may interfere with blood coagulation. Shivering can increase oxygen consumption 300% to 600%. Hypothermia and alkalosis will doubly affect the oxygen dissociation curve. Hyperthermia will greatly increase the oxygen consumption.
- Suction and drainage for evidence of bleeding
- Urinary output
- Cardiac output evaluates the condition of the myocardium.

Bay J, Nunn, JF, Prys–Roberts C: Factors influencing arterial Po_2 during recovery from anaesthesia, Br J Anaesth 40:398, 1968

Kaplan JA: Cardiac Anesthesia, pp 405–413. New York, Grune & Stratton, 1979

Prys–Roberts C: Postanesthetic shivering in common and uncommon problems. In Jenkins MT (ed): Anesthesiology, Vol. 3. Clinical Anesthesia Series, Philadelpha, FA Davis, 1968

D.3. Discuss postoperative ventilation.

This patient, and most patients who have undergone cardiopulmonary bypass, should be mechanically ventilated for 12 to 24 hours or until there is evidence that the cardiorespiratory system can function without support. This patient showed signs of pulmonary overload preoperatively and should benefit from mechanic ventilation. Ventilator volumes can be set at 10 cc/kg with a rate of 10 and an F_1O_2 of 60% until blood gases can be obtained. The rate, volume, and F_IO_2 are adjusted accordingly. PEEP is added if necessary, but can have deleterious effects on the cardiac output. Sedation and muscle relaxants may be needed to prevent reaction on the endotracheal tube. Respiratory support can be discontinued when the following occur:

- Blood gases and chemistries are within acceptable range
- Patient is awake
- Blood pressure is adequate and the rate and rhythm of the heart are normal
- Bleeding is minimal
- Temperature is 36°C or more
- Chest x-ray shows no pneumothorax or severe atelectasis

Kaplan JA: Cardiac Anesthesia, pp 473–477. New York, Grune & Stratton, 1979

9 Pacemaker

Fun–Sun F. Yao

A 76-year-old man was scheduled for insertion of a permanent transvenous pacemaker. He had an anterior myocardial infarction 8 months ago. His blood pressure was 120/80 torr; heart rate, 40 per minute. He is currently taking propranolol, digoxin, furosemide, and isosorbide.

A. Medical Disease and Differential Diagnosis

1. What is the possible ECG rhythm when the heart rate is 40 per minute?
2. What is the problem of complete atrioventricular block?
3. What are the common causes of heart block?
4. What are the indications for permanent pacemakers?
5. What is sick sinus syndrome?
6. How would you diagnose first, second, and third-degree AV block, left anterior fascicular hemiblock, and left posterior fascicular hemiblock?
7. How many types of pacemakers are there? How do they work?
8. How would you know if it is atrial, ventricular, or AV sequential pacing?
9. What are the advantages and disadvantages of atrial pacing?
10. What are the indications for AV sequential pacemakers?
11. In a permanent pacemaker battery, what are the usual values for pulse amplitude, pulse width, pulse rate, and sensing threshold?
12. What is hysteresis rate?
13. How do you set the external pacemaker to test the pacing threshold, sensing R wave, and diaphragmatic pacing?
14. What are the acceptable values of pacing threshold, sensing R wave, and resistance?
15. What are the usual life spans of pacemakers?
16. How do you know if the implanted demand pacemaker is working?

B. Preoperative Evaluation and Preparation

1. What kind of work-up would you like the patient to have?

C. Intraoperative Management

1. Would you give general or local anesthesia for insertion of transvenous pacemaker? Why?
2. If it is an epicardial electrode, would you give local or general anesthesia?
3. What premedication would you give for local anesthesia?
4. What drugs and equipment would you like to have on hand in the operating room?
5. How do you sedate the patient?
6. After the endocardial pacemaker was inserted, the ECG pattern changed from left bundle branch block to right bundle branch block. What is the possible diagnosis?

D. Postoperative Management

1. What are the complications of transvenous implantation of pacemakers?
2. What are the causes of pacemaker failure?
3. What kinds of environmental electromagnetic interference may affect the function of a demand pacemaker?
4. Two months later, the patient came back for transurethral resection of the prostate because of prostatic hypertrophy. How would you prevent interference to the pacemaker from the electrocautery?
5. How do you detect inhibition of pacemaker function?

A. Medical Disease and Differential Diagnosis

A.1. What is the possible ECG rhythm when the heart rate is 40 per minute?

Bradycardia may come from any part of the conduction system including sinus bradycardia, nodal bradycardia, second-degree or third-degree AV block, atrial fibrillation with slow ventricular rate, and idioventricular rhythm.

Braunwald E: Heart Disease, pp 744–777. Philadelphia, WB Saunders, 1980

A.2. What is the problem of complete AV block?

Complete heart block is the failure of the electrical activity from the atrium to progress through the AV node into the His-Purkinje system. When an impulse is not initiated immediately in the bundle of His, arrest occurs for a brief period and Stokes–Adams syndrome occurs, which causes lightheadedness, dizziness, or loss of consciousness, sometimes accompanied by convulsions. During bradycardia, cardiac output is maintained by an increasing stroke volume. When the stroke volume is maximally increased, any further decrease in the heart rate will compromise cardiac output and cause circulatory failure.

Kaplan JA: Cardiac Anesthesia, pp 347–367. New York, Grune & Stratton, 1979

A.3. What are the common causes of heart block?

Organic Disease
- Disease affecting primary conduction tissue
  - Lenegre's disease: sclerodegenerative process of the terminal portions of His bundles
  - Lev's disease: fibrous encroachment of the proximal His conduction pathway
- Disease affecting cardiac tissue
  - Coronary artery disease with ischemia or infarction
  - Cardiomyopathy
  - Myocarditis
- Surgically produced
- Congenital block

Functional Disturbances
- Increased vagal tone
- Drug therapy with quinidine, digitalis, procainamide, propranolol, potassium

Wynande JE: Anesthesia for patients with heart block and artificial cardiac pacemakers. Anesth Analg 55:626–631, 1976

A.4. What are the indications for permanent pacemakers?

Artificial pacing is indicated for treatment of persistent bradycardia of any origin if it compromises hemodynamics or if bradycardia documented to predispose to ventricular irritability manifested by premature beats or ventricular tachycarida. Clinically, the following types of arrhythmias are common indications for pacemakers:

- Sinoatrial (SA) node: sick sinus syndrome, bradytachyarrhythmia, or bradycardia
- AV node: second-degree or third-degree AV block
- Bifascicular or trifascicular block
  - Right bundle branch block and left anterior hemiblock
  - Right bundle branch block and left posterior hemiblock
  - Alternating left bundle branch block and right bundle branch block
  - Left bundle branch block and first-degree AV block
- Occasionally pacemakers are used to treat drug-resistant or DC shock-resistant tachyarrhythmias.

Simon AB: Perioperative management of the pacemaker patient. Anesthesiology 46: 127–131, 1977

Wynande JE: Anesthesia for patients with heart block and artificial cardiac pacemakers. Anesth Analg 55:626–631, 1976

A.5. What is sick sinus syndrome?

Sick sinus syndrome describes an array of clinical disorders of sinus node function characterized by intrinsic inadequacy of the sinus node to perform its pacemaking function due to automatic dysfunction or failure of sinus node impulse to activate the rest of the atrium. The brady–tachycardia syndrome is a common form of sick sinus syndrome. It is one of the most common indications for pacemakers and is characterized by the following:

- Unexpected persistent severe sinus bradycardia
- Episodes of sinus arrest or block
- Paroxysmal or chronic atrial fibrillation or atrial flutter
- Slow return to sinus rhythm following cardioversion
- Lack of increase in sinus rate above 90 beats per minute following intravenous administration of atropine 1.5 to 2.0 mg.

Braunwald E: Heart Disease, pp 680–681. Philadelphia, WB Saunders, 1980

Ferrer MI: The sick sinus syndrome. Circulation 47:635–641, 1973

A.6. How would you diagnose first, second, and third-degree AV block, left anterior fascicular hemiblock, and left posterior-fascicular hemiblock?

First-degree AV block is characterized by a P–R interval of more than 0.20 seconds. Second-degree AV block is subdivided into two types. Mobitz type 1, or Wenckebach block, is characterized by a progressively lengthening P–R interval which occurs until an impulse is not conducted and a beat is dropped. Mobitz type II block is characterized by a sudden dropping of the QRS complex, with no progressive lengthening of the P–R interval occuring. Third-degree AV block, also called complete heart block, occurs when all electrical activity from the atrium fails to progress into the Purkinje system. The atrial and ventricular contractions have no relationship with each other. The QRS complex is normal in complete AV nodal block. The QRS complex with complete infranodal block is frequently wide, and the ventricular rate is slow, averaging 40 beats per minute. Left anterior superior hemiblock is indicated when ECG shows right bundle branch block and left axis deviation. Complete right bundle branch block with right axis deviation is indicative of right bundle branch block and left posterior inferior hemiblock.

Kaplan JA: Cardiac Anesthesia, pp 347–367. Grune & Stratton, 1979

Wynande JE: Anesthesia for patients with heart block and artificial cardiac pacemakers. Anesth Analg (Cleve) 55:626–631, 1976

A.7. How many types of pacemakers are there? How do they work?

There are 3 types of pacers: asynchronous, synchronous, and AV sequential.

- Asynchronous or fixed-rate pacemakers discharge at a preset rate that is independent of the inherent heart rate. They can be atrial or ventricular. Competition and ventricular fibrillation are the potential complications when normal heart rate reappears.
- Synchronous or demand pacemakers discharge at a preset rate only when the spontaneous heart rate drops below the preset rate. There are three types of synchronous pacers: ventricular-inhibited, ventricular-triggered, and atrial. The ventricular-inhibited pacer is the most popular type and is suppressed by normal electrical activity of the QRS complex. The ventricular-triggered pacers sense the QRS complex and then discharge into the absolute refractory period; therefore, they do not trigger another contraction. Atrial synchronous pacers function through a double electrode system. When the P wave is sensed, the ventricle is stimulated to contract. When the P wave is not sensed, the ventricle is paced at the preset rate.
- AV sequential pacing usually uses two electrodes, one in the atrial appendage and one in the right ventricular apex. The atrium is stimulated to contract first; then, after an adjustable P–R interval, the ventricle is stimulated to contract. The atrial sequential ventricular-inhibited pacer is a combination of atrial, ventricular, sequential, and demand pacing. It may be totally dormant, may stimulate only the atrium, or may stimulate both atria and ventricles with a preset sequence.

Braunwald E: Heart Disease, p. 744–777. Philadelphia, WB Saunders, 1980

Kaplan JA: Cardiac Anesthesia, pp 350–351. New York, Grune & Stratton, 1979

A.8. How would you know if it is atrial, ventricular, or AV sequential pacing?

In atrial pacing, an electrical spike appears before the P wave and the QRS complex is usually normal. In ventricular pacing, the electrical spike is followed immediately by a widened QRS complex. In AV sequential pacing, there are two spikes, one before the P wave and another preceding the QRS complex.

Braunwald E: Heart Disease, pp 744–777. Philadelphia, WB Saunders, 1980

A.9. What are the advantages and disadvantages of atrial pacing?

Atrial pacing increases cardiac output 26% over the cardiac output during ventricular pacing, because atrial contraction contributes 15% to 25% of the preload to the ventricle. It has been shown that coronary blood flow increases and coronary resistance decreases during atrial pacing. Atrial pacing is useless if atrioventricular block is present.

Yoshida S et al: Coronary hemodynamics during successive elevation of heart rate by pacing in subjects with angina pectoris. Circulation 44:1062, 1971

A.10. What are the indications for AV sequential pacemakers?

AV sequential pacing increases cardiac output 34% over the cardiac output during ventricular pacing. When ventricular pacing cannot maintain adequate cardiac output, and atrial pacing is not justified as in complete AV block, AV sequential pacing is indicated.

Hartzler G et al: Hemodynamic benefits of AV sequential pacing after cardiac surgery. Am J Cardiol 40:323, 1977

A.11. In a permanent pacemaker battery, what are the usual values for pulse amplitude, pulse width, pulse rate, and sensing threshold?

The specifications of pacemakers differ slightly from one model to the other. The pulse amplitude or the output of stimulation usually is 4.8 to 5.0 volts or 9.6 to 10 milliamps. The pulse width or the duration of stimulation is usually preset at 0.5 to 0.8 milliseconds. The pulse rate or the frequency of stimulation is usually set at 70 beats per minute. The sensing threshold or sensitivity is around 2.0 to 3.5 mv. The specifications may be programmed to suit special situations of each individual patient in a programmable pacemaker. The sensing threshold is the minimal electrical output from the heart to suppress the demand pacemaker.

Braunwald E: Heart Disease, pp 744–777. Philadelphia, WB Saunders, 1980

A.12. What is the hysteresis rate?

Some types of pacemakers have a built in hysteresis rate below the demand pacing rate. If the hysteresis rate is 60/m and the pacing rate is 70/m, the pacemaker will discharge at 70/m when the spontaneous cardiac rate falls below 60/m.

Technical Manual for Spectrax® Multiprogrammable Pulse Generator. Models 5984/5985, Minneapolis, Medtronic Inc, March, 1980

A.13. How do you set the external pacemaker to test the pacing threshold, sensing R–wave, and diaphragmatic pacing?

Any kind of electrical stimulation should have the following three components: strength (pulse amplitude), duration (pulse width), and frequency (pulse interval or rate). The pulse rate should be set approximately 10% higher than the patient's intrinsic heart rate in order to overdrive the heart. If the patient is in complete heart block, the rate is set to a physiological level, 70 to 80 beats per minute. The pulse width depends on the factory preset value of the pacemaker generator to be implanted. It should be set at either the same number or slightly lower than the factory preset value in order to assure that the implanted generator will work.

The pulse width of new generators is usually preset at 0.5 to 0.6 msec. The energy output of each impulse depends on the product of pulse amplitude and pulse width. If we test the pacing threshold with pulse width higher than that of the generator to be implanted, the generator may not work because of low energy output. The pulse amplitude is set at 10 milliamps or 5 volts, which is the output of internal pacemaker to be implanted. Decrease the output until the ventricle is no longer paced, then increase the output until pacing begins. The pacing threshold is the minimal output necessary to pace the ventricle. It may be represented by voltage or current. Resistance may be obtained from Ohm's Law, dividing voltage by current. In the Medtronic 5300 Pacing System Analyzer, the R–wave may be tested by turning the control function to R–wave and pushing the R–wave test button. The number of millivolts in the QRS complex, sensed by the pacemaker, passing from the ventricle through the electrode is essential for the demand type of pacemaker. Low pacing threshold, low resistance, and a high sensing R-wave indicate a satisfactory position of the pacing electrode. Diaphragmatic pacing may be detected by increasing the pacing output to 5 to 10 volts or 10 milliamps and watching diaphragm movements and hiccups while the patient is asked to breathe deeply.

Kaplan JA: Cardiac Anesthesia, pp 347–367. New York, Grune & Stratton, 1979

A.14. What are the acceptable values of pacing threshold, sensing R-wave, and resistance?

Since the implant generators have a maximal initial output of 5 volts or 10 milliamps, the pacing threshold cannot exceed the above values. The acceptable values are below 1.0 milliamps or 0.5 to 1.0 volts in acute or initial implants and up to 2.0 to 3.5 milliamps or 2.0 to 3.5 volts in chronic implants. There is an initial sharp rise in the pacing threshold, during the first 2 weeks, of up to 10 times the acute level because of tissue reaction around the tip of electrode. Then it falls to 2 to 3 times the acute level from the scar formation. In the chronic state, it remains essentially at the same level in 80% of patients; only 20% of patients exhibit a late rise in threshold. The sensing R-wave should be at least 4 to 5 millivolts amplitude to inhibit or trigger a demand pacemaker because the preset sensitivity is around 2.0 to 4.0 millivolts. Resistance should be between 500 to 1000 Ohms.

Braunwald E: Heart Disease, pp 744–777. Philadelphia, WB Saunders, 1980

A.15. What are the usual life spans of pacemakers?

The mercury–zinc pacemakers have a life span of 18 to 36 months, whereas the lithium-powered pacemakers can last 6 to 8 years.

Braunwald E: Heart Disease, pp 744–777. Philadelphia, WB Saunders, 1980

A.16. How do you know if the implanted demand pacemaker is working?

We must slow the intrinsic heart rate to a rate below that of the pacemaker by carotid massage or a Valsalva maneuver. If the rate does not slow down enough for the pacemaker to take over the ventricle, a magnet can be applied over the pacemaker to convert it to the fixed rate mode, and captured beats can be observed by watching the ECG and palpating the pulse.

Kaplan JA: Cardiac Anesthesia, pp 347–367. New York, Grune & Stratton, 1979

B. Preoperative Evaluation and Preparation

B.1. What kind of work-up would you like the patient to have?

Preoperative evaluation should include the routine systemic work-up and more attention should be paid to cardiovascular disorders. The systemic routine includes complete blood count, urinalysis, coagulation screening with prothrombin time and partial thromboplastin time, serum electrolytes, BUN, blood sugar, chest x-ray, and ECG. Special attention should be paid to the history, symptoms, and signs of myocardial infarction, congestive heart failure, and arrhythmia. Serum electrolytes, especially potassium level, must be in the normal range. Blood pressure and consciousness level are checked to assure adequate perfusion before implantation of the pacemaker.

Simon AB: Perioperative management of the pacemaker patient. Anesthesiology 46: 127–131, 1977

C. Intraoperative Management

C.1. Would you give general or local anesthesia for insertion of a transvenous pacemaker? Why?

We prefer local anesthesia because patients who have heart block with symptoms and are given general anesthesia may develop cardiac standstill, ventricular tachycardia, or ventricular fibrillation. During local anesthesia, we can request that patients cough to check for the possibility of electrode dislodge or breathe deeply to test diaphragmatic pacing.

Wynande JE: Anesthesia for patients with heart block and artificial cardiac pacemakers. Anesth Analg (Cleve) 55:626–631, 1976

C.2. If it is a epicardial electrode, would you give local or general anesthesia?

Although local anesthesia with sedation has been used successfully for transthoracic implantation of epicardial electrodes, general anesthesia is commonly administered at Cornell Medical Center. If a complete block or severe bradycardia is present before the induction of general anesthesia, it is necessary to insert a transvenous temporary pacemaker under local anesthesia. When the patient is in sinus rhythm at the time of induction, a temporary pacer probably is not indicated. If a complete block suddenly develops after induction, isoproterenol may be given.

Kaplan JA (ed): Cardiac Anesthesia, p 357. New York, Grune & Stratton, 1979

Wynande JE: Anesthesia for patients with heart block and artificial cardiac pacemakers. Anesth Analg 55:626–631, 1976

C.3. What would you give for premedication for local anesthesia?

We prefer light sedation with pentobarbital, 1.5 mg/kg, intramuscularly. Because most of the patients with pacemakers are elderly and have cardiac disease, heavy sedation should be avoided to prevent cardiopulmonary depression.

C.4. What drugs and equipment would you like to have on hand in the operating room?

A complete array of drugs and equipment must be ready for cardiopulmonary resuscitation. The minimal requirements include a finger on the pulse, ECG monitor, a DC defibrillator, and the usual drugs for resuscitation. Atropine and isoproterenol are used to treat bradycardia. Lidocaine or a DC defibrillator is necessary to treat ventricular arrhythmia during the insertion of endocardial electrodes.

Wyande JE: Anesthesia for patients with heart block and artificial cardiac pacemakers. Anesth Analg (Cleve) 55:626–631, 1976

C.5. How do you sedate the patient?

We usually titrate small doses of short acting sedatives such as thiopental sodium in 25 mg increments or diazepam in 1 to 2 mg increments. Fentanyl in 0.025 mg increments is used to supplement the local anesthesia. Oxygen is given by mask to prevent hypoxia from sedation. Hypoventilation is avoided by reminding the patient to take deep breaths intermittently. A precordial stethoscope is applied over the right chest to monitor respiration.

C.6. After the endocardial pacemaker was inserted in our patient, the ECG pattern suddenly changed from left bundle branch block to right bundle branch block. What is the possible diagnosis?

The endocardial electrode has perforated the interventricular septum and paces the left ventricle. When the electrode is in the right ventricle, the ECG pattern is usually that of left bundle branch block.

Chung EK: Artificial Cardiac Pacing, p 338. Baltimore, Williams & Wilkins, 1978

D. Postoperative Management

D.1. What are the complications of transvenous implantation of pacemakers?

The complications are displacement of electrode, inability to pace or sense, skin erosion, infection, myocardial perforation, ventricular fibrillation, diaphragm stimulation, endocarditis, increased threshold, and cardiac tamponade.

Mansour K et al: Cardiac pacemakers: Comparing epicardial and pervenous pacing. Geriatrics 28:151, 1973

D.2. What are the causes of pacemaker failure?

Failure of pacing may be due to battery failure, disruption of electrodes, or failure of capture at a myocardial level.

- Battery failure: exhausted battery, leak in seal, suppression, runaway pacemaker
- Disruption of electrode: broken wire
- Failure of capture: increasing threshold, myocardium perforation

Kaplan, JA: Cardiac Anesthesia, p 356. New York, Grune & Stratton, 1979

D.3. What kinds of environmental electromagnetic interference may affect the function of a demand pacemaker?

- Microwave oven: The patient should not approach within three feet of an operating microwave oven.
- Diathermy: contraindicated
- Electrocautery: Do not use within 15 cm of the implanted pulse generator.
- Electric razor: Do not use on the skin area over the implant site.
- Amateur radio transmitting equipment: Linear power amplifiers are contraindicated.
- Power transmission lines: High voltage electric fields produced by 765 KV power lines should be avoided.

Braunwald E: Heart Disease, p 771. Philadelphia, WB Saunders, 1980

D.4. Two months later, the patient came back for transurethral resection of the prostate because of prostatic hypertrophy. How would you prevent interference to the pacemaker from the electrocautery?

- The grounding plate of the cautery should be placed as close to the operative site as possible and as far from the pacemaker as possible.
- The cautery should not be used within 15 cm of the pacemaker not only because it may interfere with the battery circuitry, but also because if the cautery should come in contact with a break in the insulation of the electrode, it may cauterize the myocardium at the tip of the electrode, rendering it insensitive to pacing impulses.

- The use of cautery should be limited to 1-second bursts every 10 seconds to prevent repetitive asystolic periods.
- If the pacemaker is inhibited by the cautery, a high-powered magnet should be applied over the demand pacemaker to convert it to fixed-rate mode.

Simon AB: Perioperative management of the pacemaker patient. Anesthesiology 46: 127–131, 1977

Wynande JE: Anesthesia for patients with heart block and artificial cardiac pacemakers. Anesth Analg (Cleve) 55:626–631, 1976

D.5. How do you detect inhibition of pacemaker function?

During electrocautery, the ECG is frequently useless because of interference. The best monitor available to determine if inhibition is taking place is a hand on the pulse. The precordial or esophageal stethoscope, or blood pressure is also acceptable.

Kaplan JA: Cardiac Anesthesia, pp 347–367. New York, Grune & Stratton, 1979

10 Abdominal Aortic Aneurysm

Vinod Malhotra

A 64-year-old man with a history of frequent angina and two episodes of myocardial infarction 1 year ago is scheduled for elective abdominal aortic aneurysm resection. He smokes two packs of cigarettes a day and has a long history of emphysema. BP 164/90; PR 70; RR 10; Hct. 48.

A. Medical Disease and Differential Diagnosis

1. What are the major problems in this patient?
2. What are the problems associated with previous history of myocardial infarction?
3. What is the incidence of perioperative myocardial infarction?
4. What is the peak time of reinfarction in the perioperative period?
5. What is the mortality rate from perioperative recurrent myocardial infarction?
6. What are the factors that are associated with increased incidence of reinfarction?
7. What is the risk of perioperative myocardial infarction in patients with prior coronary artery bypass graft (CABG)?
8. What are the perioperative problems associated with hypertension?
9. What are the perioperative problems associated with chronic obstructive pulmonary disease?
10. What are some of the other commonly associated problems you wish to know about in this patient?
11. What relevant information about the aneurysms do you want to know?

B. Preoperative Evaluation and Preparation

1. What laboratory tests do you wish to obtain?
2. What values of pulmonary function tests do you expect in this patient?

3. What is your interpretation of the arterial blood gases—pH 7.38, PO_2 68, PCO_2 52, CO_2 32?
4. What is creatinine clearance?
5. How will you prepare this patient for surgery?
6. What premedication will you order?

C. Intraoperative Management

1. What monitors will you employ during the case?
2. What is your choice of anesthetic technique and agent?
3. What are the hemodynamic changes during aortic clamping?

D. Postoperative Management

1. What are the common postoperative problems that you may encounter in this type of patient?

A. Medical Disease and Differential Diagnosis

A.1. What are the major problems in this patient?

The major presenting problems in this patient are as follows: coronary artery disease, evidenced by history of myocardial infarction; myocardial ischemic episodes, indicated by frequent angina; hypertension, atherosclerosis, and chronic obstructive pulmonary disease. All these factors support an increased risk for anesthesia.

A.2. What are the problems associated with previous history of myocardial infarction.

In patients with previous history of myocardial infarction there is a greater risk of perioperative recurrent myocardial infarction, which carries a high mortality. Despite the sophistication in anesthetic techniques and intensive care, there has not been any significant change in the statistics over the past 20 years.

Steen PA, Tinker JH, Tarhan S: Myocardial reinfarction after anesthesia and surgery. JAMA 239:2566–2570, 1978

Topkins MJ, Artusio JF: Myocardial infarction and surgery: A five year study. Anesth Analg (Cleve) 43:716–720, 1964

A.3. What is the incidence of perioperative myocardial infarction?

In the general population, the incidence of perioperative myocardial infarction is 0.13%. However, the incidence of recurrent myocardial infarction in patients with history of previous myocardial infarction increases to 6%.

Steen PA, Tinker JH, Tarhan S: Myocardial reinfarction after anesthesia and surgery. JAMA 239:2566–2570, 1978

Tarhan S, Moffitt EA, Taylor WF et al: Myocardial infarction after anesthesia. JAMA 220:1451, 1972

Topkins MJ, Artusio JF: Myocardial infarction and surgery: A five year study. Anesth Analg (Cleve) 43:716–720, 1964

A.4. What is the peak time of reinfarction in the perioperative period?

The peak time for recurrence of myocardial infarction in the perioperative period is between 3 and 5 days postoperatively. Intraoperative myocardial infarction occurs in less than $1/5$ of the cases.

Vandam LD: To make the Patient Ready for Anesthesia: Medical Care of the Surgical Patient, p 6. Menlo Park, CA, Addison–Wesley Publishing Co, 1980

A.5. What is the mortality rate from perioperative recurrent myocardial infarction?

The mortality is still very high and in the range of 70%.

Steen PA, Tinker JH, Tarhan S: Myocardial reinfarction after anesthesia and surgery. JAMA 239:2566–2570, 1978

A.6. What are the factors that are associated with increased incidence of myocardial reinfarction?

Of the several factors, the time interval between the previous infarction and the current surgery is, perhaps, the most important determinant of the rate of reinfarction (see Table 10–1). Other factors associated with increased risk of reinfarction include the following: preoperative hypertension, prolonged intraoperative hypotension, upper abdominal, intrathoracic, or aortic surgery—procedures requiring more than 3 hours. Factors that have been shown to cause statistically insignificant changes in the risk of reinfarction include age, sex, diabetes, angina, intraoperative hypertension, anesthetic technique, anesthetic agent, duration of anesthesia at operative sites other than upper abdominal, intrathoracic, and major vascular and ICU care.

Table 10–1. Incidence of perioperative reinfarction in relation to the interval since previous myocardial infarction

TIME ELAPSED SINCE MYOCARDIAL INFARCTION (MONTHS)	PERIOPERATIVE REINFARCTION RATE (%)
0–3	27
3–6	11
6–	4–5

Steen PA, Tinker JH, Tarhan S: Myocardial reinfarction after anesthesia and surgery. JAMA 239:2566–2570, 1978

A.7. What is the risk of perioperative myocardial infarction in patients with prior coronary artery bypass graft (CABG)?

The risk of myocardial infarction in patients with prior coronary artery bypass graft is relatively low. In a recent study involving 168 operative procedures on patients with CABG, no myocardial infarctions were reported. On the other hand, in patients with angiographically documented three-vessel coronary artery disease, the risk factor is similar to previous myocardial infarction.

Brown BR: Anesthesia and Patient With Heart Disease: Contemporary Anesthesia Practice, p 71. Philadelphia, FA Davis, 1980

A.8. What are the perioperative problems associated with hypertension?

Mild Hypertension

The patient with diastolic pressures of 90 to 100 torr usually presents only a slightly higher risk than the healthy individual. The anesthetic morbidity and mortality is mainly due to atherosclerotic phenomena. In this group, there is no significant difference between treated and untreated groups.

Moderate Hypertension

Patients with sustained diastolic pressures of 100 to 115 torr usually present with organ involvement and present a higher risk. Compared to the treated patients, the untreated patients are at a threefold risk of developing major complications such as cerebrovascular accident, myocardial infarction, or congestive heart failure.

Severe Hypertension

By definition patients with a diastolic pressure between 115 to 130 torr present a significantly high risk for anesthesia and surgery. Major problems during anesthesia include cerebrovascular accidents, myocardial infarction, congestive heart failure, and acute renal failure. No untreated patient in this category should be anesthetized for any elective surgical procedure.

Brown BR: Anesthesia and Patient With Heart Disease: Contemporary Anesthesia Practice, pp 91–92. Philadelphia, FA Davis, 1980

Goldman L, Caldera DL: Risk of general anesthesia and elective operation in the hypertensive patient. Anesthesiology 50:6-285–292, 1979

Prys–Roberts C, Melode R, Foex P: Studies of anesthesia in relation to hypertension: Cardiovascular responses of treated and untreated patients. Br J Anesth 43:112–137, 1971

A.9. What are the perioperative problems associated with chronic obstructive pulmonary disease?

Patients with COPD (chronic bronchitis, asthma, and emphysema) present a higher risk for postoperative respiratory complications. Respiratory failure is a major cause of postoperative death. Postoperative atelectasis, pulmonary infection, and respiratory failure are the common problems in this group of patients. These patients already possess varying degrees of hypoxemia, hypercapnia, hypoventilation, V/Q abnormalities, increased mucous secretions, bronchospasm, or small airway obstruction, and acute or chronic infection. Surgery and anesthesia further reduce the already poor pulmonary reserves (see Table 10–2). Depending upon the severity of the disease, the postoperative problems may vary.

Table 10–2. Respiratory changes following upper abdominal surgery

Respiratory rate	↓
Tidal volume	↓
Vital capacity	↓↓
FEV_1	↓↓
Compliance	↓
FRC	↓
Surfactant	↓
V/Q abnormality	↑
Secretions	↑

Mild COPD
The patient with mild disease usually has a decreased vital capacity and forced expiratory volume in one second (FEV_1) greater than 50% of predicted. Arterial blood gases are normal at rest, but exercise may produce slight hypoxemia. These patients present only a slightly higher risk of pulmonary complications.

Moderately Severe COPD
This type of patient has a markedly decreased vital capacity, a maximum mid-expiratory flow rate (MMEFR) of less than 0.75 l/sec and FEV_1 of less than 50% of predicted. The arterial blood gases are abnormal. Following adequate pulmonary therapy, an improvement is usually seen in pulmonary function tests and arterial blood gases, indicative of a reversible component in the existent pulmonary disease. The postoperative mortality in this group is about 8%. The incidence of postoperative pulmonary complication in the well treated patient in this group is about 25% and increases twofold to threefold in the untreated patient.

Severe COPD
This is the "pulmonary cripple" with severe reduction in pulmonary function. FEV_1 is about 25% of predicted or lower. Arterial blood gases show hypoxemia and hypercapnia and the patient is on the borderline of respiratory failure. This patient presents a significant risk of postoperative respiratory failure and death. Postoperative ventilatory care in an intensive care unit is usually required, and weaning from the ventilator is difficult. In this patient, the benefit of surgery should be carefully weighed against the risks of anesthesia and surgery.

Cheney FW: Effects of surgery on pulmonary function. ASA Refresher Courses in Anesthesiology 6:31–42, 1978

Heironimus TW: The anesthetic management of the pulmonary cripple. ASA Refresher Courses in Anesthesiology 3:89–102, 1975

Tarhan S, Moffitt, EA, Sessler AD et al: Risk of anesthesia and surgery in patients with chronic bronchitis and chronic obstructive pulmonary disease. Surgery 74:720–726, 1973

Vandam LD: To Make the Patient Ready for Anesthesia: Medical Care of the Surgical Patient. Menlo Park, CA, Addison–Wesley Publishing Co, pp 41–42, 1980

A.10. What are some of the other commonly associated problems you wish to know about in this patient?

The abdominal aortic aneurysm is usually just one of the manifestations of a systemic etiopathology (i.e., arteriosclerosis). Therefore, one should look for signs of arteriosclerotic involvement of other arteries and organ systems. In addition to the already discussed issues of coronary artery disease and hypertension, one should look for involvement of the carotid arteries, the renal arteries, and the iliac artery (see Table 10–3). A history of renal dysfunction or a stroke is important preoperative information.

Schwartz: SI: Principles of Surgery, p 959. New York, McGraw–Hill, 1979

Table 10–3. Incidence of clinically significant arterial disease in patients with aortic aneurysm

ARTERY CLINICALLY INVOLVED	FREQUENCY (%)	ORGAN DYSFUNCTION
Coronary	30	Myocardial ischemia, infarction
Carotid	7	Cerebrovascular accident
Renal	2	Decreased renal function (also hypertensive renal disease)
Iliac	16	Peripheral arterial insufficiency

A.11. What relevant information about the aneurysm do you want to know?

It is important to know the size and location of the aneurysm. In 1% to 2% of the cases, the renal artery is involved in the aneurysm. One should also get information regarding any other aneurysms present elsewhere. DeBakey and associates found concomitant thoracic aneurysms in 4% of patients with abdominal aortic aneurysm.

Schwartz SI: Principles of Surgery, p 959. New York, McGraw–Hill, 1979

B. Preoperative Evaluation and Preparation

B.1. What laboratory tests do you wish to obtain?

The following laboratory test should be performed in this patient: complete blood count; urinalysis; serum electroytes; blood urea nitrogen;

serum creatinine; creatinine clearence (if serum creatinine is elevated or renal dysfunction is suspected); coagulation study—platelet count, prothrombin time, partial thromboplastin time; chest x-ray; arterial blood gases; screening spirometry.

Vandam LD: To Make the Patient Ready for Anesthesia: Medical Care of the Surgical Patient, pp 41–42, 65, 149. Menlo Park, CA, Addison–Welsey Publishing Co, 1980

B.2. What values of pulmonary function tests do you expect in this patient?

The patient's respiratory problem is emphysema. Therefore, the significant derangement will be that of obstructive airway disease manifested in flow studies (see Table 10–4). Depending on the reversible component of the disease (i.e., bronchospasm) bronchodilators will improve the pulmonary flow rates. Other tests that are helpful include flow volume curves and measurement of closing volumes.

Heironimus TW: The anesthetic management of the pulmonary cripple. ASA Refresher Courses in Anesthesiology 3:89–102, 1975

West JB: Pulmonary Pathophysiology—The Essentials, pp 3–12. Baltimore, William & Wilkins, 1980

B.3. What is your interpretation of the arterial blood gases–pH 7.38, PO_2 68 torr, PCO_2 52 torr, CO_2 32 mEq/L?

The arterial blood gas analysis indicates primary respiratory acidosis along with compensatory metabolic alkalosis. Hypoxemia is also evident, which together with hypercapnia, correlates well with the clinical picture of significant respiratory disease.

B.4. What is creatinine clearance?

Creatinine clearance is a measure of glomerular filtration rate. It is a sensitive test of renal function. It is calculated as follows:

$$\text{Creatine clearance} = \frac{U}{P} \times V$$

U = urinary concentration of creatinine (mg/100ml)
P = plasma concentration of creatinine (mg/100ml)
V = urine volume (ml/min)

A 24-hour creatinine clearance is a more accurate method of determining the values, compared with a 2-hour creatinine clearance. Normal values are: 85–125ml/min in women, 95–140ml/min in men. Creatinine clearance decreases with advancing age and the value approaches 70 at age 70.

Vandam LD: To Make the Patient Ready for Anesthesia: Medical Care of the Surgical Patient, p 66. Menlo Park, CA, Addison–Wesley Publishing Co, 1980

Table 10-4. Pulmonary function test findings in chronic obstructive pulmonary disease

TEST	OBSTRUCTIVE DISEASE	APPROXIMATE NORMAL VALUES
Total lung (TLC) capacity	↑	6 liters
Vital capacity (VC)	normal or ↓	5 liters
Functional residual capacity (FRC)	↑	3 liters
Forced expiratory vol 1 second (FEV_1)	↓↓	> 72% of VC
Forced expiratory volume—3 seconds (FEV_3)	↓↓	> 92% of VC
Maximum mid expiratory flow rate (MMEFR) or FEV_{25-75}	↓↓	2.5L/sec
Maximum ventilatory volume	↓↓	125 L/min

B.5. How will you prepare this patient for surgery?

The objective in preparing the patient for an operative procedure is to achieve medical stability. Therefore, the problems that should be addressed and well controlled preoperatively are the following: blood pressure, intravascular volume, myocardial perfusion and performance, and respiratory therapy.

Blood Pressure

Adequate blood pressure control should be achieved and recorded. This may require the use of diuretics, vasopressors, or vasodilators.

Intravascular Volume

Intravascular volume restoration is usually required following the use of vasopressors or vasodilators. This will minimize the fluctuations in blood pressure intraoperatively.

Myocardial Perfusion and Performance

Every effort should be made to reduce myocardial oxygen demand and improve myocardial blood flow. This will require a reduction in afterload, preload, and heart rate. B-blockers and nitroglycerin should be instituted as necessary. Dosages may have to be readjusted.

Respiratory Therapy

Adequate preparation of the respiratory system is mandatory to minimize the incidence of postoperative respiratory complications. To improve pulmonary function, the following is necessary:

- Treatment of any acute infection
- Treatment of chronic pulmonary infection
- Bronchodilator therapy to relieve bronchospasm
- Chest physiotherapy to clear secretions
- Treatment of cor pulmonale by oxygen, ventilation, and drugs
- Voluntary coughing and deep breathing
- Respiratory therapy
- Good hydration

- Correction of electrolyte and acid base balance
- Spirometry and arterial blood gases should be repeated following this regimen.

Brown BR: Anesthesia and Patients with Heart Disease: Contemporary Anesthesia Practice, pp 10–15. Philadelphia, FA Davis, 1980

Heironimus TW: The anesthetic management of the pulmonary cripple. ASA Refresher Courses in Anesthesiology 3:89–102, 1975

Vandam LD: To Make the Patient Ready for Anesthesia: Medical Care of the Surgical Patient, pp 10–15. Menlo Park, CA, Addison–Wesley Publishing Co, 1980

B.6. What premedication will you order?

An adequate premedication includes atropine and a barbiturate. Atropine should be avoided in patients suspected of being dehydrated or having thick tenacious secretions because it will further dry the endobronchial secretions. Sedation should be light to avoid respiratory depression.

Vandam LD: To Make the Patient Ready for Anesthesia: Medical Care of the Surgical Patient, pp 22, 34. Menlo Park, CA, Addison–Wesley Publishing Co, 1980

C. Intraoperative Management

C.1. What monitors will you employ during the case?

This patient should be monitored with the following:

- Electrocardiogram, using a V_5 lead
- Arterial blood pressure, using an indwelling radial arterial catheter
- Pulmonary capillary wedge pressure
- Temperature
- Precordial or esophageal stethoscope
- Arterial blood gases through the indwelling catheter
- Indwelling Foley catheter

C.2. What is your choice of anesthetic technique and agent?

A general inhalation anesthetic with endotracheal intubation and controlled ventilation is as good a choice as any other technique. There is little difference between various techniques and agents when correlated with incidence of respiratory complications. During aortic surgery, the circulatory changes which occur during and after the cross clamping are similar when different anesthetic agents and techniques are compared. The important factor is the prevention, early recognition, and proper treatment of circulatory and respiratory problems intra- and postoperatively.

Bartkowski RR, Ankburg SJ, Greenhow DE et al: Comparing Anesthetic Technique During Aortic Cross-Clamp Anesthesiology. 51:S136, 1979

Heironimus TW: The anesthetic management of the pulmonary cripple. ASA Refresher Courses in Anesthesiology 3:93–94, 1975

Tarhan S, Moffitt EA, Sessler AD et al: Risk of anesthesia and surgery in patients with chronic bronchitis and chronic obstructive pulmonary disease. Surgery 74:721–723, 1973

C.3. What are the hemodynamic changes during aortic clamping?

Significant hemodynamic changes may occur following aortic cross clamping. These include increases in blood pressure, central venous pressure, and pulmonary artery pressure. The increase in afterload may result in myocardial ischemia and left ventricular failure. These changes are attenuated in well treated patients and one may not see any significant changes in these parameters. Judicious use of depth of anesthesia, intravascular volume control, and vasodilators following cross-clamping, will further limit any changes. Following unclamping, significant hypotension may occur due to decreased afterload and peripheral vascular resistance. Increased metabolic oxygen consumption and metabolic acidosis is apparent following unclamping and persists for 20 to 30 minutes thereafter. At this point, again, the hypotension can be avoided by volume loading during cross-clamp, decreasing the depth of anesthesia, and using vasopresors, if required.

Attia RR, Murphy JD, Snider M et al: Myocardial ischemia due to infrarenal aortic cross-clamping during aortic surgery in patients with severe coronary–artery disease. Circulation 53:961–965, 1976

Bush HL, LoGerfo FW, Weisel RD et al: Assessment of myocardial performance and optimal volume loading during elective abdominal aortic aneurysm resection. Arch Surg 112:1304–1305, 1977

Meloche R, Pottecher T, Aude J et al: Hemodynamic changes due to clamping of the abdominal aorta. Can Anaesth Soc J 24:2034, 1977

Thompson D, Neglen P, Eklof B: Central hemodynamic changes during aortic reconstructive surgery: Effects of adrenergic blockade and temporary shunt. Anesthesiology 51:S125, 1979

Silverstein P, Calder D, Cullen DJ et al: Avoiding the hemodynamic consequences of aortic cross-clamping and unclamping. Anesthesiology 50:465–466, 1979

D. Postoperative Management

D.1. What are the common postoperative problems that you may encounter in this type of patient?

The post-anesthesia recovery period is crucial in these patients and the common problems include the following:

Ventilatory Inadequacy
- Severe COPD
- Respiratory depression from general anesthesia
- Respiratory depression due to narcotic analgesia
- Major upper abdominal surgery restricting pulmonary function
- Gastric distension
- Possible fluid accumulation under the diaphragm

- Circulatory instability
- Electrolyte or acid base imbalance secondary to clamping and massive fluid replacement

Circulatory Instability
- Circulation may be still unstable, since autonomic activity increases during emergence from anesthesia.
- Hypertension and vasoconstriction occur from pain and shivering from cold.
- Hypotension may also occur during this period.

Coagulation
- Problems secondary to massive blood transfusion and heparinization

Electrolyte imbalance or *acid–base derangement*

Hypothermia due to elderly patient with poor thermoregulation, long surgery with exposed body cavity, and massive transfusion of banked blood

Cullen DJ: Anesthesia and monitoring for abdominal aortic surgery. ASA Refresher Course in Anaesthesiology 118:5–6, 1980

Section Three
The Gastrointestinal System

11 Intestinal Obstruction

Joseph F. Artusio, Jr

A 45-year-old man, with a history of vomiting for 72 hours, had abdominal pain, a swollen abdomen, and had not passed flatus for the same period of time. There is a nasogastric tube in place. T 39°C; P 120; BP 85/65; Hct 48

A. Medical Disease and Differential Diagnosis

1. Briefly outline the differential diagnosis of the acute abdomen.
2. What are the causes of intestinal obstruction?
3. Is there any difference in import whether the obstruction is located in the small bowel or large bowel?
4. Outline the methods of abdominal decompression.
5. What are the effects of bowel distention?
6. How would you describe the fluid shifts that occur during small bowel intestinal obstruction?
7. What hemodynamic changes occur related to intestinal obstruction?
8. Can there be actual losses of red cell mass?
9. Are there any systemic effects from the absorption of bacteria and bacterial products?

B. Preoperative Evaluation and Preparation

1. Is it important to decompress the abdomen prior to surgical intervention? Why?
   What are the respiratory implications?
   What are the implications of the tense abdominal wall?
2. What do you use as a guide to fluid volume replacement?
3. What principles would you use when choosing drugs for premedication of this patient?

C. Intraoperative Management

1. What dangers are present during the induction of anesthesia? How are they planned for?
2. In what position would you intubate this patient? Would you use Sellick's maneuver?
3. What agents and techniques would you use for this operation?

D. Postoperative Management

1. Are there any postoperative respiratory problems not associated with aspiration?
2. If the patient did aspirate gastric contents, what are the possible sequelae of this event? What is the treatment?
3. What is gram negative sepsis? What is the clinical picture and how would you treat it?

A. Medical Disease and Differential Diagnosis

A.1. Briefly outline the differential diagnosis of the acute abdomen.

The acute abdomen is usually manifest by pain emanating from the peritoneum, hollow intestinal viscera, mesentery, or pelvic organs. The pain may be caused by inflammation or by a mechanical process such as obstruction, acute distention, or vascular disturbances. There are many extraperitoneal causes for the acute abdomen which manifest themselves by abdominal pain, but are actually due to intrathoracic, neurogenic, vascular, or metabolic causes.

Isselbacher KJ et al: Harrison's Principles of Internal Medicine, 9th ed, pp 34–37. New York, McGraw–Hill, 1980

A.2. What are the causes of intestinal obstruction?

The most common causes of mechanical intestinal obstruction are adhesions, hernia, and neoplasms of the bowel. Obstruction interferes with the normal progression of intestinal contents. The term mechanical intestinal obstruction denotes an actual physical barrier that blocks the intestinal lumen. The term ileus is now used to connote failure of downward progress of bowel contents because of disordered propulsive motility of the bowel.

Schwartz S et al: Principles of Surgery, 3rd ed, pp 1051–1052. New York, McGraw–Hill, 1979

A.3. Is there any difference in import whether the obstruction is located in the small bowel or large bowel?

Small bowel mechanical obstruction with intact blood supply allows the accumulation of fluid and gas at the point of obstruction and alters bowel motility. This leads to systemic derangements with fluid and electrolyte loss. Small bowel obstruction results in bowel distention by intestinal gas, decrease in bowel motility, and, eventually, strangulated obstruction due to the occlusion of the blood supply to the obstructed segment of bowel.

Obstruction of the large bowel, with the exception of volvulus, usually does not strangulate. Since the colon is principally a storage organ with relatively minor absorptive and secretory functions, fluid and electrolyte sequestration progresses more slowly. The systemic derangement is therefore of a less magnitude and urgency than in small bowel mechanical obstruction. Progressive distention is the most dangerous aspect of nonstrangulative colon obstruction. If the ileocecal valve is competent, then the colon essentially becomes a closed loop—closed below the obstructing lesion and above by the competent valve. If the obstruction is not relieved, distention progresses into rupture of the colon. The cecum is usually the site of rupture.

Schwartz S et al: Principles of Surgery, 3rd ed, pp 1052–1055. New York, McGraw–Hill, 1979

A.4. Outline the methods of abdominal decompression.

The abdomen may be decompressed by placing a tube in the stomach or placing a longer tube in the small intestines. The short gastric tube will empty the stomach of fluid, and it is important that the stomach be empty prior to the induction of anesthesia. This is best done by the "sump" tube, which is more efficient than the old simple Levine tube, long tubes, or Miller-Abbott tubes that are passed into the stomach and then, with a weighted balloon, passed through the pylorus into the small bowel. Although there is some controversy surrounding the use of the long intestinal tube, it is of value particularly when the intestinal obstruction is the result of inflammation that is expected to subside under conservative therapy. Otherwise, it is necessary to use surgery to relieve the obstruction.

Schwartz S et al: Principles of Surgery, 3rd ed, p 1058. New York, McGraw-Hill, 1979

A.5. What are the effects of bowel distention?

If a distended bowel is allowed to remain distended for a long period of time, it will produce sufficient decrease in blood supply to cause a strangulated obstruction. The accumulation of fluid and gas in the obstructed bowel and the altered motility seen in mechanical obstruction may be overshadowed by blockage of the venous outflow from the strangulated segment, with subsequent extravasation of blood and fluid into the bowel wall. In addition to a loss of blood and plasmalike fluid, the gangrenous bowel leaks toxic material into the peritoneal cavity. These are exotoxins, endotoxins, and toxic hemin breakdown products.

Schwartz S et al: Principles of Surgery, 3rd ed, p 1054. New York, McGraw–Hill, 1979

A.6. How would you describe the fluid shifts that occur during small bowel intestinal obstruction?

Normally, 7 liters of fluid are secreted daily into the upper intestinal tract. The secretions include saliva (1500 cc), gastric juice (2500 cc), bile (300 cc), pancreatic juice (750 cc), and succus entericus (1000–3000 cc). Normally, these fluid secretions are absorbed so that only 400 cc passes the ileocecal valve. In small bowel obstruction, the normal absorption of secreted fluids into the circulation is subject to interference so that fluids rapidly accumulate above the obstructed segment of bowel. In early small bowel obstruction, 1500 cc of fluid accumulates in the bowel. If intestinal obstruction is well established and is associated with vomiting, 3000 cc of fluid is present in the small bowel. When hypotension and tachycardia are present, indicating circulatory instability, 6000 cc of fluids is in the gut. Small bowel obstruction, with its associated vomiting, results in a loss of gastric juice. The decrease in chloride ions in the blood may result in metabolic alkalosis. However, metabolic acidosis is more common, due to dehydration, starvation, ketosis, and loss of secretions. The most consistent finding is a loss of isotonic salt water, which produces an isotonic contraction of the extracellular fluid volume. The resulting loss of the extracellular fluid causes disturbances in acid–base balance and loss of potassium. Monitoring consists of serial determinations of sodium, potassium, chloride, and CO_2. Corrective quantities of electrolytes are added to fluid replacement until normal electrolyte values are achieved. Serial hematocrit determinations are also good monitors of fluid loss, a rise in hematocrit is proportionate to fluid loss. If hematocrit has risen to 55%, approximately 40% of plasma and extracellular fluid volume has been lost.

Glenn F et al: Surgery in the Aged, p 252. New York, McGraw–Hill, 1960

Schwartz S et al: Principles of Surgery, 3rd ed, pp 1056, 1058. New York, McGraw–Hill, 1979

A.7. What hemodynamic changes occur related to intestinal obstruction?

If fluid and electrolyte losses are not corrected, central venous pressure will fall. Hypotension and tachycardia will follow as the vascular volume decreases in relation to the size of the vascular bed. The shock state develops as the body calls forth sympathomimetic amines to increase cardiac output and decrease the size of the vascular bed. Hyponatremia will aggravate hypovolemic hypotension and confusion and somnolence will ensue. Hypopotassemia will be manifested in delayed ventricular conduction, ST–T segment changes and ventricular arrhythmia will follow. All these fluid and electrolyte deficits can be corrected by the judicious use of balanced salt solution, monitoring CVP, blood pressure, ECG and urinary output.

Isselbacher KJ et al: Harrison's Principles of Internal Medicine, 9th ed, pp 176–177. New York, McGraw–Hill, 1980

Miller RD: Anesthesia, pp 59, 61. New York, Churchill Livingstone, 1981

A.8. Can there be actual losses of red cell mass?

Yes. In long-standing intestinal obstruction, especially when associated with strangulation, increased permeability of the bowel wall occurs, with loss of red cells into the bowel and peritoneal cavity. Whole blood or packed cells may be needed to restore circulating red blood cells.

Schwartz S et al: Principles of Surgery, 3rd ed, p 1054. New York, McGraw–Hill, 1979

A.9. Are there any systemic effects from the absorption of bacteria and bacterial products?

The normal mucosa is impermeable to bacteria and toxins produced by bacterial degradation, but permeability is affected when there is impairment of blood supply in a strangulated segment of bowel. Thus, toxic absorption can result in septic shock from transperitoneal absorption of toxins.

Schwartz S et al: Principles of Surgery, 3rd ed, pp 1054, 1058–1059. New York, McGraw–Hill, 1979

B. Preoperative Evaluation and Preparation

B.1. Is it important to decompress the abdomen prior to surgical intervention? Why?

Yes. Because of the respiratory and circulatory complications that ensue.

What are the respiratory implications?

The distended bowel produces pressure on the diaphragm, which limits its downward progression and produces inadequate ventilation. The decrease in tidal volume and a decrease in functional residual capacity result in a low PO_2 and an elevated PCO_2. It is especially true if the stomach is also distended. An additional reason for gastric decompression is the removal of fluid and air from the stomach to lessen the likelihood of aspiration of gastric contents into the tracheobronchial tree during the induction of anesthesia. A long-standing obstruction and its associated prolonged respiratory inadequacy will result in a gasping, dusky, cyanotic, semicomatose patient.

Dripps RD, Eckenhoff JE, Vandam LD: Introduction to Anesthesia. The Principles of Safe Practice, 5th ed, pp 427–428. Philadelphia, WB Saunders, 1977

Miller RD: Anesthesia, pp 710–711. New York, Churchill Livingstone, 1981

What are the implications of the tense abdominal wall?

There are several implications of the tense abdominal wall. The first is related to the higher incidence of reverse peristalsis. Second, the stretched abdominal wall requires deeper anesthesia and more muscle relaxant to provide adequate operating conditions. These implications may increase morbidity. The undecompressed abdomen has a significant effect on venous return by two mechanisms. First, distention decreases negative intrathoracic pressure and decreases venous return. The second is due to direct vena caval compression from intraperitoneal tension. In long-standing intestinal obstruction, a large volume of intraperitoneal fluid may be present in the abdominal cavity. At the time of the surgical incision care must be taken to prevent the fluid from escaping rapidly from the abdomen. This will minimize severe hypotension. As fluid is slowly released from the abdominal cavity, the blood pressure should be checked frequently and fluid released at a rate that does not produce hypotension.

B.2. What do you use as a guide to fluid volume replacement?

Fluid losses can be calculated knowing that the body turns over 17 to 18 liters of fluid a day, made up of intestinal secretions, urine excreted by the kidneys, fluid loss through the feces, and insensible loss from the lungs and skin. The obstructive factors cause extracellular fluid loss into the gut, outlined in answer to question A.6. The above losses may be 4500 to 9000 cc of functional fluid loss. Added to this volume is the loss due to vomiting and gastric or intestinal suctioning. If there is significant edema of the bowel wall, and leakage of fluid into the peritoneal cavity due to peritonitis, an additional 7 liters of fluid may be sequestered in the peritoneal space. Measurement of central venous pressure, hourly urine output, blood pressure, and heart rate can be used to guide fluid replacement.

Schwartz S et al: Principles of Surgery, 3rd ed, p 1058. New York, McGraw–Hill, 1979

B.3. What principles would you use when choosing drugs for premedication of this patient?

Because these individuals may have a diminished respiratory reserve due to the distended abdomen, any premedication that depresses respiratory drive will diminish the ability of the patient to ventilate. This will exaggerate preexistent hypoxia and hypercarbia. The use of 100 mg of pentobarbital sodium will provide mild sedation for the anxious patient with minimal effect on ventilation. Narcotic analgesics should be avoided, in spite of the fact that the patient may be in considerable pain associated with the abdominal distention. The use of atropine or other anticholinergic drugs has some value in protecting the heart from potent vagal stimulation associated with the use of vagomimetic drugs and endotracheal intubation. In those patients with preexisting tachycardia or hyperthermia, atropine or glycopyrrolate is omitted. Some physicians have advocated the use of antacids to increase the pH of gastric contents prior to the induction of anesthesia, but this may stimulate vomiting. Antacids themselves, if aspirated, can produce pulmonary irritation.

Miller RD: Anesthesia, pp 97, 101–102. New York, Churchill Livingstone, 1981

Dripps RD, Eckenhoff JE, Vandam LD: Introduction to Anesthesia. The Principles of Safe Practice, 5th ed, pp 44–45. Philadelphia, WB Saunders, 1977

C. Intraoperative Management

C.1. What dangers are present during the induction of anesthesia? How are they planned for?

The greatest danger during the induction of anesthesia is vomiting or regurgitation of gastric contents into the pharynx and into the tracheobronchial tree. To aid in preventing this complication, have an assistant present during induction and together plan the safest method for intubation, so it can be accomplished quickly without aspiration. In our opinion, the first choice, particularly in the cooperative individual, is the awake intubation. Most patients will cooperate if the danger of aspiration is explained. If the awake intubation is chosen, the patient's lips and tongue and upper oral pharynx should be sprayed with a topical anesthetic. When this is accomplished, additional spray further down into the pharynx can be done, but care must be taken to avoid the laryngeal mechanism. Do not anesthetize the larynx because the defense mechanism of laryngeal closure will be lost in the event that regurgitation or vomiting occurs. When topical anesthesia is accomplished, then intubation usually is readily performed and the patient can be anesthetized rapidly with an intravenous hypnotic agent followed by a potent inhalation anesthetic agent. If the patient is uncooperative, there may be more trauma and a greater danger of aspiration with the awake intubation. Under these circumstances, a rapid sequence induction is the next line of defense against aspiration. If a rapid sequence induction is planned, the patient should be denitrogenated with 100% oxygen and precurarized with 3 to 6 mg of d-tubocurarine to prevent vigorous fasciculations following succinylcholine injection. Fasciculations may increase intraabdominal pressure and induce regurgitation. After 3 to 5 minutes of preoxygenation and precurarization, the patient is intubated following an injection of thiopental sodium and succinylcholine. If the patient's circulation is still unstable following fluid and electrolyte resuscitation, ketamine is to be preferred over thiopental sodium for the rapid sequence induction.

Miller RD: Anesthesia, pp 1250–1251. New York, Churchill Livingstone, 1981

C.2. In what position would you intubate this patient? Would you use Sellick's maneuver?

There is an advantage to intubating the patient in the semi-sitting position, five degrees higher than the parallel so that gravity will aid in keeping gastrointestinal contents within the stomach. Some experts advise that the patient be intubated in the supine position for fear that if the patient did vomit and he was in the semi-sitting position, he would have a greater tendency to aspirate. However, we believe the slightly elevated position of the torso is preferable. We would use Sellick's maneuver (the compression of the cricoid cartilage against the esophagus), which aids in preventing aspiration. Whether we use topical anesthesia for the awake intubation, or use the rapid sequence technique just prior to passing the endotracheal tube through the glottis and into the trachea, Sellick's maneuver can be a significant help. Although there has been some caution about using Sellick's maneuver in the vomiting patient, for fear of rupture of the esophagus, we have never seen this complication. We have, on the other hand, certainly seen Sellick's maneuver prevent aspiration into the tracheobronchial tree.

Dripps RD, Eckenhoff JE, Vandam LD: Introduction to Anesthesia. The Principles of Safe Practice, 5th ed, p 132. Philadelphia, WB Saunders, 1977

C.3. What agents and techniques would you use for this operation?

Our technique of choice would be a potent inhalation anesthetic agent. We would favor isoflurane as the inhalation anesthetic. It allows rapid change in depth and a good degree of peripheral large muscle relaxation. This reduces the total quantity of muscle relaxants needed to accomplish adequate operating conditions. The inhalation anesthetic is exhaled rather rapidly following surgery, and one can plan for the muscle relaxant to be at the end of its time action curve. If residual muscle relaxant is present, it may be reversed by a suitable reversal drug. Upper airway reflexes will have returned, eliminating the danger of aspiration.

Dripps RD, Eckenhoff JE, Vandam LD: Introduction to Anesthesia. The Principles of Safe Practice, 5th ed, p 132. Philadelphia, WB Saunders, 1977

Miller RD: Anesthesia, pp 501–502. New York, Churchill Livingstone, 1981

D. Postoperative Management

D.1. Can there be any postoperative respiratory problems not associated with aspiration?

Yes. The postoperative respiratory problems are those related to hypoventilation. Although the intestinal obstruction has been relieved, there may still be significant abdominal distention that will inhibit diaphragmatic motion and the patient may develop hypoxia and hypercarbia. For these reasons, the endotracheal tube may be left in place to decrease anatomical dead space and make it possible to ventilate the patient during the immediate postanesthesia period. Leaving the endotracheal tube in place is also desirable for those patients with previous respiratory disease, or in the morbidly obese individual. In both of these situations, the respiratory support will decrease residual atelectasis in the basilar portions of the lung. This will decrease any pulmonary shunt and lessen the need for a high inspired oxygen concentration (F_IO_2). For those patients not requiring ventilatory support, a T-piece attached to the endotracheal tube

Intestinal Obstruction · 169

will increase the F_1O_2 to maintain the PO_2 at an acceptable level. As the patient gradually regains respiratory adequacy (as shown by measuring inspiratory force and vital capacity), ventilation returns to normal and the patient can be extubated.

Miller RD: Anesthesia, pp 1345–1347. New York, Churchill Livingstone, 1981

D.2. If the patient did aspirate gastric contents, what are the possible sequelae of this event? What is the treatment?

If the patient did aspirate gastric contents, and the *p*H of the aspirate was less than 2.5, it is likely that respiratory distress will ensue. The low *p*H or the high hydrogen ion content of the gastric aspirate produces a burn of the lung and tracheobronchial tree. The tracheobronchial burn allows transudation of plasma out of the cells into the interstitial spaces and produces interstitial pulmonary edema. If this process continues, frank pulmonary edema will result. The treatment is to keep the patient intubated, and well ventilated, and follow the arterial blood gases. Depending on the arterial blood gases, regulation of the F_1O_2 and the amount of ventilation to maintain a PO_2 and PCO_2 within normal limits will be necessary. If the F_1O_2 has to be maintained above 60%, the use of positive end expiratory pressure (PEEP) may be necessary to recruit alveoli and improve oxygen diffusion. The best PEEP will have the least effect on venous return and at the same time allow F_1O_2 to be reduced to a safe level (40% or lower), thus decreasing the likelihood of oxygen toxicity. It is important to realize that although a patient may look well and have a clear chest without rhonchi or wheezes in the immediate postanesthesia period following aspiration, respiratory distress may still develop. It may take as long as 6 to 12 hours before the syndrome becomes manifest. The patient should be observed closely during the immediate postoperative period and well into the first 24 hours post-op, before you can feel comfortable that the adult respiratory distress syndrome will not ensue. The use of steroids is controversial. Culture of aspirate and bronchial secretions has to be obtained before administration of broad spectrum antibiotics.

Dripps RD, Eckenhoff JE, Vandam LD: Introduction to Anesthesia. The Principles of Safe Practice, 5th ed, pp 427–428, 518–519. Philadelphia, WB Saunders, 1977

Miller RD: Anesthesia, pp 1253–1254. New York, Churchill Livingstone, 1981

D.3. What is gram negative sepsis? What is the clinical picture and how would you treat it?

Gram negative sepsis is a shock state associated with toxins from the cell walls of gram negative organisms circulating in the blood. In a normovolemic patient, early septic shock is characterized by hypotension, high cardiac output, normal or increased blood volume, normal or high central venous pressure, low peripheral resistance, warm dry extremities, hyperventilation, and respiratory alkalosis. The clinical picture prior to the sepsis, especially in those patients who were hypovolemic (particularly with strangulation obstruction of the small bowel) may be quite similiar to hypovolemic hypotension associated with a peripheral vasoconstriction response by the body to maintain the circulating blood volume. It must be treated by the judicious use of fluids to maintain kidney perfusion and urinary output, and by appropriate antibiotics that will overcome the gram negative organisms. If therapy is delayed, the patient will develop cardiac and circulatory failure with a low fixed cardiac output and metabolic acidosis. Circulatory monitoring is necessary, using a Swan–Ganz catheter to determine the function of the central pump. Hemodynamic data may be calculated and appropriate drugs used to achieve the best cardiac output.

Schwartz S et al: Principles of Surgery, 3rd ed, pp 174–179. New York, McGraw–Hill, 1979

12 Esophageal Varices

Alan Van Poznak

A 47-year-old man has cirrhosis of the liver. Bleeding esophageal varices are now controlled with an esophageal pressure balloon. He is scheduled for portacaval anastomosis. Blood pressure, 90/60; pulse, 105; temperature, 39C; respiratory rate, 36; hematocrit 29.

A. Medical Disease and Differential Diagnosis

1. What is the major pathological derangement producing esophageal varices?
2. What produces an increase in portal pressure? What are the normal anastomoses of the portal system?
3. What is the normal portal pressure?
4. Why does cirrhosis produce a rise in portal pressure?
5. What are the dangers of the esophageal balloon?

B. Preoperative Evaluation and Preparation

1. How would you prepare the patient for surgery? What fluids would you use?
2. What premedication would you choose?

C. Intraoperative Management

1. How would you conduct the anesthesia induction?
2. Would you intubate this patient? How? What technique would you use?
3. What anesthetic regimen would you choose? Why?
4. What are the significant monitors to use during the surgery?
5. What are the anesthesia implications of the necessary intraabdominal manipulations?
6. What are the implications of clamping the inferior vena cava?

172 · Anesthesiology

D. Postoperative Management

1. Are there any postoperative complications that are more common with portacaval anastomosis?

A. Medical Disease and Differential Diagnosis

A.1. What is the major pathological derangement producing esophageal varices?

The major pathological derangement producing esophageal varices is obstruction to the flow of blood in the hepatic portal veins. This obstruction is most commonly caused by cirrhosis of the liver.

Baker L, Smith C, Lieberman G: The natural history of esophageal varices. Am J Med 26:228, 1959

Schwartz SI: Principles of Surgery, 3rd ed, p 1287. New York, McGraw–Hill, 1979

A.2. What produces an increase in portal pressure? What are the normal anastomoses of the portal system?

Because the blood is partially blocked from its normal channels of flow, it seeks alternate routes of lower pressure. These can be found in the areas of the gastrointestinal tract where the portal venous drainage and the systemic venous drainage share common territory. These areas include the esophageal veins, the hemorrhoidal veins, and the paraumbilical veins, which are the normal anastomoses of the portal system.

Schwartz SI: Principles of Surgery, 3rd ed, p 1291. New York, McGraw–Hill, 1979

A.3. What is the normal portal pressure?

The normal portal pressure is less than 250 mm of water with a mean value of 215 mm of water.

Schwartz SI: Principles of Surgery, 3rd ed, p 1290. New York, McGraw–Hill, 1979

A.4. Why does cirrhosis produce a rise in portal pressure?

The implicated pathogenic factors include the following:
- Hepatic fibrosis with compression of portal venules
- Compression by regenerative nodules
- Increased arterial blood flow
- Fatty infiltration and acute inflammation
- Intrahepatic vascular obstruction

Any of these factors will obstruct flow, leading to a rise in pressure in the vessels proximal to the point of obstruction.

Child CG III: Hepatic Circulation and Portal Hypertension. Philadelphia, WB Saunders, 1954

Schwartz SI: Principles of Surgery, 3rd ed, p 1290. New York, McGraw–Hill, 1979

A.5. *What are the dangers of the esophageal balloon?*

The principal dangers of the esophageal balloon are associated with incorrect placement, inadequate or excessive inflation of either or both of the balloon components, or displacement of the balloon from an initially correct position. Complications associated with this technique include aspiration, asphyxiation, rupture of the esophagus, and ulceration at the site of tamponade.

Reynolds TB, Freedman T, Winsor W: Results of the treatment of bleeding esophageal varices with balloon tamponade. Am J Med Sci 224:500, 1952

Schwartz SI: Principles of Surgery, 3rd ed, pp 1293, 1314. New York, McGraw–Hill, 1979

B. Preoperative Evaluation and Preparation

B.1. *How would you prepare the patient for surgery? What fluids would you use?*

Preparation for surgery must take into account the facts that this patient is anemic, febrile, tachycardic, hypotensive, and dyspneic. In addition to the anemia, there may be a considerable reduction of circulating blood volume and hypoproteinemia. In the face of these facts, it is well to transfuse with fresh whole blood not only to increase the oxygen carrying capacity, but also to compensate for inadequate plasma proteins, and possibly deficient clotting factors in the blood. Fresh whole blood also contains less ammonia than stored blood, and lessens the danger of hepatic coma from excessive blood ammonia levels. Because of the nutritional problems of these patients, it is reasonable to consider using 10% dextrose as an intravenous fluid. The source of the fever should be sought and appropriate therapy instituted. Consideration should be given to the use of hypothermia. Gastric lavage of the stomach with chilled saline may act to slow or stop bleeding, and will also reduce body temperature. When gastric lavage is performed, the airway should be appropriately protected.

Schwartz SI: Principles of Surgery, 3rd ed, p 1294. New York, McGraw–Hill, 1979

B.2. *What premedication would you choose?*

I would use no premedication, unless I saw a specific indication. These patients may be stuporous or comatose, requiring no sedation. Should the patient be awake, I would use only minimal doses of sedatives or narcotics for control of anxiety or pain, respectively. If the patient is awake with an esophageal balloon or traction, there may be considerable pain, which should have been titrated with small doses of intravenous narcotics to the point of reasonable comfort. Since the patient has fever and tachycardia, I would not routinely use atropine, but would have it ready for intravenous administration if need for its use should arise.

C. Intraoperative Management

C.1. How would you conduct the anesthesia induction?

I would induce anesthesia with careful regard to the stomach full of blood and the precarious cardiovascular status. The airway must be rapidly secured, but without excessive risk to the circulatory system. If the patient was stuporous or comatose, I would proceed directly to intubation. If the patient was awake, I would consider using a small dose of ketamine, which would secure unconsciousness with minimal depression of the cardiovascular system. A large dose of thiopental should be avoided.

C.2. Would you intubate this patient? How? What technique would you use?

Intubation is mandatory, preferably by the oral route, and accomplished with the use of minimal amounts of drugs depressant to either central nervous system or neuromuscular function. Awake intubation should be done if possible, using local topical anesthesia and minimal sedation. If abolition of consciousness is required, a small dose of ketamine may be useful. Muscle relaxants may be used if required, but remember that when using succinylcholine in these patients their plasma cholinesterase may be reduced by severe liver disease, thereby prolonging the duration of action of the drug. Nondepolarizing relaxants such as d-tubocurarine can also be used, but their action may be erratic and reversal with neostigmine is difficult, probably due to distortions in the patient's electrolyte and protein status.

C.3. What anesthetic regimen would you choose? Why?

Light general inhalation anesthesia with nitrous oxide-oxygen and added small percentages of isoflurane would be my choice, coupled with small doses of d-turocurarine as needed. Ventilation would be assisted or controlled. I would choose isoflurane because of its minimal biotransformation, minimal liver toxicity, and minimal kidney toxicity. It also augments the actions of nondepolarizing relaxants, making it possible to use far less d-tubocurarine than would be otherwise required.

C.4. What are the significant monitors to use during the surgery?

In addition to blood pressure, EKG, and oxygen monitors, it would be good to follow central venous pressure. An intraarterial line could also be used, not only for continuous monitoring of arterial pressure, but also for serial determinations of arterial blood gases and electrolytes.

C.5. What are the anesthesia implications of the necessary intraabdominal manipulations?

The anesthesiologist must be prepared to provide adequate muscle relaxation, and must also be prepared for sudden changes in cardiovascular status. A rapid release of ascitic fluid may cause a sudden fall in blood pressure.

Madden JL, Lone JM Jr, Gerold FP, Ravid JM: The pathogenesis of ascites and a consideration of its treatment. Surg Gynecol Obstet 99:385, 1954

C.6. What are the implications of clamping the inferior vena cava?

The immediate effect will be to reduce the amount of blood returning to the right atrium. If cardiac filling is significantly decreased, there will be a corresponding fall in cardiac output. Judicious management with intravenous fluids and possibly vasopressors is demanded at this point. The anesthesiologist must be careful not to overload with fluids because congestive heart failure may be produced when the clamps are removed from the anastomosis and a very large volume of blood is suddenly presented to the right side of the heart.

D. Postoperative Management

D.1. Are there any postoperative complications that are more common with portacaval anastomosis?

The surgery of portal hypertension can reduce the hazards of death by exsanguination, but it has little or no effect on the progress of the underlying hepatic disease. Two prominent postoperative complications that may be seen following portacaval anastomosis are hepatic coma and fulminant hepatic and renal failure. Hepatic coma is treated by a variety of methods all designed to reduce the blood level of ammonia. Fulminant hepatic and renal failure have been treated by cross-circulation with humans or baboons, with some slight success.

Brown H, Trey C, McDermott WV Jr: Lactulose treatment of hepatic encephalopathy in outpatients. Arch Surg 102:25, 1971

Fischer JE, James HJ: Treatment of hepatic coma and hepatorenal syndrome: Mechanism of action of L-dopa and Aramine. Am J Surg 123:222, 1972

Garrett JC, Voorhees AB Jr, Sommers SC: Renal Failure following Portasystemic Shunt in Patients with Cirrhosis of the Liver. Ann Surg 172:218, 1970

Schwartz SI: Complication of Portal–Systemic Shunting Procedures. In Beebe H (ed): Complications of Vascular Disease, Philadelphia, JB Lippincott, 1973

Schwartz SI: Principles of Surgery, 3rd ed, pp 1295, 1309. New York, McGraw–Hill, 1979

13 Pyloric Stenosis

Vinod Malhotra

This 3-week-old first-born male infant has projecticle vomiting, which contains the ingested formula but no bile. His body weight is 2.5 kg. Serum electrolytes: K, 2.2 mEq/L; Cl, 86 mEq/L. Blood pH is 7.68.

A. Medical Disease and Differential Diagnosis

1. What is the diagnosis in this patient?
2. What is the differential diagnosis of pyloric stenosis?
3. What are the metabolic problems in this newborn, secondary to his disease?
4. What are the adverse effects of metabolic alkalosis?
5. How would you treat this infant?
6. How would you determine fluid replacement in a newborn and what fluids would you use?
7. How would you correct metabolic alkalosis in this patient?

B. Preoperative Evaluation and Preparation

1. How would you evaluate this patient preoperativeley?
2. How would you prepare this patient rapidly for emergency surgery? Is surgical intervention an acute emergency in this case?
3. How would you prepare this patient for anesthesia?

C. Intraoperative Management

1. What anesthetic techniques or agents would you employ?
2. What induction–intubation sequence would you use?
3. What are the anatomical characteristics of the airway in the newborn and how do they differ from that in the adult?
4. How do you determine the size of the endotracheal tube in pediatric patients?

5. What anesthesia system would you use and why?
6. What are the advantages and disadvantages of commonly employed non-rebreathing systems?
7. How would you monitor this patient intraoperatively?

D. Postoperative Management

1. What are the complications that may occur in the postanesthesia recovery period?
2. How would you treat postextubation "croup" in this infant?

A. Medical Disease and Differential Diagnosis.

A.1. What is the diagnosis in this patient?

The most likely diagnosis in this patient is pyloric stenosis. The factors that favor the diagnosis are as follows:

- Age—3 weeks (average age at onset)
  (Range 5 days to 5 months)
- Male child (male:female ratio = 4:1)
- Projectile vomiting (characteristic)
- Contents—ingested formula, no bile

The resultant biochemical abnormality in this patient is a hypokalemic, hypochloremic alkalosis.

Nelson WE, Vaughan VC, McKay RJ: Textbook of Pediatrics, 10th ed, p 821. Philadelphia, WB Saunders, 1975

Smith RM: Anesthesia for Infants and Children, 4th ed, p 324. St Louis, CV Mosby, 1980

A.2. What is the differential diagnosis of pyloric stenosis?

Pyloric stenosis is distinguished from other congenital anomalies which cause obstruction of the alimentary tract in the newborn. These include the following: chalasia of the esophagus, hiatus hernia, duodenal atresia, jejunal atresia, ileal atresia, pancreatic annulus, malrotation of the gut, intraabdominal hernias, extraabdominal hernias, and Meckel's diverticulum. Pathognomonic features of pyloric stenosis include absence of bile-staining of the vomitus and the presence of visible gastric peristaltic waves on abdominal examination along with a palpable pyloric mass.

Nelson WE, Vaughan VC, McKay RJ: Textbook of Pediatrics, 10th ed, p 821. Philadelphia, WB Saunders, 1975

A.3. What are the metabolic problems in this newborn, secondary to his disease?

Metabolic changes occur secondary to protracted vomiting and comprise the characteristic hypokalemic, hypochloremic alkalosis, as evident in this patient. Hyponatremia, although present, may not be manifested in serum value determinations, due to severe dehydration. Compensatory respiratory acidosis is a frequent finding, and results from hypoventilation that may be marked and associated with periods of apnea. In severe dehydration leading to circulatory shock, the lack of adequate perfusion, coupled with impaired renal and hepatic function, may produce an entirely different picture of metabolic acidosis with hyperventilation, resulting in respiratory alkalosis. Therefore, depending on the severity and duration of the vomiting and the type of replenishment of fluids, one can encounter wide variations in findings on arterial blood gas and electrolyte determinations. However, the most frequent findings are hypokalemia, hyponatremia, hypochloremia, and primary metabolic alkalosis with secondary respiratory acidosis. These findings are summarized in Table 13–1.

Table 13–1. Metabolic findings in the newborn, secondary to pyloric stenosis

SEVERITY OF DEHYDRATION	ARTERIAL BLOOD GASES				SERUM ELECTROLYTES			
	pH	PCO_2	CO_2	PO_2	Na	K	Cl	HCO_3
Mild	↑	↑	↑	↔	↓ (↔)	↓	↓↓	↑
Moderate	↑↑	↑↑	↑↑	↔	↓	↓↓	↓↓↓	↑↑
Severe circulatory shock	↓↓	↓	↓↓	↓	↓	↓↓	↓↓↓	↓↓

(↔) = no change; ↑/↓ = slight change; ↑↑/↓↓ = moderate change; ↑↑↑/↓↓↓ = marked change

A.4. What are the adverse effects of metabolic alkalosis?

- An increase in pH results in the shifting of the oxygen dissocation curve to the left, thereby binding more oxygen to the hemoglobin and unloading less oxygen at the tissue level. This phenomenon assumes even more importance in newborns because at 3 weeks they still have up to 70% fetal hemoglobin with an already low value of P_{50} (*i.e.*, 20 to 22 torr).
- Respiratory compensation is affected by hypoventilation with resultant increased potential for atelectasis, as well as periods of apnea.
- Decrease in ionized calcium
- Increased potential for seizures

Jenkins MT: Common and Uncommon Problems in Anesthesiology—Clinical Anesthesia, Vol 3, p 284. Philadelphia, FA Davis, 1968

Rothstein P: Respiratory physiology in the pediatric patient. ASA Refresher Courses in Anesthesiology 8:155–166, 1980

West JB: Respiratory Physiology—The Essentials, 2nd ed, p 76. Baltimore, Williams & Wilkins, 1979

A.5. How would you treat this infant?

Medical management of the infant with pyloric stenosis is of acute urgency and should be undertaken early and vigorously. The principles of management can be grouped under the following three categories: supportive therapy, to stabilize the patient; diagnostic tests, to confirm the diagnosis and to monitor therapy; and surgery as the corrective therapy.

Supportive Therapy
- Circulatory support
- Correction of electrolyte derangement
- Prevention of aspiration

Fluids

The infant with pyloric stenosis is hypovolemic and dehydrated secondary to repeated vomiting. The severity of dehydration may vary from a mild hypovolemia to circulatory shock. The following parameters are good indicators of the severity of dehydration.

- Physical appearance—skin turgor, parched mucous membranes, sunken fontanelle, sunken eyeballs
- Blood pressure—decreased
- Pulse—increased
- Urine output—decreased
- Weight—(birth and present) and weight loss

Quantitative assessment of these parameters gives a fair estimate of the amount of total body fluid depletion.

A wide bore intravenous cannula should be placed and an infusion started immediately to correct the deficits and provide maintenance fluids.

Electrolytes

The patient is alkalotic, hypokalemic, hypochloremic, and hyponatremic and must be provided with the necessary ions to replenish the deficit. Albumin or Ringer's lactate might be used to treat the shock first. Next, the deficit should be corrected, a 0.45% to 0.9% saline is adequate for this purpose. Potassium must be added to this to correct hypokalemia and aid in the correction of alkalosis. However, the infusion of potassium should be withheld until satisfactory renal function is established. Maintenance fluid should be added to this regimen, and for this purpose 5% dextrose in 0.225% saline is usually adequate.

Prevention of Aspiration

A nasogastric tube should be inserted to thoroughly empty the stomach and the upper airway reflexes should be preserved.

Diagnostic Tests
- To assess the severity of the fluid and electrolyte derangement and to monitor therapy, the following should be evaluated: complete blood count, serum electrolytes, blood gases, BUN, urinalysis, and ECG (for marked hypokalemia).
- To confirm the diagnosis—barium swallow

Surgery

Pyloromyotomy is the only definitive treatment for these infants. It should be carried out early, but only after the patient has been stabilized satisfactorily.

Jenkins MT: Common and Uncommon Problems in Anesthesiology—Clinical Anesthesia, Vol 3, pp 277–279. Philadelphia, FA Davis, 1968

Nelson WE, Vaughan VC, McKay RJ: Textbook of Pediatrics, 10th ed, p 822. Philadelphia, WB Saunders, 1975

Smith RM: Anesthesia for Infants and Children, 4th ed, p 580. St. Louis, CV Mosby, 1980

A.6. *How would you determine fluid replacement in a newborn and what fluids would you use?*

The general principles of fluid therapy are based on the following: maintenance, correct deficits, and replace losses.

Maintenance Fluids—in the newborn are as follows:
- First 48 hours of life—75 cc/kg/day or 3 cc/kg/hr
- 2 days to one month—150 cc/kg/day or 5 cc/kg/hr
- 1 month onwards (up to 10 kg)—100 cc/kg/day or 4 cc/kg/hr

The maintenance fluids take into account the fluid losses occurring normally through the kidney, bowel, skin, and lungs. At birth, the kidney is still undergoing maturation and there exists what may be called a glomerulotubular imbalance. What this implies is that some mature glomeruli may be connected to immature tubules and vice versa. Hence, the kidney is functionally limited at birth, but undergoes rapid maturation during the first week of life.

Electrolytes

The newborn is an obligate sodium loser as well as a poor tolerator of excessive sodium overload. The maintenance electrolytes are as follows:
- Sodium—3–5 mEq/kg/day
- Potassium—2–3 mEq/kg/day
- Chloride—1–3 mEq/kg/day

Correct Deficits

Deficits take into account the previous unreplaced losses due to a period of nothing by mouth; dehydration secondary to increased losses, (*e.g.*, vomiting, diarrhea, and increased body temperature). The amount of deficit can be assessed by physical examination (see Table 13-2), body weight loss, and hematocrit.

Replace Losses

This covers ongoing abnormal losses not covered by maintenance fluids, and intraoperatively it covers evaporative losses from the operating site, third spacing, and losses from the lungs if dry gases are used in nonrebreathing circuits (see Table 13-3).

Table 13-2. Estimation of the degree of dehydration in a newborn

	MILD	MODERATE	SEVERE
Percent fluid loss	5	10	15–20
Skin turgor	Poor	Very poor	Parched
Mucous membrane and tongue	Dry	Dry	Parched
Other	—	Sunken fontanelle	Sunken eyes
Urine	Concentrated, oliguria	Oliguria with maximal concentration	Oliguria to anuria
Pulse	Normal	Tachycardia	Marked tachycardia
Blood pressure	Normal	Hypotension	Marked hypotension to shock

Table 13-3. Fluid requirement to replace intraoperative fluid losses (except blood loss) in the newborn

	FLUID REPLACEMENT ml/kg/hr
Minor surgery (e.g., herniorrhaphy)	1–3
Moderate surgery (e.g., pyloromyotomy)	3–5
Major surgery (e.g., intestinal)	5–7
Respiratory water loss due to dry gases	2

Ahlgren EW: Rational fluid therapy for children. ASA Refresher Courses in Anesthesiology 7:1–12, 1979

Berry FA: Pediatric fluid and electrolyte therapy. ASA Refresher Courses in Anesthesiology 3:1–10, 1975

Smith RM: Anesthesia for Infants and Children, 4th ed. St Louis, CV Mosby, 1980

A.7. How would you correct metabolic alkalosis in this patient?

To correct the metabolic alkalosis in this patient the underlying electrolyte derangements must be corrected; namely, hyponatremia, hypokalemia, and hypochloremia. We correct the deficits by using calculated volumes of 5% dextrose in normal saline or Ringer's lactate solution. This helps to restore sodium and chloride mainly. Dextrose, 5%, with ¼ strength normal saline, may be used to provide maintenance fluids. Once renal function is established, potassium supplements are added to the infusion. Depending on the deficit, this therapy may take anywhere from 12 to 72 hours. In severely alkalotic patients, HCl and NH_4Cl have been used to correct the derangement. However, we have rarely found it necessary.

Jenkins MT: Common and Uncommon Problems in Anesthesiology—Clinical Anesthesia, Vol 3, pp 280–284. Philadelpha, FA Davis, 1968

Smith RM: Anesthesia for Infants and Children, 4th ed, pp 580–581. St Louis, CV Mosby, 1980

B. Preoperative Evaluation and Preparation

B.1. How would you evaluate this patient preoperatively?

The following information is necessary in evaluating this patient.

History
- Onset of illness, frequency and amount of vomiting, last feeding, diarrhea, urine output, activity of the newborn (active or lethargic), birth weight

Physical examination
- Present body weight (to determine weight loss), temperature, signs of dehydration (skin turgor, mucus membranes, fontanelles, eyeballs, blood pressure, pulse, color and volume of urine), muscle tone, level of consciounsess

Laboratory findings
- Complete blood count, electrolytes—BUN and blood sugar, urinalysis, arterial blood gases

Based on the data available, we can determine the fluid and electrolyte status of the patient and correct these accordingly to stablize for surgery and anesthesia.

Jenkins MT: Common and Uncommon Problems in Anesthesiology—Clinical Anesthesia, Vol 3, pp 277–278. Philadelphia, FA Davis, 1968

B.2. How would you prepare this patient rapidly for emergency surgery? Is surgical intervention an acute emergency in this case?

Surgical intervention is never an acute emergency in hypertrophic pyloric stenosis. Therefore, no newborn should be subjected to the additional hazards of anesthesia and surgery until stabilized medically. Medical intervention is of acute urgency to stabilize the patient.

Jenkins MT: Common and Uncommon Problems in Anesthesiology—Clinical Anesthesia, Vol 3, p 277. Philadelphia, FA Davis, 1968

Smith RM: Anesthesia for Infants and Children, 4th ed, p 325. St Louis, CV Mosby, 1980

B.3. How would you prepare the patient for anesthesia?

The fluid and electrolyte replacement must be accomplished satisfactorily and this may take anywhere from 12 to 72 hours depending on the patient's status.

The next step is to empty the stomach through a wide lumen nasogastric tube and lavage out any barium left over after the x-ray studies. We find that we can use a bigger lumen tube and ensure better emptying if we pass the tube orally. Premedication is usually atropine 0.01 to 0.02 mg/kg intramuscularly. Very light or no sedation is ordered to prevent loss of airway reflexes and aspiration.

Smith RM: Anesthesia for Infants and Children, 4th ed, p 326. St Louis, CV Mosby, 1980

C. Intraoperative Management

C.1. What anesthetic techniques or agents would you employ?

We have found that using inhalation anesthesia, such as halothane, with the trachea intubated, is most satisfactory. Halothane provides a rapid, smooth, and easy induction in these patients. Intubation of the trachea is performed to minimize the risk of aspiration. The use of muscle relaxants for this procedure is rarely, if ever, necessary and the patient is extubated when he regains consciousness and airway reflex at the end of the case in the operating room.

Jenkins MT: Common and Uncommon Problems in Anesthesiology—Clinical Anesthesia, Vol 3, p 285. Philadelphia, FA Davis, 1968

Smith RM: Anesthesia for Infants and Children, 4th ed, pp 326–327. St Louis, CV Mosby, 1980

C.2. What induction–intubation sequence would you use?

The patient is induced with a mixture of 50% O_2 and 50% N_2O and 1.5% to 3% halothane, with spontaneous ventilation and gentle assist as respiration is depressed. The trachea is intubated without the use of a muscle relaxant once the proper depth of anesthesia is obtained. If one employs the intravenous technique of anesthesia, the rapid induction–intubation sequence is recommended. Awake intubation may be accomplished in skillful hands for a lethargic neonate or a very sick infant. However, the stabilized baby is usually fit and healthy, and we feel that awake intubation in the active infant is more traumatic than beneficial.

Jenkins MT: Common and Uncommon Problems in Anesthesiology—Clinical Anesthesia, Vol 3, pp 284–286. Philadelphia, FA Davis, 1968

Smith RM: Anesthesia for Infants and Children, 4th ed, p 326. St Louis, CV Mosby, 1980

C.3. What are the anatomical characteristics of the airway in the newborn and how do they differ from that in the adult?

The special characteristics of the upper airway in the newborn are as follows:

- Nasopharynx—narrow nasal passages, obligate nasal breather
- Oropharynx—large tongue, long and pendulous epiglottis
- Larynx—the distinctive features are shown in Table 13–4

It is apparent, therefore, that the newborn who has low respiratory reserves can get airway obstruction easily. He may present problems during intubation and he tolerates airway trauma poorly.

Applebaum EL, Bruce DL: Tracheal Intubation, p 17. Philadelphia, WB Saunders, 1976

Smith RM: Anesthesia for Infants and Children, 4th ed, pp 15–16. St Louis, CV Mosby, 1980

Table 13-4. Comparative anatomy of the larynx and trachea in the newborn and the adult

ANATOMICAL FEATURES	NEWBORN	ADULT
Size	4 cm	10–13 cm
Shape	Funnel	Cylindrical
Position of glottis	C_{3-4}	C_6
Narrowest point	1 cm below vocal cords	At vocal cords
Vocal cords	Slanting anteriorly	Transverse or slight slanting posteriorly
Mucous membrane	Loose (swells easily)	More firmly bound

C.4. How do you determine the size of the endotracheal tube in pediatric patients?

The two parameters of endotracheal tube sizes are the tube length and diameter depending on the age of the child, as shown in the following table. However, these are approximate sizes and one must have one size bigger and one size smaller tube available when selecting any size tube. A simple way to remember these numbers is to know the sizes at newborn, 6 months, and 1 year of age. Between 2 and 12 years the following guides may be used (see Table 13–5).

$$\text{Tube length in cms. (ages 2-12 yrs).} = 14 + \frac{\text{Age}}{2}$$

$$\text{Tube internal diameter (mm)} = 4 + \frac{\text{Age}}{4}$$

$$\text{Tube diameter (French)} = 18 + \text{Age}$$

$$\text{External circumference (French)} = \text{I D (mm)} \times 4 + 2$$

(French size means external circumference in millimeter which equals π times external diameter. $\pi = 3.1416$)

Applebaum EL, Bruce DL: Tracheal Intubation, p 36. Philadelphia, WB Saunders, 1976

Smith RM: Anesthesia for Infants and Children, 4th ed, p 175. St Louis, CV Mosby, 1980

Table 13-5. Estimated tube sizes for the pediatric patient

AGE	LENGTH (cm)	INTERNAL DIAMETER (mm)	FRENCH SIZES
Newborn	10	3.0	14
6 mos	12	3.5	16
1 yr	14	4.0	18
2 yr	15	4.5	20
4 yr	16	5.0	22
6 yr	17	5.5	24
8 yr	18	6.0	26
10 yr	19	6.5	28
12 yr	20	7.0	30

C.5. What anesthesia system would you use and why?

We employ the circle system with light circuit and modified—Y adapter. The adapter we use is the Keats modification of Rackow's Columbia Pediatric valve. The circle system is more advantageous because it maintains heat and humidification better and offers the freedom of choosing varying fresh gas flows. The controversy about the increased resistance in the adult circuit system is discounted by the fact that the respiration is assisted or controlled intraoperatively.

Smith RM: Anesthesia for Infants and Children, 4th ed, pp 132–133. St Louis, CV Mosby, 1980

C.6. What are the advantages and disadvantages of commonly employed nonrebreathing systems?

The most commonly used nonrebreathing system, the Jackson–Rees modification of Ayre's T–piece, offers the following:

Advantages
- Minimal dead space
- No valves, low resistance
- Lightweight
- Reservoir bag to assist ventilation
- Good appreciation of patient's respiratory exchange

Disadvantages
- High flows of fresh gas required
- Low flows may allow rebreathing of gases without CO_2 absorption
- Loss of heat and humidity due to high flow of cold, dry gases
- Scavenging problems of waste gases

Dorsch JA, Dorsch SE: Understanding Anesthesia Equipment, p 172. Baltimore, William & Wilkins, 1975

Smith RM: Anesthesia for Infants and Children, 4th ed, pp 132–135. St Louis, CV Mosby, 1980

C.7. How would you monitor this patient intraoperatively?

Monitoring should include blood pressure, EKG, rectal temperature, and precordial stethoscope.

Smith RM: Anesthesia for Infants and Children, 4th ed, pp 196, 327. St Louis, CV Mosby, 1980

D. Postoperative Management

D.1. What are the complications that may occur in the postanesthesia recovery period?

The patient should be carefully observed for signs of respiratory depression and periods of apnea secondary to a combination of metabolic alkalosis, general anesthesia, and decreased body temperature. Hypoventilation predisposes to atelectasis. Patients should be awake and responsive to avoid aspiration. Postextubation "croup" is a potentially dangerous complication in this age group.

Jenkins MT: Common and Uncommon Problems in Anesthesiology—Clinical Anesthesia, Vol 3, p 286. Philadelpha, FA Davis, 1968

Smith RM: Anesthesia for Infants and Children, 4th ed, p 327. CV Mosby, 1980

D.2. How would you treat postextubation "croup"?

Treatment of the potentially catastrophic postextubation laryngeal edema should be immediate, vigorous, and carried out under direct observation of the anesthesiologist. It consists of the following:

- Increasing inspired oxygen concentration (50% to 60%)
- Humidification of inspired gases
- Adequate hydration using parenteral fluids
- Light sedation to calm the patient and allow for cooperation in therapy. Avoid any significant respiratory depression.
- Epinephrine through hand-held nebulizer and mask, 50 µg/kg/min of active isomer
  - Racemic epinephrine (2.25%) diluted in 5 ml saline solution
    Dose—0.05 ml/kg delivered in 10 minutes
  - Aqueous epinephrine (0.1%) diluted in 5 ml saline solution
    Dose—0.1% 0.5 ml/kg delivered in 10 minutes

The treatment should be given over 10 minutes and may be repeated every 30 minutes, as necessary.

   Rebound phenomenon may be expected about 2 hours after cessation of this therapy.

- Steroids. Dexamesthasone, 4 mg intravenously, if the patient is less than 1 year of age; 8 mg IV if the patient is more than 1 year of age.
- Reintubation—if signs of deterioration or hypoxia appear
- Tracheostomy, if necessary. Rarely, subglottic edema may be so rapid and so severe that tracheostomy is the only choice.

The age group most likely to manifest this complication is from 1 to 4 years. At most risk is an infant under 1 year of age, mainly because of the size of the airway. Fortunately, this entity is most amenable to early and vigorous intervention and should always be treated as an emergency requiring the continued presence and evaluation by a physician who is adept at securing an airway for the child.

Deming MV, Oech SR: Steroid and antihistaminic therapy for postintubation subglottic edema in infants and children. Anesthesiology 22:933–935, 1961

Downes JJ, Godiuez RI: Acute upper-airway obstruction in the child. ASA Refresher Courses in Anesthesiology 8:29–48, 1980

Koka BU, Jeon IS, Andrea JM: Postintubation group in children. Anesth Analg (Cleve) 56:501–505, 1977

Section Four
The Nervous System

14 Brain Tumor and Craniotomy

Alan Van Poznak

The patient is a 67-year-old man in mild, congestive heart failure. He has had one month of increasing lethargy, headache, aphasia, and right sided weakness. Moderate bilateral papilledema is present. Arteriogram and CT scan suggest a left convexity meningioma that involves the superior sagittal sinus.

A. Medical Disease and Differential Diagnosis

1. What are the determinants of intracranial pressure under normal healthy conditions?
2. By what mechanisms may the presence of a brain tumor change the intracranial pressure?
3. What are the determinants of cerebral blood flow under normal healthy conditions?
4. How may intracranial diseases modify cerebral blood flow? Discuss cerebral steal syndromes.
5. What are the special dangers of posterior cranial fossa pathology?

B. Preoperative Evaluation and Preparation

1. How would you prepare the patient for surgery? Discuss medical management, fluids, and drugs.
2. What premedication would you choose?

C. Intraoperative Management

1. How would you conduct the anesthesia induction?
2. What special dangers are there during induction?
3. What are the significant monitors to use during surgery?
4. Discuss air embolism—its cause, symptoms, recognition, avoidance, and treatment.

5. What are the special problems associated with large meningiomas?
6. What are the two special requirements of anesthesia for brain tumor removal?
7. Enumerate four techniques with which one can make room for the surgeon to work in the head.
8. How does hyperventilation increase the room within the head?
9. How much hyperventilation is desirable?
10. If a little hyperventilation is good, will a lot be better?
11. What is the claimed danger of extreme hyperventilation?
12. What do you think about this?
13. Vigorously hyperventilated patients take longer to awaken. What else besides hypoxia could cause this?
14. Should all brain tumor patients be hyperventilated?
15. Why are hypertonic solutions used?
16. Why do hypertonic solutions have a preferential effect on the brain?
17. What percentage of total cardiac output is the cerebral blood flow?
18. What hypertonic solution is currently in use?
19. What is the dose?
20. Can excessive mannitol draw so much water from the heart cells that irreversible cardiac arrest ensues?
21. Give four reasons why intraoperative fluid restriction is desirable?
22. How can one increase the chances of successful spinal fluid drainage?
23. What four factors should be sequentially considered for the safe induction of hypotension during craniotomy?
24. Why is it important to follow the above sequence?
25. What are the effects of anesthetic agents on intracranial pressure?

D. Postoperative Management

1. Discuss the more common early postoperative problems following craniotomy.
2. How does anesthesia management for carotid endarterectomy differ significantly from craniotomy management?
3. Discuss special problems that may be seen after posterior cranial fossa procedures.

A. Medical Disease and Differential Diagnosis

A.1. What are the determinants of intracranial pressure under normal healthy conditions?

The intracranial pressure is ultimately determined by the volume relationships between the intracranial contents and the enclosure around them. Intracranial contents are largely fluid and therefore almost incompressible. The cranial enclosure is largely a rigid bony box in the adult, although it does have areas of lesser rigidity, such as various foramina and membranes. In the infant with open fontanelles and open skull sutures, the enclosure is far more compliant. The accumulation of blood, cerebrospinal fluid, tumor tissue, or other substances within the adult cranium will at first cause only a slight pressure rise. However, when the compliance of the system has been exceeded, the accumulation of only a very little more fluid or tumor will result in a very sharp rise in pressure. These relationships between the cranium and its contents are known as the Monro–Kellie hypothesis, which in its original form regarded the cranium as a rigid bony box. The principal determinants of the intracranial pressure under normal healthy conditions are the cerebral and spinal cord blood flow and cerebrospinal fluid mechanisms.

Kety SS, Schmidt CF: The nitrous oxide method for the quantitative determination of cerebral blood flow in man: Theory, procedure, and normal values. J Clin Invest 27:476, 1948

Lassen NA, Munck O: The cerebral blood flow in man determined by the use of radioactive krypton. Acta Physiol Scand 33:30, 1955

A.2. By what mechanisms may the presence of a brain tumor change the intracranial pressure?

A brain tumor may initially be so small as to have no effect on intracranial pressure. This is because there may be a compensatory reduction in the volume of cerebrospinal fluid. With continued enlargement of the tumor, the ability of other structures to compensate will be exceeded, and intracranial pressure will begin to rise. This rise is caused in part by the bulk of the tumor, but is also caused by the increase in cerebral blood flow in the areas surrounding the tumor and by cerebral edema in adjacent normal brain. If venous thrombosis results, there can be an abrupt rise in intracranial pressure. If local tissue pressure exceeds perfusion pressure of the arterioles supplying the area, there can be hypoxic injury of local tissue, with endothelial injury and increased transudation across the capillary membrane.

Marmarou A, Shulman K, LaMorgese J: Compartmental analysis of compliance and outflow resistance of the cerebrospinal fluid system. J Neurosurg 43:523–534, 1975

Marmarou A, Shulman K, Rosende RM: A nonlinear analysis of the cerebrospinal fluid system and intracranial pressure dynamics. J Neurosurg 48:332–344, 1978

A.3. What are the determinants of cerebral blood flow under normal healthy conditions?

Under normal healthy conditions, cerebral blood flow is determined by the perfusion pressure, the brain extracellular fluid PTT, and the nerve cell activity. The cerebral blood flow tends to be held constant by the process of autoregulation within limits of about 40 to 130 mm Hg mean arterial blood pressure. Outside of these limits, cerebral blood flow tends to become more pressure-dependent as autoregulation becomes less effective.

Haggendal E, Lofgren J, Nilsson NJ, Zwetnow NN: Effects of varied cerebrospinal fluid pressure on cerebral blood flow in dogs. Acta Physiol Scand 79:262, 1970

Lassen NA: Cerebral blood flow and oxygen consumption in man. Physiol Rev 39:183, 1959

A.4. How may intracranial diseases modify cerebral blood flow? Discuss cerebral steal syndromes.

Intracranial disease may modify cerebral blood flow by producing brain tissue regions with vasodilatation and high cerebral blood flow. This phenomenon is called "luxury perfusion." It may allow shunt of blood away from normal areas of brain with intact autoregulation, producing what is known as "cerebral steal." The phenomenon of "inverse steal" may be seen when hyperventilation produces vasoconstriction in normal, but not in damaged brain tissue.

Haggendal E, Lofgren J, Nilsson NJ, Zwetnow NN: Effects of varied cerebrospinal fluid pressure on cerebral blood flow in dogs. Acta Physiol Scand 79:262, 1970

Symon L, Pasztor E, Dorsch NWC, Branston NM: Physiological responses of local areas of the cerebral circulation in experimental primates determined by the method of hydrogen clearance. Stroke 4:632, 1973

A.5. What are the special dangers of posterior cranial fossa pathology?

The special dangers of posterior fossa pathology include compression of the lower cranial nerves in the brainstem with resultant difficulty in maintaining an open airway free of secretions. In addition, compression of respiratory and vasomotor centers in the medulla may produce severe compromise of cardiorespiratory function.

Cherniak JS, Longobardo GS: Cheyne–Stokes breathing: An instability in physiologic control. N Engl J Med 288:952, 1973

Strandgaard S, MacKenzie ET, Sengupta D et al: Upper limits of autoregulation of cerebral blood flow in the baboon. Circ Res 34:435, 1974

B. Preoperative Evaluation and Preparation

B.1. How would you prepare the patient for surgery? Discuss medical management, fluids, and drugs.

Preparation for surgery would include control of the congestive heart failure with whatever means were appropriate, including digitalization, diuretics, antihypertensives, and antiarrhythmic drugs as needed for the particular situation.

B.2. What premedication would you choose?

Choice of premedication should be limited to whatever dose of sedative is required for control of anxiety, if present. Since the patient is not in pain, narcotics are not needed; their respiratory depressant effect may dangerously elevate the intracranial pressure. Atropine may be given as a

Brain Tumor and Craniotomy · 193

premedicant intramuscularly or intravenously just prior to anesthetic induction.

C. Intraoperative Management

C.1. How would you conduct the anesthesia induction?

Regardless of the method chosen, the anesthesiologist should avoid hypoxia or hypercarbia. Hyperventilation prior to intubation and use of potent inhalation anesthetics is desirable. A thiopental–muscle relaxant sequence would be a thoroughly acceptable technique.

Sharpiro HM: Intracranial hypotension: Therapeutic and anesthetic considerations. Anesthesiology 43:445, 1975

C.2. What special dangers are there during induction?

The special dangers of induction are hypoxia, hypercarbia, and wide swings in blood pressure.

Shapiro W, Wasserman AJ, Patterson JL: Human cerebrovascular response to combined hypoxia and hypercapnia. Circ Res 19:903, 1966

Woolman H, Smith TC, Stephen GW et al: Effects of extremes of respiratory and metabolic alkalosis of cerebral blood flow in man. J Appl Physiol 24:60, 1968

C.3. What are the significant monitors to use during surgery?

Significant monitors include blood pressure, ECG, P_{CO_2}, precordial Doppler, temperature, and O_2 monitors.

C.4. Discuss air embolism–its cause, symptoms, recognition, avoidance, and treatment.

Air embolism can occur when atmospheric air enters an open vein in the operative area. Dangerous conditions develop if the amount of air is sufficient to interfere with the ability of the right heart to pump blood to the lungs. Air in the pulmonary capillaries can cause reflex pulmonary vasoconstriction, further decreasing the already compromised pulmonary function. Precordial Doppler monitoring is the most efficient way of recognizing a small amount of air in the heart. Avoidance of air embolism is most easily done by proper positioning of the patient so that there is always a small positive pressure in the veins of the operative site. If blood is coming out, air can't be going in. Expansion of intravascular volume and controlled ventilation with positive end expiratory pressure also help to maintain a continuous positive pressure in the veins of the operative site. The best treatment of this condition is not as good as prevention, but includes such measures as large-bore right atrial catheters, Swan–Ganz catheters, and the rapid employment of steep head–down tilt to force the foamy blood from the right atrium. Paradoxical passage of air through a patent foramen ovale into the left heart and systemic circulation is another esoteric rare complication of air embolism.

Brechner VL, Bethune WM, Soldo NJ: Pathological physiology of air embolsim. Anesthesiology 28:240, 1967

Chandler W, Demcheff S, Taren J: Acute pulmonary edema following venous air embolism during a neurosurgical procedure. J Neurosurg 40:400, 1974

Steffey EP, Gauger GE, Eger EI: Cardiovascular effects of venous air embolism during air and oxygen breathing. Anesth Analg (Cleve) 53:599, 1974

C.5. What are the special problems associated with large meningiomas?

Meningiomas arise from dural cells, and may invade or compress the venous sinuses that are formed by dural duplications. The special hazards are venous thrombosis, bleeding, and air embolism, as mentioned above.

C.6. What are the two special requirements of anesthesia for brain tumor removal?

- Make room for the surgeon to work in the head
- Control excessive bleeding

Adams, RW, Gronert GA, Sundt TM et al: Halothane, hypocapnia, and cerebrospinal fluid pressure in neurosurgery. Anesthesiology 37:510, 1972

Kety SS, Schmidt CF: The determination of cerebral blood flow in man by the use of nitrous oxide in low concentrations. Am J Physiol 143:53, 1945

C.7. Enumerate four techniques with which one can make room for the surgeon to work in the head.

- Hyperventilation
- Hypertonic intravenous fluids
- Spinal fluid removal
- Controlled hypotension

Miller JD, Leech P: Effects of mannitol and steroid therapy on intracranial volume–pressure relationships in patients. J Neurosurg 42:274–281, 1975

Waltz AG: Effects of blood pressure on blood flow in ischemic and nonischemic cerebral cortex. Neurology (NY) 18:613, 1968

C.8. How does hyperventilation increase the room within the head?

Reduction of P_{CO_2} decreases vascular engorgement and brain bulk.

Plum F, Siesjo BK: Recent advances in CSF physiology. Anesthesiology 42:708, 1975

C.9. How much hyperventilation is desirable?

To an end-expiratory CO_2 of approximately 4%, corresponding to a P_{CO_2} of approximately 30 torr.

Rossanda M, Collice M, Porta M, Beselli L: Intracranial hypertension in head injury: clinical significance and relation to respiration. In Lundberg M, Penten U, Brock M: Intracranial Pressure II p 475. New York, Springer Verlag, 1975

C.10. If a little hyperventilation is good, will a lot be better?

Not necessarily. There is a reasonable limit to the reduction of brain bulk that can be produced by hyperventilation. In addition, some have pointed out a theoretical danger of extreme hyperventilation.

Kogure K, Scheinberg P, Reinmuth OM et al: Mechanisms of cerebral vasodilation in hypoxia. J Appl Physiol 29:223, 1970

C.11. What is the claimed danger of extreme hyperventilation?

Hypoxia caused by extreme cerebral vasoconstriction.

Siesjo BK, Nielsen L: The influence of arterial hypoxemia upon labile phosphates and upon extracellular and intracellular lactate and pyruvate concentration in the rat brain. Scand J Clin Lab Invest 27:83, 1971

C.12. What do you think about this?

It is something to argue about. Harp and Wollman have presented a review of the conflicting claims.

Harp JR, Wollman H: Cerebral metabolic effects of hyperventilation and deliberate hypotension. Br J Anaesth 43:256, 1973

C.13. Vigorously hyperventilated patients take longer to awaken. What else besides hypoxia could cause this?

Hyperventilation lowers PCO_2 and raises pH, causing a fall in ionized calcium that is needed for proper synaptic function. The time required for restoration of ionized calcium to optimum levels could explain the prolonged awakening time.

Christensen MS, Brodersen P, Olesen J et al: Cerebral apoplexy (stroke) treated with or without prolonged artificial hyperventilation: Cerebrospinal fluid acid–base balance and intracranial pressure. Stroke 4:620, 1973

C.14. Should all brain tumor patients be hyperventilated?

No. Sometimes the neurosurgeon will prefer spontaneous respiration if he must work near the medulla. All factors should be considered.

C.15. Why are hypertonic solutions used?

To draw water from the cells by their osmotic effect.

Rottenbert DA, Hurwitz BJ, Posner JB: The effect of oral glycerol on intraventricular pressure in man. Neurology 27:360, 1977

Weed LH, McKibben PS: Pressure changes in the cerebrospinal fluid following intravenous injection of solutions of various concentrations. Am J Physiol 48:512–530, 1919

C.16. Why do hypertonic solutions have a preferential effect on the brain?

Because the brain receives a relatively large percentage of the cardiac output.

C.17. What percentage of total cardiac output is the cerebral blood flow?

Approximately 15%.

Cottrell JE, Turndorf H: Anesthesia and Neurosurgery, p 2. St Louis, CV Mosby, 1980

C.18. What hypertonic solution is currently in use?

Mannitol, 20%.

Rottenbert DA, Hurwitz BJ, Posner JB: The effect of oral glycerol on intraventricular pressure in man. Neurology 27:360, 1977

C.19. What is the dose?

From 2/3 to 1 1/2 gram per kilogram body weight.

Miller JD, Leech P: Effects of mannitol and steroid therapy on intracranial volume–pressure relationship in patients. J Neurosurg 42:274–281, 1975

C.20. Can excessive mannitol draw so much water from the heart cells that irreversible cardiac arrest ensues?

Yes.

Rottenbert DA, Hurwitz BJ, Posner JB: The effect of oral glycerol on intraventricular pressure in man. Neurology 27:360, 1977

C.21. Give four reasons why intraoperative fluid restriction is desirable.

- A given dose of mannitol will exert a greater osmotic effect if put into a smaller circulating blood volume.
- If circulating volume has been expanded with isotonic fluids, the addition of mannitol to patients with marginally compensated circulation may increase circulatory failure. Pulmonary edema may occur before the kidneys can remove the excess water from the circulation.
- Restriction of intraoperative intravenous fluids facilitates the management of induced hypotension.
- The probability of postoperative cerebral edema, a major neurosurgical concern, is lessened by intraoperative fluid restriction. You can't have edema without water.

C.22. How can one increase the chances of successful spinal fluid drainage?

By proper positioning of the patient for lumbar puncture: hip and shoulders vertical on the table, large bore needles entered horizontally in the midline. Let fluid drip into a sterile syringe barrel. Don't exert strong negative pressure with a syringe. You may draw tissue against the level of the needle and jam the system.

C.23. What four factors should be sequentially considered for the safe induction of hypotension during craniotomy?

- Depth of anesthesia

- Tilt of operating table
- Relative blood volume of patient
- Use of drugs

Van Poznak A, Jenkins MT, Artusio JF Jr: Anesthesia for Surgery of the Pituitary Gland. Clinical Anesthesia, Vol 3, Chap. 8, pp 118–125. Philadelphia, FA Davis, 1963

C.24. Why is it important to follow the above sequence?

The depth of anesthesia and tilt of the table may be sufficient to establish reduction of both arterial and venous pressures in the brain. In such cases, drugs are rarely needed, and then only in small amounts, thus minimizing the likelihood of toxic reactions. Should excessive hypotension occur, it can usually be easily reversed by lessening the doses of inhalation agent and lessening the tilt of the table. Conversely, if the anesthetic depth and table tilt are minimal, then more hypotensive drug will be required and there will be a greater probability of toxic accumulation. Should excessive hypotension occur, further lessening of anesthetic depth may invite coughing on the endotracheal tube, which can be disastrous if the dura has been opened. If the table is brought level or head down, profuse venous bleeding may occur.

Van Poznak A, Jenkins MT, Artusio JF Jr: Anesthesia for surgery of the pituitary gland. Clinical Anesthesia, Vol 3, Chap 8, pp 118–125. Philadelphia, FA Davis, 1963

C.25. What are the effects of anesthetic agents on intracranial pressure?

All potent inhalation anesthetic agents increase cerebral blood flow. This will cause an increase in intracranial pressure. If a mass lesion is present, there may be a dangerously sharp increase in intracranial pressure when a potent inhalation anesthetic such as halothane is added to the inspired mixture. Much of this pressure rise can be prevented by hyperventilation of the patient to reduce the PCO_2 prior to adding halothane to the inspired mixture.

    Enflurane and isoflurane, while qualitatively similar to halothane in their effects on intracerebral blood flow, do not seem to produce as much of a rise in intracranial pressure in either normal or diseased states. Some authors have felt that extreme hyperventilation is not necessary before adding enflurane or isoflurane to the inspired mixture and that it is sufficient to ventilate the patient to a $PaCO_2$ of about 30 torr. Nitrous oxide has also been reported to increase cerebral blood flow, but not nearly as much as the potent volatile inhalation anesthetics.

    Barbiturates decrease cerebral blood flow and may also produce a selective cerebral vasoconstriction, according to some authors. This effect, along with a reduction in $CMRO_2$, has made barbiturates such as thiopental desirable not only for neurosurgical anesthesia, but also for attempts at mimimizing brain damage after cerebral trauma or hypoxic insult. Although laboratory studies on animals have shown a protective effect when given prior to global cerebral ischemic insult, clinical studies have been less clear cut in demonstrating a protective or therapeutic effect if the barbiturate has been given after the ischemic or hypoxic event has occurred.

Narcotics such as morphine or fentanyl reduce neuronal activity and blood pressure, but they also decrease ventilatory drive. In the spontaneously ventilating patient, the $PaCO_2$ will rise, thereby causing an increase in cerebral blood flow and an increase in intracranial pressure. For this reason, narcotics should be used cautiously if at all in spontaneously ventilating patients with brain tumors or other intracranial lesions. If respiration is assisted or controlled to hold the $PaCO_2$ to an acceptably low level, narcotic analgesics can be safely used.

Ketamine increases cerebral blood flow and increases intracranial pressure. Despite these effects, ketamine is a useful drug in small doses during neuroradiological diagnostic procedures.

Succinylcholine and other depolarizing neuromuscular blocking drugs may transiently increase intracranial pressure during the period of fasciculation, but not afterwards, provided that respiration is adequately controlled. Pancuronium and d-tubocurarine likewise have no effects on intracranial pressure in the presence of adequately controlled respiration.

Cottrell JE, Turndorf H: Anesthesia and Neurosurgery, pp 15–17. St Louis, CV Mosby, 1980

D. Postoperative Management

D.1. Discuss the more common early postoperative problems following craniotomy.

The principal postoperative problems following craniotomy relate partly to mechanical manipulations by the surgeon and chemical manipulations by the anesthesiologist. In order to allow early assessment of neurological function, one should choose anesthetic drugs that are rapidly excreted or metabolized, or can be readily reversed. Temperature should be near normal. Intravenous fluids should be restricted to lessen the probability of cerebral edema, which can be a major early postoperative complication. Intracranial pressure monitoring has been advocated by some authors.

James HE, Bruno LA, Schut L: Intracranial subarachnoid pressure monitoring in children. Surg Neurol 3:313, 1975

Johnston IH, Jennett B: The place of continuous intracranial pressure monitoring in neurosurgical practice. Acta Neurochir (Wien) 29:53, 1973

D.2. How does anesthesia management for carotid endarterectomy differ significantly from craniotomy management?

Carotid endarterectomy anesthesia management is significantly different in that it is desirable to optimize cerebral blood flow rather than reduce it, as is usually done in anesthesia management for craniotomy.

Wade JG: Carotid endarterectomy: The anesthetic challenge. ASA Refresher Courses in Anesthesiology 6:145–152, 1978

D.3. Discuss special problems that may be seen after posterior cranial fossa procedure.

Following posterior fossa craniotomies, special problems may arise from brain stem edema or hematoma, which may compress respiratory centers or lower cranial nerve nucleic; causing difficulty in swallowing, holding the airway open for managing secretions such as saliva or mucous.

Cottrell JE, Turndorf H: Anesthesia and Neurosurgery, pp 176–178. St Louis, CV Mosby, 1980

15 Carotid Endarterectomy

Alan Van Poznak

The patient is a 60-year-old man with cerebral vascular insufficiency. During the past year he has had two transient ischemic attacks. He gives a history of mild angina on effort. Neurological examination today is within normal limits. Blood pressure 160/90, pulse 72.

A. Medical and Differential Diagnosis

1. What are the possible causes of transient ischemic attacks (TIA)?
2. How might obstructed blood flow be determined?
3. What are the risks of these determinations?
4. What are the risks if nothing is done?
5. What is meant by the term "luxury perfusion"?
6. What is meant by the term "intracerebral steal"?
7. What is the "inverse steal" or "Robin Hood" syndrome?
8. What is the arterial circle of Willis?

B. Preoperative Evaluation and Preparation

1. What is normal cerebral blood flow (CBF)?
2. What is critically low cerebral blood flow as measured by EEG?
3. What is normal brain P_{O_2} and P_{CO_2}?
4. What is critically low P_{O_2} in brain?
5. What is autoregulation?
6. Do premature infants have good cerebral autoregulation?
7. How does P_{CO_2} affect autoregulation?
8. How do anesthetic agents affect autoregulation?
9. What are the principal determinants of cerebral blood flow?
10. How would you premedicate this patient?

C. Intraoperative Management

1. Enumerate the factors affecting the induction of anesthesia.
2. Outline an induction technique that would be least disturbing to this patient.
3. Discuss control of blood pressure and P_{CO_2}.
4. Would you use a respirator? Give reasons.
5. What is the mechanism of action of heparin and of protamine?
6. How can one be certain of the adequacy of cerebral perfusion at the time the carotid artery is clamped?

D. Postoperative Management

1. What early postoperative complications would you watch for very carefully?
2. What would you do about them?
3. What might cause hypertension and tachycardia in the early postoperative period?

A. Medical Disease and Differential Diagnosis.

A.1. What are the possible causes of transient ischemic attacks (TIA)?

They are almost exclusively due to atherosclerotic thrombosis causing transient focal ischemia. About 2/3 of all patients with TIA are men or hypertensive, or both.

Toole JF, Yuson CP, Janeway R: Transient ischemic attacks: A study of 225 patients. Neurology 28:746, 1978

Ueda K, Toole JF, McHenry LC: Carotid and vertebral transient ischemic attacks: Clinical and angiographic correlation. Neurology 29:1094, 1978

A.2. How might obstructed blood flow be determined?

- By the presence of carotid bruit in the neck
- By evidence of impaired flow on examination with a Doppler principle flow detector
- By evidence of occlusion of the internal carotid artery in the neck as determined by palpation, auscultation, and ophthalmodynamometry
- By evidence of impaired flow by angiography

Toole JF, Yuson CP, Janeway R: Transient ischemic attacks: A study of 225 patients. Neurology 28:746, 1978

A.3. What are the risks of these determinations?

Almost none on physical examination by the first three above mentioned signs. Angiography carried a 5% to 10% risk of transient complications and a 2% to 3% risk of permanent deficit.

Faught E, Trader SD, Hanna GR: Cerebral complications of arteriography for transient ischemia and stroke. Neurology 29:4, 1979

A.4. What are the risks if nothing is done?

Approximately 20% of infarcts that follow TIA occur within a month after the first attack and about 50% within a year.

Mohr JP et al: The Harvard Cooperative Stroke Registry: A prospective registry of patients hospitalized with stroke. Neurology 28:754, 1978

Whisnant JP, Matsumoto N, Elverback LR: Transient cerebral ischemic attacks in a community: Rochester, Minnesota, 1955 through 1969. Mayo Clin Proc 48:194, 1973

A.5. What is meant by the term "luxury perfusion"?

Luxury perfusion is blood flow that is in excess of metabolic need (increased CBF/CMR O_2 ratio). It is most frequently observed in tissues surrounding tumors or areas of infarction, and has also been observed in brain tissue that has been manipulated during surgery.

Brock N, Luyendijk W (ed): In Progress in Brain Research—Cerebral Circulation, p 125. New York, Elsevier–Dutton, 1968

Paulson OB: Cerebral apoplexy (stroke): Pathogenesis, pathophysiology and therapy as illustrated by regional blood flow measurements in the brain. Stroke 2:327–360, 1971

A.6. What is meant by the term "intracerebral steal"?

Intracerebral steal is a paradoxical response to CO_2 in which hypercapnia decreased the blood flow in an ischemic area. It may be the consequence of the vasodilator action of CO_2 on the normal arterioles at the periphery of the lesion.

Paulson OB: Cerebral apoplexy (stroke): Pathogenesis, pathophysiology and therapy as illustrated by regional blood flow measurements in the brain. Stroke 2:327–360, 1971

A.7. What is the "inverse steal" or "Robin Hood" syndrome?

This is a paradoxical effect of hypocapnia producing increased blood flow to ischemic areas. Vasoconstriction is assumed to occur in adjacent normal arterioles, thereby causing a local increase in perfusion pressure and augmenting collateral flow to the abnormal area.

Betz E: Cerebral blood flow: Its measurement and regulation. Physiol Rev 52:595–630, 1972

A.8. What is the arterial circle of Willis?

The cerebral arteries are derived from the internal carotid and vertebral arteries. They form a remarkable anastomosis at the base of the brain known as the arterial circle of Willis. The circle is formed anteriorly by the two anterior cerebral arteries that are connected together by the anterior communicating artery and posteriorly by the two posterior cerebral arteries, which are connected by the two posterior communicating arteries to internal carotid arteries (Fig. 15–1).

Goss CM: Gray's Anatomy, 29th ed, p 599. Philadelphia, Lea & Febiger, 1973

B. Preoperative Evaluation and Preparation

B.1. What is normal cerebral blood flow (CBF)?

Approximately 50 ml per 100 grams per minute for the entire brain. However, blood flow is about four times higher in gray matter than it is in white matter, the flows being respectively 80 ml and 20 ml per 100 grams per minute.

Kety SS, Schmidt CF: The nitrous oxide method for the quantitative determination of cerebral blood flow in man: Theory, procedure and normal values. J Clin Invest 27:476, 1948

Lassen NA, Munch O: The cerebral blood flow in man determined by the use of radioactive krypton. Acta Physiol Scand 33:30, 1955

B.2. What is critically low cerebral blood flow as measured by EEG?

Approximately 20 ml/100 g/min.

Sundt TM, Sharbrough FW, Anderson RE et al: Cerebral blood flow measurements and electroencephalograms during carotid endarterectomy. J Neurosurg 41:310, 1974

Trojaborg W, Boysen G: Relation between EEG, regional cerebral blood flow and internal carotid artery pressure during carotid endarterectomy. Electroencephalogr Clin Neurophysiol 34:61, 1973

B.3. What is normal brain PO_2 and PCO_2?

For oxygen, approximately 100 torr. For CO_2 approximately 40 torr.

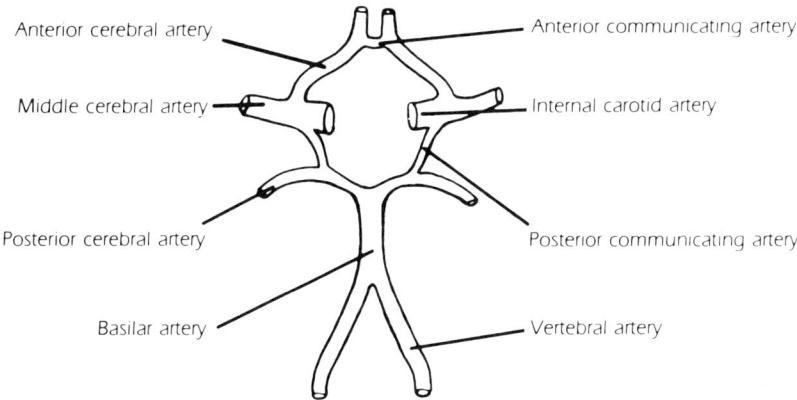

Fig. 15-1. Arterial circle of Willis

Harp JR, Wollman H: Cerebral metabolic effects of hyperventilation and deliberate hypotension. Br J Anaesth 45:256, 1973

Kogure K, Scheinberg P, Reinmuth OM et al: Mechanisms of cerebral vasodilatation in hypoxia. J Appl Physiol 29:223, 1979

B.4. What is critically low PO_2 in brain?

Approximately 50 mm Hg.

Kogure K, Scheinberg P, Reinmuth OM et al: Mechanisms of cerebral vasodilatation in hypoxia. J Appl Physiol 29:223, 1970

B.5. What is autoregulation?

The tendency of a tissue to maintain normal blood flow despite variations in blood pressure.

Haggendal E, Lofgren J, Nilsson NJ et al: Effects of varied cerebrospinal fluid pressure on cerebral blood flow in dogs. Acta Physiol Scand 79:262, 1970

Symon L, Pasztor E, Dorsch NWC et al: Physiological responses of local areas of the cerebral circulation in experimental primates determined by the method of hydrogen clearance. Stroke 4:632, 1973

B.6. Do premature infants have good cerebral autoregulation?

Probably not.

B.7. How does PCO_2 affect autoregulation?

CBF changes about 4% for each mm Hg change in arterial PCO_2.

Skinhoj E, Paulson OB: Carbon dioxide and cerebral circulatory control: Evidence of a nonfocal site of action of carbon dioxide on cerebral circulation. Arch Neurol 20:249, 1969

B.8. How do anesthetic agents affect autoregulation?

They decrease it, with the exception of nitrous oxide.

Morita H, Bleyarnt AL, Stezoski SW et al: The effect of halothane anesthesia on cerebral blood flow, autoregulation and cerebral metabolism of oxygen and glucose. Abstracts of Scientific Papers presented at the annual meeting of the American Society of Anesthesiologists, pp 63–64, 1974

Murphy FL, Kennell EM, Johnston RE et al: The effects of enflurane, isoflurane and halothane on cerebral blood flow and metabolism in man. Abstracts of Scientific Papers presented at the annual meeting of the American Society of Anesthesiologists, p 62, 1974

B.9. What are the principal determinants of cerebral blood flow?

Nerve cell activity, perfusion pressure, PCO_2, pH, PO_2, and neurogenic influences.

Cottrell JE, Turndorf H: Anesthesia and Neurosurgery, pp 3–11. St Louis, CV Mosby, 1980

B.10. How would you premedicate this patient?

Lightly, using only enough barbiturate, benzodiazepine, or other tranquilizer to control whatever anxiety might be present. In the absence of pain there is no need for narcotic analgesics.

C. Intraoperative Management

C.1. Enumerate the factors affecting the induction of anesthesia.

Anxiety, pain, reflexes causing hypertension or hypotension, drugs causing marked changes in blood pressure, carbon dioxide, and oxygen levels.

Cottrell JE, Turndorf H: Anesthesia and Neurosurgery, pp 4–10. St Louis, CV Mosby, 1980

C.2. Outline an induction technique that would be least disturbing to this patient?

A moderate (approximately 2–3 mg per kg) dose of intravenous thiobarbiturate to avoid sharp falls in blood pressure. A small dose of intravenous ketamine (approximately 1 mg per kg) may be used with the barbiturate. After thorough oxygenation, succinylcholine, 1 mg per kg is given, and an endotracheal tube is placed. Nitrous oxide, oxygen, and enflurane are then ventilated into the patient until adequate spontaneous respiration returns.

C.3. Discuss control of blood pressure and Pco_2.

It is best to stay in the patient's normal range. Hypotension may cause inadequate cerebral or myocardial perfusion, leading to stroke or myocardial infarction. Extreme hypertension may cause cerebral hemorrhage, and may dangerously increase the myocardial work load. Hypercapnia may increase cerebral perfusion, but the dangers of various steal syndromes and luxury perfusion must be considered. Hypocapnia, if extreme, may bring a risk of hypoxia, according to some authors.

Christensen MD, Hoedt–Rasmussen K, Lassen NA: Cerebral vasodilatation by halothane anesthesia in man and its potentiation by hypotension and hypercapnia. Br J Anaesth 39:927, 1967

Wollman H, Alexander SC, Cohen PJ et al: Cerebral circulation of man during halothane anesthesia: Effects of hypocarbia and of d-tubocurarine. Anesthesiology 25:180, 1964

Wollman H, Smith TC, Chase PE et al: Cerebral circulation during general anesthesia and hyperventilation in man: Thiopental induction to nitrous oxide and d-tubocurarine. Anesthesiology 26:329, 1965

C.4. Would you use a respirator? Give reasons.

Spontaneous respiration with slightly elevated Pco_2 is often entirely satisfactory. If a respirator is used, CO_2 monitoring would seem to be desirable to avoid extremes of hypocarbia or hypercarbia, either of which may be harmful.

C.5. What is the mechanism of action of heparin and of protamine?

Heparin acts indirectly by means of a plasma cofactor, antithrombin III, that neutralizes several activated clotting factors XII a, karrikrein, XIa IXa, Xa, IIa, and XIIIa. Protamine combines ionically with heparin to form a stable complex that is devoid of anticoagulant activity.

Goodman LS, Gilman A: The Pharmacological Basis of Therapeutics, 6th ed, pp 1349–1352. New York, Macmillan, 1980

C.6. How can one be certain if the adequacy of cerebral perfusion at the time the carotid artery is clamped?

There is no simple answer to this question. Numerous approaches have been attempted, and each has its problems. Some of the methods are as follows:

- Monitoring jugular venous oxygen saturation. Although this reflects the relationship between total cerebral blood flow and total cerebral oxygen consumption, it is not a reliable method of determining regional cerebral ischemia.
- Electroencephalograms. This is a reliable index of cerebral metabolism. It is sensitive to perfusion, oxygenation, depth of anesthesia, temperature, pH, $PACO_2$, and PAO_2. If normal temperature, normal blood gases, and light anesthesia is held constant, the EEG is a dependable monitor of adequacy of cerebral perfusion.
- Regional cerebral blood flow measurement. While this is a reliable research tool, it is not available in most operating rooms.
- Stump pressure. This is the pressure measured in the ipsilateral carotid artery, and reflects the pressure in the circle of Willis. A stump pressure of 60 torr usually will provide adequate perfusion of normal brain during general anesthesia.
- Use of shunts. There is much variation among surgeons regarding the use of shunts. Some surgeons always use them, some occasionally, some never. A rational approach would be to monitor the EEG during several minutes of temporary carotid occlusions. If no EEG deterioration occurs, a shunt is probably not needed. If EEG deterioration occurs, the temporary clamp is removed to allow the EEG to return to baseline form, after which a shunt is inserted. Vasopressors may be of some value in increasing cerebral perfusion, but their use is not without danger to both the brain and the heart.

Wade JG: Carotid endarterectomy: The anesthetic challenge. ASA Refresher Courses in Anesthesiology 6:150–153, 1978

D. Postoperative Management

D.1. What early postoperative complications would you watch for very carefully?

- Bleeding from the operative site

- Development of hemiparesis, aphasia, or coma
- Signs of myocardial infarction

Wade JG: Carotid endarterectomy: The anesthetic challenge. ASA Refresher Courses in Anesthesiology 6:150–153, 1978

D.2. What would you do about them?

Keep close communication with surgeon and internist, and be ready to take prompt corrective action.

D.3. What might cause hypertension and tachycardia in the early postoperative period?

Section of the carotid sinus nerve, especially after endarterectomy on the second side. Also, uncontrolled pain, and a forgotten vasopressor drug still running.

Wade JG: Carotid endarterectomy: The anesthetic challenge. ASA Refresher Courses in Anesthesiology 6:150–153, 1978

16 Spinal Cord Tumor

Alan Van Poznak

The patient is a 59-year-old man with metastatic melanoma to the cervical and lumbar spine. He has progressive quadriparesis. Bone scan showed increased uptake at C 3–4–5–6. Myelogram showed blockage at C 4–5. He is scheduled for laminectomy C 3–4–5–6 and posterior fusion with iliac bone graft. He appears short of breath at rest. He has only diaphragmatic breathing.

A. Medical Disease and Differential Diagnosis

1. What are the particular dangers of anesthesia and surgery for this patient?

B. Preoperative Evaluation and Preparation

1. What are some important factors in the preoperative evaluation of this patient?
2. How would you premedicate this patient?

C. Intraoperative Management

1. What monitoring procedures would you use for this operation on this patient?
2. How can you detect air embolism? What is the treatment?
3. How would you induce anesthesia and intubate the patient?
4. How would you maintain anesthesia?
5. In a patient with a spinal cord lesion above T 7, what important cause of sudden hypertension must be considered during surgery below the level of the spinal cord lesion?
6. What intraoperative complications may be reasonably expected from surgery near the upper part of the cervical spinal cord?

D. Postoperative Management

1. What is the principal postoperative complication peculiar to this type of surgery? How do you manage it?

A. Medical Disease and Differential Diagnosis

A.1. What are the particular dangers of anesthesia and surgery for this patient?

The particular surgical danger is that of additional damage to a spinal cord whose function has been seriously compromised by metastatic tumor. The particular anesthetic dangers relate to surgery on an ill patient who is to be placed in the sitting position. These anesthetic dangers are both respiratory and circulatory, and the special danger is that of air embolism.

Albin MS, Jannetta PJ, Maroon JC et al: Anesthesia in the sitting position, p 755. Proceeding of the fourth World Congress of Anesthesiologists, Congr Amsterdam, Excerpta Medica, 1974

Lassen NA: Control of the cerebral circulation in health and disease. Circ Res 34:749, 1974

Maroon JC, Albin MS, Carroll R: Venous air embolism in neurosurgery. Presented at the annual meeting of the American Association of Neurological Surgeons, Toronto, April, 1977

Wilkins RH, Albin MS: An unusual entrance site of venous air embolism during operations in the sitting position. Surg Neurol 7:71, 1977

B. Preoperative Evaluation and Preparation

B.1. What are some important factors in the preoperative evaluation of this patient?

One can suspect a possible pneumonia from the patient's vital signs. The temperature is elevated, the patient is short of breath, and there appears to be only diaphragmatic breathing. Obviously, more information is needed. A chest x-ray and preoperative blood gas values would be helpful, as well as pulmonary function tests. The source of the fever should be determined. It could be from causes other than pneumonia, and these should be sought. If possible, an antibiotic and another appropriate treatment should be carried out prior to surgery. If the urgency for decompression of the spinal cord will not allow a delay, then means to control the fever should be prepared for use during surgery. The low blood pressure and rapid pulse are also warnings of potential trouble. These may result from the anemia and hypovolemia that occur late in the course of many malignant diseases. In addition, there could be an expansion of the vascular tree caused by interruption of sympathetic nerve transmission from tumor compression of the spinal cord. In either case, the size of the vascular tree is disproportionate to its contents. The induction of further disproportion through cardiovascular effects of general anesthetics and head-up tilt could prove disastrous. For this reason, correction of preoperative hypovolemia and anemia is needed. One should also remember that patients with chronic illness may have a reduced blood volume even though the hemoglobin and hematocrit values are not severely reduced.

The hypotension may also be caused by relative adrenal insufficiency. If so, it may be worsened by the stress of anesthesia and surgery. Steroid preparation should be considered in cases where pituitary or adrenal insufficiency is suspected. Many malignant tumors have been known to metastasize to both these important endocrine areas.

B.2. *How would you premedicate this patient?*

Premedication, if used at all, should be limited to whatever dose of sedative is necessary to control the patient's anxiety. Often the preoperative visit by the anesthesiologist is the best medicine for this purpose. If physical pain is present, it should be controlled by an appropriately timed dose of analgesic narcotic. Opinions vary regarding the merits of preanesthetic anticholinergic agents. Since irritating inhalation agents are no longer used, the antisecretory effect is usually not needed. To accelerate the heart rate in this already tachycardic patient seems unwise. I would prefer to give atropine only when it is needed, and then in small incremental intravenous doses.

C. Intraoperative Management

C.1. *What monitoring procedures would you use for this operation on this patient?*

In addition to blood pressure, finger perfusion, and ECG monitoring, I would use a precordial Doppler bubble detector, and would also weigh the merits of a right atrial catheter and an arterial catheter. I would also use a continuous end-expiratory CO_2 monitor, if available. Surgery in the sitting position invites air embolism if venous channels are opened in areas of negative venous pressure. Since the normal right atrial pressure is 8 to 10 cm of water there will be positive pressure in veins that are not more than this height above the heart. By adjustment of the tilt of the operating table, it is often possible to lessen the height differential between head and heart. This can also be done by avoiding too erect a sitting position when setting up the case. Venous pressure in the neck and head can also be increased by blood volume augmentation, and by the use of positive end-expiratory pressure (PEEP). The clinical aphorism for judging the safety and adequacy of the system is idiot-simple. Look at the veins in the surgical field. If blood is coming out, then air can't be going in.

To prevent sudden generation of negative pressure within the veins, it is better to have the patient on controlled rather than spontaneous ventilation.

Spinal Cord Tumor · 211

C.2. How can you detect air embolism? What is the treatment?

Should air unexpectedly enter the veins, its presence will be immediately audible on the precordial Doppler monitor. If the amount of air is sufficient to interfere with the pumping action of the heart, there will be a fall in the expired CO_2 and a decrease in the cardiac output, as measured by the arterial line or the finger pulse monitor. An attempt can be made to remove the air through the previously placed right atrial catheter, or the table may be rapidly lowered to the head-down position to force the bubbles from the heart out through the superior vena cava and retrograde up the neck veins to exit at the surgical site. Repositioning of the patient on the table is theoretically desirable, but is not practical in neurosurgical work because of the complexities of fixation and positioning, which would take too long to dismantle to be of practical benefit. My personal preference for the finger pulse monitor is based on many years of experience. It is simple, safe, non-invasive, and is the first portion of the circulatory system to shut down in the event of trouble. I have never had damage to the brain or myocardium from inadequate perfusion as long as the finger pulse monitor showed adequate perfusion. From this long experience comes another aphorism: if you are perfusing the finger, then you are perfusing the heart, brain, and other vital organs. Either I am correct in this assumption, or else I have been a lucky fool for a long time.

Aidinis SJ, Lafferty J, Shapiro HM: Intracranial responses to PEEP. Anesthesiology 45:275, 1976

C.3. How would you induce anesthesia and intubate the patient?

Induction of anesthesia may be done using a thiobarbiturate–succinylcholine sequence. If there is question of cervical spine instability, particular care should be taken with positioning the head for endotracheal intubation, and afterwards, until the head is securely fixed in a Mayfield head holder or other suitable device.

C.4. How would you maintain anesthesia?

Maintenance of anesthesia may be accomplished with inhalation agents such as enflurane or isoflurane, or with nitrous oxide–oxygen, narcotic, and muscle relaxant. Ventilation is preferably controlled, for reasons mentioned above. Fluid and blood administration should be sufficient to compensate for the head-up tilt and the Valsalva effect of the ventilator.

C.5. In a patient with a spinal cord lesion above T 7, what important cause of sudden hypertension must be considered during surgery below the level of the spinal cord lesion?

Autonomic hyperreflexia must be an important consideration in the differential diagnosis of hypertension in a patient with a spinal cord lesion above T 7 during surgery below the level of the lesion. Although numerous methods of treatment have been advocated, general or spinal anesthesia is usually quite effective in blocking the hypertensive response to surgical stimulation.

Lambert DH, Deane RS, Mazuzan JE Jr: Anesthesia and the control of blood pressure in patients with spinal cord injury. Anesth Analg (Cleve) 61:344–348, 1982

C.6. What intraoperative complications may be reasonably expected from surgery near the upper part of the cervical spinal cord?

The cervical spinal cord contains the motor neurons for the diaphragm at C 3–4–5. In addition, there are numerous autonomic pathways. It is reasonable to expect changes in respiration, blood pressure, and heart rate. One should be prepared to assist or control respiration, and support blood pressure and heart rate in the event of hypotension or bradycardia.

Hunter AR: Neurosurgical Anesthesia, 2nd ed, pp 309–323. New York, Oxford University Press, 1975

D. Postoperative Management

D.1. What is the principal postoperative complication peculiar to this type of surgery? How do you manage it?

Edema of the cervical spinal cord near the operative area may develop insidiously during the early postoperative period. If the patient has been extubated and is breathing spontaneously, a gradual development of respiratory insufficiency may develop as edema spreads upward along the spinal cord to involve the respiratory centers. This condition may develop without initial significant impairment of consciousness. In addition, there may be impairment of function of the ninth and tenth cranial nerves, so that the patient has difficulty coughing, and swallowing his salivary secretions.

For the above reasons, it is important to monitor brain stem function in terms of respiration and ability to cough and swallow. Should these brain stem functions become impaired, as evidenced clinically or by serial arterial blood gas determinations, consider reintubating or performing a tracheotomy until the period of postoperative edema has passed, which is usually 48 to 72 hours. Other useful measures to lessen edema during this period include steroids and hypertonic solutions such as mannitol.

McComish PB, Bodley PO: Anaesthesia for Neurological Surgery. Chicago, Year Book Medical Publishers, 1971

17 Reflex Sympathetic Dystrophy

Vinod Malhotra

A 35-year-old man complained of diffuse burning pain in the left arm for the last 6 months following blunt trauma. His left hand feels colder than the right and occasionaly the fingertips turn blue.

A. Medical Disease and Differential Diagnosis

1. What is the most likely diagnosis in this man?
2. What is reflex sympathetic dystrophy?
3. How does causalgia differ from neuralgia?

B. Treatment

1. How would you treat this patient?
2. What is the sympathetic nerve supply to the arm?
3. Where is the stellate ganglion located? What are its important anatomical relationships?
4. What are the anatomical landmarks used in the stellate ganglion block?
5. What are the clinical signs of stellate ganglion block?
6. What is Horner's syndrome?
7. Following stellate ganglion block, this patient reports no significant change in pain in the arm despite a Horner's syndrome. Is the pain psychogenic in this patient?
8. What type of nerve fibers are interrupted in a stellate ganglion block?
9. What are the two major classes of local anesthetics? Describe the major differences in their clinical pharmacology.
10. Describe some of the physiochemical properties of significance of commonly available local anesthetics.
11. How does pH affect the action of local anesthetics?

12. How does the addition of epinephrine to commercially available premixed solutions affect the efficacy of local anesthetics?
13. Does increased concentration of the local anesthetic speed the induction of a block?
14. What are the effects of local anesthetic mixtures in clinical practice?

C. Complications

1. What are the possible complications of stellate ganglion block?
2. What is the systemic toxicity of local anesthetics?
3. How do you treat the systemic toxicity of local anesthetic drugs?

A. Medical Disease and Differential Diagnosis

A.1. What is the most likely diagnosis in this man?

The most likely diagnosis in this man is posttraumatic reflex sympathetic dystrophy.

A.2. What is reflex sympathetic dystrophy?

Reflex sympathetic dystrophy is a syndrome characterized by diffuse burning pain, vasomotor and sudomotor changes, and hyperalgesia or hyperesthesia. It is usually aggravated by cold and emotional factors and follows trauma. It may progress to limb edema, muscular dysfunction and atrophy, and osteoporotic changes in the bones. Causalgia is one of the clinical entities included in this group of diseases and strictly the term should be used for the sympathetic dystrophy following blunt injury to a nerve trunk.

Cousins MJ, Bridenbaugh PO: Neural Blockade in Clinical Anesthesia and Management of Pain, p 574. Philadelphia, JB Lippincott, 1980

A.3. How does causalgia differ from neuralgia?

The major differences are indicated in Table 17-1.

Cousins MJ, Bridenbaugh PO: Neural Blockade in Clinical Anesthesia and Management of Pain, p 717. Philadelphia, JB Lippincott, 1980

Table 17-1. The differences of causalgia and neuralgia

	CAUSALGIA	NEURALGIA
Time	Pain sustained	Usually paroxysmal
Distribution	Diffuse	Follows nerve distribution
Character	Burning	Sharp, shooting
Associated findings	Vasomotor changes	Usually absent
	Sudomotor changes	Usually absent
	Trophic changes	Disuse atrophy may be seen

B. Treatment

B.1. How would you treat this patient?

We would administer a left stellate ganglion block to improve the circulation.

B.2. What is the sympathetic nerve supply to the arm?

The preganglionic sympathetic outflow to the upper extremity is derived from T 2—T 9 and these fibers synapse with postganglionic fibers in the stellate ganglion. Therefore, a stellate ganglion block interrupts sympathetic outflow to the upper extremity.

Carron H: Management of Common Pain Problems. ASA Refresher Courses in Anesthesiology 3:51–61, 1975

B.3. Where is the stellate ganglion located? What are its important anatomical relationships?

The stellate ganglion is a star shaped (hence, the name) sympathetic ganglion formed by the fusion of the inferior cervical and the first thoracic ganglia. In some instances the fusion may not occur or the shape may be different. It usually measures 2.5 cm × 1.5 cm × 0.5 cm and lies between the base of the transverse process of the seventh cervical vertebra and the neck of the first rib. It is situated behind the carotid sheath, ventral to the longus colli muscle, behind the vertebral artery and lateral to the body of the vertebra. The subclavian, the inferior thyroid and the first intercostal arteries are in close proximiity to the ganglion and so is the recurrent laryngeal nerve. The left pleura is 1 cm to 2 cm below it, whereas the right pleura is closely situated. The efferent nerves from the stellate ganglion supply the sympathetics to the head, neck, and upper extremity.

Moore DC: Regional Block, p 123. Springfield, IL, Charles C Thomas, 1978

B.4. What are the anatomical landmarks used in the stellate ganglion block?

The landmarks used in the stellate ganglion block are the jugular notch of the sternum, the sternocleidomastoid muscle, the cricoid cartilage, and Chassaignac's tubercle. In a supine patient with neck extended, a mark placed approximately 3.5 cm from the midline along the jugular notch, and the same distance above the clavicle, should overlie the transverse process of the seventh vertebra and along the medial border of the sternocleidomastoid muscle. This marking is further confirmed by palpating the cricoid cartilage, which lies at the level of the sixth cervical vertebra, and the anterior tubercle on the sixth vertebral transverse process, which is the most prominent tubercle in the neck (Chasssaignac's tubercle).

Moore DC: Regional Block, p 127. Springfield, IL, Charles C Thomas, 1978

B.5. What are the clinical signs of stellate ganglion block?

The clinical signs of a successful stellate ganglion block include the following on the ipsilateral side.

- Eye: ptosis, narrowing of palpebral fissure, miosis, enophthalmos, conjunctival injection, lacrimation
- Face and neck: anhydrosis, elevated local temperature, nasal stuffiness
- Arm: increased temperature, plethysmographic evidence of improved cutaneous blood flow

Moore DC: Regional Block, p 131. Springfield, IL, Charles C Thomas, 1978

B.6. What is Horner's syndrome?

Horner's syndrome is a clinical entity characterized by the triad of ptosis, miosis, and anhydrosis. Usually seen in association with a disease process involving the cervical sympathetics, it is a classical sign of stellate ganglion block.

Moore DC: Regional Block, p 131. Springfield, IL, Charles C Thomas, 1978

B.7. Following stellate ganglion block, this patient reports no significant change in pain in the arm despite a Horner's syndrome. Is the pain psychogenic in this patient?

Not necessarily. The Horner's syndrome indicates only the interruption of sympathetic supply to the head and neck. Unless it is accompanied by objective changes in the arm, it does not indicate sympathetic nerve block of the upper extremity.

Moore DC: Regional Block, p 131. Springfield, IL, Charles C Thomas, 1978

B.8. What type of nerve fibers are interrupted in a stellate ganglion block?

The stellate ganglion block results in interruption of the preganglionic, thinly myelinated, type B fibers, as well as the postganglionic, unmyelinated, type C fibers.

Cousins MJ, Bridenbaugh PO: Neural Blockade in Clinical Anesthesia and Management of Pain, p 122. Philadelphia, JB Lippincott, 1980

B.9. What are the two major classes of local anesthetics? Describe the major differences in their clinical pharmacology.

The two major categories of clinically employed local anesthetics are esters and amides. The esters are hydrolyzed in the plasma by pseudocholinesterase; the amides are biotransformed in the liver. Although infrequent, local anesthetic toxicity is encountered more commonly in the ester group because of the para-aminobenzoic acid moiety. True allergic reactions to amides are rare. In most instances, they are due to preservatives in the solution. In each of the two groups of local anesthetics there are drugs

B.10. Describe some of the physiochemical properties of significance of commonly available local anesthetics.

Ionization and protein binding are the two physiochemical properties of local anesthetics that are of most clinical significance. The commonly used local anesthetics are weakly basic tertiary amines that are lipid soluble and unstable in water. They are dispensed as acidic salts, since the ionized form is soluble in water and stable. Therefore, the aqueous solution contains the ionized (cation) form of the local anesthetic in dissociation equilibrium with the unionized (free base) form depending on the pH of the medium.

$$R \equiv NH^+ \rightleftharpoons R \equiv N + H^+$$
$$\text{Cation} \quad \text{Base}$$

The degree of ionization is determined by the pH of the solution and the pKa of the local anesthetic.

$$pKa = pH - \log \frac{\text{nonionized base}}{\text{cation}}$$

The pKa of most local anesthetics is greater than 7.4 (see Table 17–2). The free base, being lipid soluble, is important for diffusion of the anesthetic across membranes, whereas the cationic form is mainly responsible for neural blockade, owing to its binding to the neural membrane. Protein binding of the drug will affect its local binding and diffusion as well as systemic elimination. With the exception of procaine and chloroprocaine, the commonly employed local anesthetics are highly protein bound (see Table 17–2).

Cousins MJ, Bridenbaugh PO: Neural Blockade in Clinical Anesthesia and Management of Pain, pp 45–51. Philadelphia, JB Lippincott, 1980

Table 17-2. Physiochemical properties of commonly used local anesthetics

LOCAL ANESTHETIC	pKa	PROTEIN BINDING (%)
Esters		
Procaine	8.9	5.8%
Chloroprocaine	8.7	—
Tetracaine	8.5	75.6
Amides		
Lidocaine	7.9	64.3
Mepivacaine	7.6	77.5
Bupivacaine	8.1	95.6
Etidocaine	7.7	94

B.11. How does pH affect the action of local anesthetics?

$$R \equiv NH^+ \rightleftharpoons R \equiv N + H^+$$
$$\text{Cation} \qquad \text{Base}$$

The degree of ionization of a local anesthetic is dependent on the pH of the solution. As the pH is lowered, more of the drug is ionized to the cationic form, which is poorly diffusible across the nerve membranes, thereby reducing the efficacy of the block. This is seen clinically when local anesthetics are injected into an infected region where the tissue pH is low. The concentration of local anesthetic base determines the quantity of local anesthetic which reaches the nerve membrane. The relative proportion of base is increased by raising the pH of the solution; alkalinizing a local anesthetic solution enhances drug penetration.

De Jong RH: Fundamentals of local anesthesia: Applied physiology. ASA Refresher Courses in Anesthesiology 2:49–64, 1974

B.12. How does the addition of epinephrine to commercially available premixed solutions affect the efficacy of local anesthetics?

The addition of epinephrine to a local anesthetic increases the duration and intensity of a block. However, in commercially available premixed solutions containing epinephrine, antioxidants are added to preserve epinephrine and the result is a lowered buffered pH of the solution. This lowering of pH can result in decreased efficacy of the local anesthetic. Best results are achieved by adding the desired concentration of epinephrine to the local anesthetic solution just prior to injection.

De Jong RH: Fundamentals of local anesthesia: Applied physiology. ASA Refresher Courses in Anesthesiology 2:49–64, 1974

Moore, DC: The pH of local anesthetic solutions: Technical communication. Anesth Analg (Cleve) 60, No. 11:833–834, 1981

B.13. Does increased concentration of the local anesthetic speed the induction of a block?

The rate of onset of local anesthesia bears a linear relationship with the logarithm of the dose. Therefore, an increase in concentration produces only a modest decrease in time of onset.

Cousins MJ, Bridenbaugh PO: Neural Blockade in Clinical Anesthesia and Management of Pain, pp 54–55. Philadelphia, JB Lippincott, 1980

De Jong RH: Fundamentals of local anesthesia: Applied physiology. ASA Refresher Courses in Anesthesiology 2:49–64, 1974

B.14. What are the effects of local anesthetic mixtures in clinical practice?

A combination of two local anesthetics may be used to try to achieve a decrease in time of onset and latency along with an increase in duration of the block. Depending on the site of the block, this may not be achieved each time.

The toxic effects of the two agents are essentially additive. It has also been shown that peak blood levels of two different agents, used concomitantly in a mixture, may occur at different intervals. The amide local anesthetics can inhibit the rate of hydrolysis of chloroprocaine. Occasionaly unsatisfactory anesthesia produced by chloroprocaine and bupivacaine has been attributed to the low pH of chloroprocaine (3.7) increasing the ionized fraction of bupivacaine.

Cohen SE: The Rational Use of Local Anesthetic Mixtures. Regional Anesthesia, 4, No. 3:11–12, 1979

Munson ES, Paul WL, Embro WJ: Central nervous system toxicity of local anesthetic mixtures in monkeys. ASA Refresher Course in Anesthesiology, pp 53–54, 1976

Raj PP, Rosenblatt R, Miller J: Dynamics of local anesthetic compounds in regional anesthesia. Anesth Analg (Cleve) 56:110–117, 1977

C. Complications

C.1. What are the possible complications of stellate ganglion block?

Although complications appear infrequently, the more common complications of this block are as follows:

- Intraarterial injection—toxic reaction, hematoma
- Recurrent laryngeal nerve paralysis—hoarseness of voice
- Brachial plexus block—motor weakness
- Pneumothorax—respiratory distress

A rare complication that may occur is an accidental subarachnoid injection.

Cousins MJ, Bridenbaugh PO: Neural Blockade in Clinical Anesthesia and Management of Pain, p 539. Philadelphia, JB Lippincott, 1980

Moore DC: Regional Block, pp 131–134. Springfield, IL, Charles C Thomas, 1978

C.2. What is the systemic toxicity of local anesthetics?

The systemic toxic effects of local anesthetics are related to their blood levels and are manifested mainly in the central nervous system and the cardiovascular system. As a rule, the central nervous system effects precede the cardiovascular system toxic manifestations.

Central Nervous System Effects

Light-headedness, dizziness, tinnitus, visual disturbances, drowsiness, disorientation, slurred speech, twitching of muscles, generalized grand mal seizure, EEG changes. Blood levels of local anesthetics associated with CNS changes in man are as follows:

- Procaine 20 mg/ml
- Lidocaine, mepivacaine, prilocaine, 5 to 10 mg/ml
- Tetracaine, bupivacaine, etidocaine, 1.5 to 4 mg/ml

Table 17-3. Cardiovascular effects of lidocaine

BLOOD LEVEL µg/ml LIDOCAINE	ECG CHANGES	HEMODYNAMIC EFFECTS
<5	—	—
5–10	↑ P–R interval ↑ QRS duration Sinus bradycardia	↓ Myocardial contraction ↓ Cardiac output Vasodilatation
> 10	↑ P–R interval ↑ QRS duration Sinus bradycardia A–V block Asystole	↓ Myocardial contractility ↓ Cardiac output Circulatory collapse

- Lowering the $PaCO_2$ by hyperventilation increases the convulsive threshhold dose of a local anesthetic drug

Cardiovascular Effects
See Table 17–3

Covino BG: Pharmacology and physiology of local anesthetics. ASA Refresher Courses in Anesthesiology 5:33–46, 1977

C.3. How do you treat the systemic toxicity of local anesthetic drugs?

The principles of treatment include the following:
- Secure and maintain airway
- Ensure adequate oxygenation and ventilation
- Control seizures with the following:
- Diazepam 0.1 to 0.2 mg/kg, intravenously
- Thiopental sodium 1 to 2 mg/kg, intravenously
- Circulatory support

Covino BG: Pharmacology and physiology of local anesthetics. ASA Refresher Courses in Anesthesiology 5:33–46, 1977

Section Five
The Endocrine System

18 Thyrotoxicosis
Joseph F. Artusio, Jr.

A 23-year-old Caucasian woman had a diffuse swelling in her neck. Her present history indicated weight loss, frequent palpitations, and an increase in sweating. She was hyperexcitable, with fine tremor seen in outstretched hands. BP 160/100; HR 120; HcT 30.

A. Medical Disease and Differential Diagnosis

1. What differential diagnosis is compatible with these symptoms?
2. What are the specific thyroid hormones and their precursors? What is their function?
3. How does the pituitary gland affect thyroid function?
4. What are the signs and symptoms of Graves' disease?
5. Discuss the possible mechanism underlying this disease.
6. What effect does this disease have on the heart?
7. Define the mechanism of heat intolerance seen with hyperthyroidism.
8. Is insomnia a prominent symptom? What is the mechanism?

B. Preoperative Evaluation and Preparation

1. What available means may we use to control this disease? What is their mechanism of action?
2. How do the alpha and beta adrenergic antagonists help control the symptoms of hyperthyroidism?
3. When is the patient with hyperthyroidism ready for surgery?
4. Outline your regimen for premedication in the euthyroid patient.
5. Is there any value in "stealing" the antithyroid resistant patient on the morning of surgery?

C. Intraoperative Management

1. What monitoring guidelines should be used prior to the administration of anesthesia?
2. What anesthetic technique would you choose?
3. Is endotracheal intubation necessary for this operation? Discuss the type and length of tube you would use.
4. What intraoperative monitors are essential for safe anesthetic management?

D. Postoperative Management

1. What are the possible causes of airway obstruction following surgery?
2. What is meant by the terms thyroid storm or thyrotoxic crisis? Outline the causes, means of diagnosis, and treatment.
3. How does thyroidectomy affect the level of plasma calcium?
4. What is tetany and how is it diagnosed? How is it treated?
5. What is Chvostek's sign? What is Trousseau's sign?

A. Medical Disease and Differential Diagnosis

A.1. What differential diagnosis is compatible with these symptoms?

Although similar symptoms may be prominent in anxiety states and in low grade chronic infections, these signs and symptoms are classical for thyrotoxicosis (Graves' disease).

Hyperthyroidism is occasionally confused with such disorders as metastatic carcinoma, cirrhosis of the liver, hyperparathyroidism, sprue, and neuromyopathies such as myasthenia gravis and muscular dystrophy. Hypokalemic periodic paralyis is more common in thyrotoxic patients, especially in the case of oriental males. Patients with pheochromocytoma may present with signs of heat intolerance, such as perspiration, tachycardia with palpitations, and a hypermetabolic state. A symmetric, diffuse goiter excludes the diagnosis of toxic multinodular goiter or toxic adenoma, both of which produce a hypermetabolic state. Very rarely, however, is thyrotoxicosis produced by thyroid-stimulating hormone (TSH) secreting tumors of the pituitary or by tumors of trophoblastic origin.

Isselbacher KJ et al: Harrison's Principles of Internal Medicine, 9th ed, p 1705. New York, McGraw–Hill, 1980

A.2. What are the specific thyroid hormones and their precursors? What is their function?

The normal function of the thyroid gland is to secrete thyroxine (T_4) and triiodothyronine (T_3), iodinated amino acids that are the active thyroid hormones. In excess, they adversely influence the metabolic processes.

For thyroid hormone synthesis to be qualitatively and quantitatively normal, there must be sufficient amounts of iodine entering into the thyroid and a concurrent synthesis of the normal receptor protein for iodine, thyroglobulin. The iodine comes from dietary intake or from deiodination of thyroid hormones, and is removed from plasma by the thyroid, the kidneys, and the salivary and gastrointestinal glands. However, net clearance is affected only by the thyroid and kidneys. Adjustments in the rate of entry of iodide into the thyroid relative to the rate of urinary excretion are mediated by changes in thyroid, rather than renal, activity.

Four steps can be delineated in the synthesis and secretion of active thyroid hormones. First, there is active inward transport of iodide into the thyroid cell. The second step in hormonal biosynthesis involves the oxidation of iodide to a higher valence form that is capable of iodinating tyrosyl residues in thyroglobulin. This high molecular glycoprotein is synthesized within the follicular epithelium. Subsequently, the iodotyrosines undergo oxidative condensation through the mediation of peroxidase, a "coupling reaction", and yield a variety of iodothyronines, including T_4 and T_3. Liberation of the active hormones into the blood, forming the third step in hormone synthesis and release, involves pinocytosis of follicular colloid at the apical margin of the cells to form colloid droplets. These fuse with thyroid lysosomes to form "phagolysosomes." The final step is the release of the now free iodothyronines, T_4 and T_3, into the blood. The reactions outlined are subject to inhibition by agents called goitrogens; due to their ability to inhibit hormone synthesis and indirectly stimulate TSH secretion, they induce goiter formation.

In the blood, T_4 and T_3 are almost entirely bound to plasma proteins. The proportion of free T_3 is normally 8 to 10 times greater than T_4. As a result, T_3 is removed from the blood much more rapidly than T_4. This accounts for its failure to contribute materially to the total hormonal iodine concentration in the blood and possibly for its more rapid onset and cessation of action. These hormones are important regulators of metabolic activity.

Isselbacher KJ et al: Harrison's Principles of Internal Medicine, 9th ed, pp 1695–1696. New York, McGraw–Hill, 1980

A.3. How does the pituitary gland affect thyroid function?

The thyroid function is affected by two general mechanisms, one suprathyroidal and the other intrathyroidal. The proximate mediator of suprathyroidal regulation is thyrotropin or thyroid-stimulating hormone (TSH), secreted by basophilic cells within the anterior pituitary. TSH stimulates thyroid hypertrophy and hyperplasia and accelerates most aspects of glandular intermediary metabolism. It enhances the synthesis of nucleic acid and protein, including thyroglobulin, and stimulates all steps in thyroid iodine metabolism leading to the synthesis and secretion of thyroid hormones. These actions are thought to be mediated, at least in part, by increased synthesis of the "second messenger", cyclic 31-51-adenosine monophosphate. Regulation of TSH secretion, in turn, is affected by two opposing influences. Thyrotropin-releasing hormone (TRH), a tripeptide amide, is secreted in the ventromedial hypothalamus. It reaches the pituitary gland by the hypophyseal portal capillary system, where it stimulates synthesis and secretion of TSH. These effects of TRH are inhibited by the extent of thyroid hormone action within the pituitary, and this is closely related to the concentration of free thyroid hormones in the blood. Therefore, negative feedback of thyroid hormones on TSH secretion occurs mainly in the pituitary gland itself.

Intrathyroid regulation of thyroid function is not as well understood. Changes in glandular organic iodine content are associated with reciprocal changes in thyroidal iodide transport activity, as well as in growth, glucose metabolism, and nucleic acid synthesis.

Isselbacher KJ et al: Harrison's Principles of Internal Medicine, 9th ed, p 1698. New York, McGraw–Hill, 1980

A.4. *What are the signs and symptoms of Graves' disease?*

Common manifestations of hyperthyroidism in Graves' disease include goiter, fine tremor of the extended fingers and tongue, increased nervousness, emotional instability, excessive sweating and heat intolerance, palpitations, hyperkinesis, and loss of weight, often despite increased appetite. Weakness is often manifested; anorexia and vomiting may occur. In people over 40 years of age, dyspnea, atrial arrhythmias, and cardiac failure occur frequently. In younger individuals, nervous symptoms dominate the clinical picture, whereas cardiovascular and myopathic symptoms predominate in older people.

The skin is warm and moist, the hair is fine and silky. Excess melanin pigmentation is not uncommon. Ocular signs include a stare with widened palpebral fissures, lid lag, lid retraction, infrequent blinking, and failure of convergence.

Cardiovascular findings include a wide pulse pressure, sinus tachycardia, atrial arrhythmias, systolic murmurs, increased intensity of the apical first sound, cardiac enlargement, and, at times, overt cardiac failure. The dermopathy of Graves' disease usually occurs on the dorsum of the legs or feet and is commonly termed localized myxedema or pretibial myxedema. About half the cases occur during the active stage of thyrotoxicosis. In the remainder, the lesions develop after treatment. The area is well demarcated from normal skin. It is raised and thickened, and may be pruritic and hyperpigmented.

Isselbacher KJ et al: Harrison's Principles of Internal Medicine, 9th ed, p 1704. New York, McGraw–Hill, 1980

A.5. Discuss the possible mechanism underlying this disease.

Graves' disease, also known as Basedow's disease, is a disorder of unknown etiology with a characteristic triad: hyperthyroidism with diffuse goiter, ophthalmopathy, and dermopathy. Although hyperthyroidism is the most common manifestation of Graves' disease, this symptom complex merely reflects the excess supply of thyroid hormone to the tissues. With respect to hyperthyroidism, it is apparent that central to this disorder is a disruption of homeostatic mechanisms that normally adjust hormone secretion to meet the needs of peripheral tissues.

Recently, there has been interest in the etiological role of a protein known as the long-acting thyroid stimulator (LATS). This protein stimulates hormonal release, increases thyroidal ^{131}I uptake, and stimulates several aspects of thyroid intermediary metabolism. It increases the activity of thyroid adenyl cyclase, and is capable of inducing thyroid hyperplasia. LATS is an immunoglobulin G and can be synthesized by the lymphocytes of patients with Graves' disease. It appears to be an antibody to some cytologic component of human thyroid. Thus, Graves' disease may be associated with an autoimmune phenomena. Despite its capacity to reproduce in the thyroid of animals many of the features of diffuse toxic goiter, titers of LATS in patients' sera do not correlate well with the presence or absence of thyrotoxicosis or its degree of severity. Some authorities believe that LATS is an epiphenomenon, and that Graves' disease is caused by cell-mediated immunity. Very little is known of the cause of the progressive infiltrative ophthalmopathy, but it may be related to another immunoglobulin. Nothing is known of the etiology of the dermopathy of Graves' disease.

Isselbacher KJ et al: Harrison's Principles of Internal Medicine, 9th ed, pp 1703–1704. New York, McGraw–Hill, 1980

A.6. What effect does this disease have on the heart?

Thyrotoxicosis imposes a burden on the heart. Hypermetabolism of the peripheral tissues increases both the metabolic and the nonmetabolic circulatory load. Direct effects of thyroid hormone on the myocardium increase the force, velocity, and rate of ventricular contraction. As a result, cardiac work and cardiac output are increased. The patient with a normal heart usually withstands this burden. However, in the patient with underlying heart disease, cardiac insufficiency may be precipitated or aggravated. This complication is more frequent in the elderly.

Patients with cardiac insufficiency related to thyrotoxicosis may have atrial fibrillation, a relatively rapid circulation time, increased cardiac output, and resistance to the usual therapeutic doses of digitalis. If cardiac decompensation occurs, treatment is carried out in the usual manner, employing larger than usual doses of digitalis. Great care must be used to avoid digitalis intoxication as the thyrotoxicosis is alleviated. Adrenergic antagonists should not be employed in the presence of cardiac failure.

Isselbacher KJ et al: Harrison's Principles of Internal Medicine, 9th ed, pp 1708–1709. New York, McGraw–Hill, 1980

A.7. Define the mechanism of heat intolerance seen with hyperthyroidism.

Due to the hypermetabolic state and increased calorigenesis, the body is using all its avenues of heat loss—conduction, radiation, and evaporation. The individual feels very uncomfortable when the environmental temperature is high, as evaporation is significantly diminished and this negates one important mechanism of heat loss.

Schwartz S: Principles of Surgery, 3rd ed, p 1554. New York, McGraw–Hill, 1979

A.8. Is insomnia a prominent symptom? What is the mechanism?

These patients are excitable, restless, hyperkinetic, and emotionally unstable. Insomnia is a prominent symptom and is due to the hyperexcitable, hypermetabolic state.

Schwartz S: Principles of Surgery, 3rd ed, p 1554. New York, McGraw–Hill, 1979

B. Preoperative Evaluation and Preparation

B.1. What available means may we use to control this disease? What is their mechanism of action?

There are two major approaches to the treatment of hyperthyroidism. Both are directed to limiting the quantity of thyroid hormones the thyroid gland can produce. The first method involves using antithyroid agents to interpose a chemical blockage, interfering with the organic binding of thyroidal iodine. The second approach is ablation of thyroid tissue, thus limiting hormone production. This is done surgically or by means of radioactive iodine. These procedures induce permanent anatomic alterations of the thyroid gland and therefore control the active phase of hyperthyroidism. Usually there is no recurrence of thyrotoxicity. However, ablation techniques may ultimately result in hypothyroidism.

Those patients managed with antithyroid drugs are frequently controlled successfully by propylthiouracil, 100 mg every 8 hours. Methimazole is at least as effective as propylthiouracil when administered in one-tenth the dose. Once the euthyroid state has been achieved, daily dosages must be reduced to prevent hypothyroidism. Usually, a 12 to 24 month course is employed and it is expected that the patient will remain in remission. Iodides are used mainly in patients with actual or impending thyrotoxic crisis or in patients with severe thyrocardiac disease. Iodides may prolong greatly the response to subsequently instituted antithyroid therapy. Therefore, iodides should be used in conjunction with other therapeutic measures. Since iodides appear to synergize with radiation in the thyroid, they are useful in controlling thyrotoxicosis following ^{131}I administration during the period in which the therapeutic effect of radioiodine has not taken place.

Isselbacher KJ: Harrison's Principles of Internal Medicine, 9th ed, pp 1705–1706. New York, McGraw–Hill, 1980

B.2. How do the alpha and beta adrenergic antagonists help control the symptoms of hyperthyroidism?

To control the adrenergic component in thyrotoxicosis, various adrenergic antagonists have been employed. The beta antagonist, propranolol, appears to be the agent of choice because it is relatively free from side effects. In doses of 40 to 120 mg daily, propranolol alleviates sweating, tremor, and tachycardia. Propranolol should be used only as an adjuvant to therapy rather than the sole therapy because the underlying metabolic abnormalities are essentially unaffected. Propranolol is contraindicated in patients with coexisting heart failure or asthma. There appears to be no therapeutic advantage to the use of alpha antagonists.

Isselbacher KJ: Harrison's Principles of Internal Medicine, 9th ed, p 1706. New York, McGraw–Hill, 1980

B.3. When is the patient with hyperthyroidism ready for surgery?

Of primary importance in the preoperative evaluation of the treated thyrotoxic patient is a history of relief of symptoms, with progressive weight gain, on near normal caloric intake. Emphasis should be on return of pulse rate to normal levels. The sleeping pulse should be below 90 beats/min. Tremor should be relieved and iodine uptake returned toward normal. The following subjective and objective findings are of importance: loss of nervousness; no requirements for sedation to sleep; normal work tolerance; no palpitations, dyspnea, or unusual fatigue on exertion; no heat intolerance; a normal pulse pressure, normal sinus rhythm, disappearance of cardiac murmurs, and decrease or disappearance of hyperreflexia.

Katz J, Benumof J, Kadis LB: Anesthesia and Uncommon Diseases, 2nd ed, pp 170–173. Philadelphia, WB Saunders, 1981

B.4. Outline your regimen for premedication in the euthyroid patient.

Although antithyroid drugs control the hyperthyroid state, those who suffer from hyperthyroidism are more excitable patients than the average patient; therefore, they require more sedation. Medication should be individualized; however, in general, we prefer to give approximately 3.5 to 4 mg/kg of pentobarbital sodium and 0.4 mg of atropine.

Katz J, Benumof J, Kadis LB: Anesthesia and Uncommon Diseases, 2nd ed, p 175. Philadelphia, WB Saunders, 1981

B.5. Is there any value in "stealing" the antithyroid resistant patient on the morning of surgery?

We believe "stealing" is the best way to begin anesthesia for these patients. Three days prior to the scheduled surgery, at approximately the same time surgery will begin, the patient receives IV fluids (*e.g.* 500 cc 5% dextrose in water). This maneuver is repeated on day two and again on day one prior to surgery. On the morning of surgery, without the patient's knowledge, a 0.4% thiopental solution replaces the 5% dextrose in water. The pentothal drip is started and takes effect very promptly and smoothly. Under this light hypnosis, the patient is moved to the operating theatre. A means of increasing the inspired oxygen concentration and producing artificial ventilation accompanies the patient to the operating room.

This technique prevents the sudden increase in sympathetic activity associated with bringing the awake patient to the operating room, and prevents the hypertension and tachycardia resulting from apprehension and anxiety.

This technique is used at the New York Hospital for patients who are resistant to antithyroid drugs.

C. Intraoperative Management

C.1. What monitoring guidelines should be used prior to the administration of anesthesia?

When a patient who is believed to be reasonably controlled with antithyroid drugs is brought to the operating room following suitable barbiturate premedication, the following guidelines should be used prior to a decision to begin the anesthesia. The blood pressure should be taken, the pulse rate counted, and the electrocardiogram evaluated on the operating room cardiac monitor. If the systolic blood pressure is above 140 torr and the heart rate above 100 beats a minute, more antithyroid therapy is in order. The surgery should probably be cancelled and the patient returned to the floor for further evaluation and treatment and returned for surgery at a later time. If the tachycardia is associated with cardiac irregularities, postponement of surgery is mandatory.

(Procedures used at New York Hospital prior to induction of anesthesia.)

C.2. What anesthetic technique would you choose?

We prefer an intravenous barbiturate induction followed by an inhalation technique. Nitrous oxide and oxygen supported with enflurane appears to be the technique that affords the greatest control of blood pressure and heart rate.

A short acting muscle relaxant such as succinylcholine, in an appropriate dose according to weight, may be used to aid in intubating the patient. During the operative procedure, a small dose of nondepolarizing relaxant helps to soften the patient's muscle tone; thus, less anesthesia is needed to maintain the anesthetic state. Topical anesthesia to the larynx and trachea prior to intubation is valuable to prevent the patient from reacting on the endotracheal tube during the early establishment of adequate depth of anesthesia for thyroidectomy. In spite of the fact that the local anesthesia wears off in a relatively short period of time, reflex activity of the upper airway appears to be obtunded for the duration of surgery unless the endotracheal tube is violently disturbed.

Miller RD: Anesthesia, 1st ed, pp 236, 241. New York, Churchill–Livingstone, 1981

C.3. Is endotracheal intubation necessary for this operation? Discuss the type and length of tube you would use.

Endotracheal intubation is an absolute necessity in thyroid surgery. The tube should be one that is difficult to kink or distort by surgical manipulation, and the tip of the tube should be below the thyroid gland itself, but above the carina. In this position, in spite of significant tracheal manipulation, the tube will not be occluded and endobronchial intubation will be avoided.

Katz J, Benumof J, Kadis LB: Anesthesia and Uncommon Diseases, 2nd ed, p 177. Philadelphia, WB Saunders, 1981

C.4. What intraoperative monitors are essential for safe anesthetic management?

Blood pressure, pulse rate, ECG, and body temperature monitoring are all necessary for this procedure. In the older patient, where there has been a history of cardiac damage, a central venous pressure catheter or a Swan–Ganz catheter may aid in fluid management and in differentiating pressures on both sides of the heart. Of course, the inherent value of this invasive technique must be weighed against the possible complications produced by the monitor itself.

Miller RD: Anesthesia, 1st ed, pp 159, 180, 1287. New York, Churchill–Livingstone, 1981

D. Postoperative Management

D.1. What are the possible causes of airway obstruction following surgery?

It is essential to watch for early signs of airway obstruction in the postoperative period. A common cause of airway obstruction in the early postoperative period is traction injury or the cutting of one of the recurrent laryngeal nerves. This usually produces slight stridor, but not significant airway obstruction. However, if there is bilateral recurrent laryngeal nerve damage, the patient will develop total airway occlusion following extubation. The patient must be reintubated immediately and a tracheostomy performed.

Another frequent cause of airway obstruction is postsurgical bleeding, particularly if the wound has been closed tightly without adequate drainage. However, in spite of a drain in the wound, an arterial bleeder could rapidly fill the neck and produce tracheal deviation and compression. The pressure on the airway must be relieved quickly by opening the neck wound, restoring the free airway, and then controlling the hemorrhage. Tracheal collapse is a rare entity these days. It is usually not associated with operations on the thyroid for thyrotoxicosis, but must be looked for in a situation where large nontoxic nodular thyroids have been present for long periods of time and have produced erosion of the tracheal wall, which becomes paper thin. Following removal of the gland, coughing, vomiting, or a deep inspiration can produce tracheal collapse, asphyxia, and death. Following surgery of the thyroid gland, a tracheostomy set should always be at the bedside in the immediate postoperative period, as the above complications can develop rapidly, and require immediate and definitive treatment.

Schwartz S: Principles of Surgery, 3rd ed, pp 1571–1572. New York, McGraw–Hill, 1979

Katz J, Benumof J, Kadis LB: Anesthesia and Uncommon Diseases, 2nd ed, p 177. Philadelphia, WB Saunders, 1981

D.2. What is meant by the terms thyroid storm or thyrotoxic crisis? Outline the causes, means of diagnosis, and treatment.

Thyroid storm occurs postoperatively in patients with preexisting thyrotoxicosis who have been inadequately treated prior to surgery. Currently, thyroid storm is a rare complication of surgical treatment, but must be watched for in the postoperative period in patients with thyrotoxicosis who have been resistant to antithyroid therapy. Causes of thyroid storm other than surgery are trauma, infection, diabetic acidosis, or toxemias of pregnancy.

When thyroid storm is related to surgical treatment, the manifestations may develop during the operative or postoperative period. The patient becomes markedly hyperthermic, with profuse sweating and tachycardia, nausea, vomiting, and abdominal pain. Initial tremor and restlessness may progress to delirium and coma. Treatment is directed at inhibiting the production of thyroid hormones and antagonizing the effects of the hormones. Large doses of sodium iodide, 1.0 to 2.5 g, should be administered intravenously and supplemented with 100 mg of cortisone. Increases in inspired oxygen concentration are indicated by serial blood gases. Fluid and electrolytes must be maintained, in view of fluid loss by sweating. A hypothermic blanket may be placed under the patient to control body temperature; propranolol can be given in doses to control beta sympathetic activity.

Schwartz S: Principles of Surgery, 3rd ed, p 1571. New York, McGraw–Hill, 1979

D.3. How does thyroidectomy affect the level of plasma calcium?

Although thyroidectomy itself does not affect the level of plasma calcium, inadvertent removal of the parathyroid glands produce acute hypoparathyroidism and the level of calcium falls sharply.

Katz J, Benumof J, Kadis LB: Anesthesia and Uncommon Diseases, 2nd ed, p 178. Philadelphia, WB Saunders, 1981

D.4. What is tetany and how is it diagnosed? How is it treated?

A decrease in concentration of free calcium ion in plasma (7 mg% or below) results in an increase in neuromuscular irritability and the syndrome of tetany. Evidence of inspiratory stridor will occur long before overt tetany is manifest. This syndrome is characterized, when fully expressed, by peripheral and perioral paresthesia, carpal spasm, pedal spasm, anxiety seizures, bronchospasm, laryngospasm, positive Chvostek's and Trousseau's signs, and lengthening of the QT interval of the electrocardiogram. Administer 10 to 30 ml of 10% calcium gluconate initially and follow by oral calcium therapy.

Schwartz S: Principles of Surgery, 3rd ed, p 1572. New York, McGraw–Hill, 1979

D.5. What is Chvostek's sign? What is Trousseau's sign?

Latent tetany may be elicited by tapping the facial nerve and producing a contraction of the facial muscle. This is Chvostek's sign. When a tourniquet or blood pressure cuff is applied to the arm for 3 minutes, and causes carpopedal spasm, this is Trousseau's sign.

Isselbacher KJ: Harrison's Principles of Internal Medicine, 9th ed, p 2070. New York, McGraw–Hill, 1980

19 Pheochromocytoma
Joseph F. Artusio, Jr.

This 35-year-old woman was to have an elective cholecystectomy for cholelithiasis following recovery from an episode of acute cholecystitis. The only positive finding was a mild hypertension of 140/95. Following premedication with pentobarbital sodium, 150 mg, and atropine, 0.4 mg, she was induced with thiopental sodium, 150 mg. In 30 seconds the blood pressure fell to 80/60. However, in the next 30 seconds the blood pressure was found to be 230/130 and pulse rate was regular at 160/min.

A. Medical Disease and Differential Diagnosis

1. What is an acceptable definition of hypertension?
2. How would you classify the various causes of hypertension?
3. What are the causes of the following events: hypertension and tachycardia; hypertension and bradycardia?
4. Trace the embryology of the adrenal gland and describe its normal anatomy.
5. Enumerate the secretions of the cortex and of the medulla of the adrenal gland, respectively.
6. What are the precursors, the synthesis, and biotransformation of epinephrine, norepinephrine, and dopamine?
7. What are the metabolic actions of the glucocorticoids and the mineral corticoids?
8. What are the usual and unusual sites for the development of pheochromocytoma? What is the cellular makeup of these tumors?
9. What symptoms herald this type of tumor? How may the diagnosis be made?

B. Preoperative Evaluation and Preparation

1. Outline an acceptable preparation for these patients prior to anesthesia and surgery.
2. How would you manage the drugs for premedication?

C. Intraoperative Management

1. How would you induce this patient?
2. During the surgical procedure, what parameters would you monitor?
3. Outline an acceptable anesthetic regimen for this patient.
4. What are the fluid and volume considerations in these patients?
5. When might you use phentolamine, propranolol or nitroprusside during surgical removal of a pheochromocytoma?
6. What are the most critical times during the operative removal of these tumors? How is each portion of the operative procedure managed?

D. Postoperative Management

1. What is the significance of postsurgical hypotension? How is it treated?
2. Can weaning from supportive drugs be a postanesthesia problem? How should it be accomplished?

A. Medical Disease and Differential Diagnosis

A.1. What is an acceptable definition of hypertension?

True systemic hypertension can be diagnosed when there is an increase in arterial pressure with elevations above accepted systolic and diastolic pressures for age, height, and weight, regardless of the primary cause. Most frequently, hypertension is related to an increase in peripheral vascular resistance. The accepted upper limit of normal blood pressure in the adult is 140/90 torr; in infants, 70/45 torr; in early childhood, 85/55 torr; and in adolescents, 100/75 torr.

Schwartz SI: Principles of Surgery, 3rd ed, p 1011. New York, McGraw–Hill, 1979

A.2. How would you classify the various causes of hypertension?

- Systolic hypertension with wide pulse pressure
- Decreased compliance of aorta (arteriosclerosis)
- Increased stroke volume
  Arteriovenous fistula, thyrotoxicosis, fever, aortic valvular insufficiency, patent ductus arteriosus
- Systolic and diastolic hypertension (increased peripheral vascular resistance)

- Renal
  Chronic pyelonephritis, acute and chronic glomerulonephritis, polycystic renal disease, renovascular stenosis or renal infarction
- Endocrine
  Oral contraceptives, adrenocortical hyperfunction, pheochromocytoma, myxedema, acromegaly
- Neurogenic
  Psychogenic, familial dysautonomia, polyneuritis, increased intracranial pressure, spinal cord section
- Miscellaneous
  Coarctation of aorta, increased intravascular volume, polyarteritis nodosa, acute intermittent porphyria, hypercalcemia, toxemia of pregnancy
- Unknown etiology
  Essential hypertension (> 90% of all cases of hypertension)

Isselbacher KJ et al: Harrison's Principles of Internal Medicine, 9th ed, p 180. New York, McGraw-Hill, 1980

A.3. What are the causes of the following events: hypertension and tachycardia; hypertension and bradycardia?

Hypertension and tachycardia are most frequently seen in hypermetabolic states such as thyrotoxicosis, fever, and in those situations where there is an acute elaboration of sympathomimetic amine, as in the alarm reaction, pain, exercise, pheochromocytoma, and the toxemias of pregnancy. Hypertension and bradycardia are more frequently seen as a reflex response to stimulation of carotid sinus receptors responding to a sudden increase in systolic blood pressure. It is also seen in acute increased intracranial pressure.

Gilman AG, Goodman LS, Gilman A: Goodman and Gilman's the Pharmacological Basis of Therapeutics, 6th ed, p 152. New York, Macmillan, 1979

Isselbacher KJ et al: Harrison's Principles of Internal Medicine, 9th ed, pp 33, 1051. New York, McGraw-Hill, 1980

A.4. Trace the embryology of the adrenal gland and describe its normal anatomy.

The adrenal cortex and medulla have separate embryologic origins. The medullary portion is derived from the chromaffin ectodermal cells of the neural crest. These cells are split off very early from the sympathetic ganglion cells, and migrate further ventrally, so as to lie ventrolateral to the aorta, where they form the paraganglia. Several such nodules near the cranial end of the gonads combine into a larger mass of cells lying between the dorsal aorta and the dorsomedial border of the mesonephros. Here, they come into approximation with a group of mesodermal cells destined to become the adrenal cortex. These latter cells drive principally from a narrow strip of coelomic mesothelium lying between the dorsal mesentery and the genital ridge. These cells, arising in numerous places in the suprarenal ridge, lose their connection with the mesothelium and form a complete layer of mesoderm around the ectodermal cells derived from the sympathetic ganglia. The chromaffin cells become enclosed within the cortex to form the medulla. The organs of Zuckerkandl are paraganglia around the aorta at the level of the kidney anterior to the inferior aorta. Accessory areas for the occurrence of pheochromocytoma are in the mediastinum, in the bladder, occasionally in the neck, in the sacrococcygeal region, anal, or in the vaginal areas.

Schwartz SI: Principles of Surgery, 3rd ed, p 1490. New York, McGraw–Hill, 1979

A.5. Enumerate the secretions of the cortex and of the medulla of the adrenal gland, respectively.

The cortex excretes the corticoid steroid and includes both the glucocorticoids and the mineral corticoids. They are the C-21 compounds, C-19 compounds, and C-18 compounds. The entire adrenal cortex contains 11- and 21-hydroxylating enzymes for the production of cortisol and other similar glucocorticoids. The zona glomerulosa contains 18-oxidase, an enzyme capable of oxidating the 18 carbon atom to produce aldosterone, the principal mineral corticoid. The two most important adrenal corticoids by far are cortisol, the major glucocorticoid and aldosterone, the major mineralocorticoid. The adrenal medulla gives rise primarily to three types of catecholamines—epinephrine, norepinephrine, and dopamine. These compounds are found in chromaffin cells of the sympathetic nervous system, which includes the adrenal medulla, aberrant tissue along the sympathetic chain, and paraganglia. Norepinephrine and dopamine are found at the endings of the postganglionic fibers of the sympathetic nervous system as well, and in the central nervous system.

Schwartz SI: Principles of Surgery, 3rd ed, pp 1491–1492, 1518. New York, McGraw–Hill, 1979

A.6. What are the precursors, the synthesis, and biotransformation of epinephrine, norepinephrine, and dopamine?

The main pathway for the formation of epinephrine begins with phenylalanine, which is hydroxylated to tyrosine and then hydroxylated to dihydroxyphenylalanine (dopa). This is acted upon by dopa decarboxylase to produce dopamine. Hydroxylation of dopamine produces norepinephrine and methylation of norepinephrine produces epinephrine. Epinephrine is metabolized by two pathways, one by catechol–O–methyltransferase (COMT) and the other by monoamine oxidase (MAO) to 3,4-dihydroxymandelic acid and then by COMT to vanillylmandelic acid (VMA). Metanephrine is converted by MAO to VMA. Norepinephrine is metabolized by MAO to 3,4-dihydroxymandelic acid or by COMT to normetanephrine. Normetanephrine is also metabolized by MAO to VMA.

Schwartz SI: Principles of Surgery, 3rd ed, pp 1519–1520. New York, McGraw–Hill, 1979

A.7. What are the metabolic actions of the glucocorticoids and the mineral corticoids?

A glucocorticoid is a C–21 steroid with predominant action on intermediary metabolism. The mineral corticoids are C–21 steroids with predominant action on the metabolism of the body minerals, sodium, and potassium. The principal glucocorticoids secreted by the normal adrenal gland are cortisol and corticosterone. The major mineral corticoid is aldosterone.

Isselbacher KJ et al: Harrison's Principles of Internal Medicine, 9th ed, pp 1715–1716. New York, McGraw–Hill, 1980

A.8. What are the usual and unusual sites for the development of pheochromocytoma? What is the cellular makeup of these tumors?

Abdominal pheochromocytomas are located commonly in the following order: the adrenal medulla, the extra-adrenal paraganglia, the organs of Zuckerkandl, and the bladder. Extra-abdominal tumors may be located in the thorax or neck. The tumors are made up of actively secreting chromaffin cells.

Schwartz SI: Principles of Surgery, 3rd ed, pp 1520, 1522. New York, McGraw–Hill, 1979

A.9. What symptoms herald this type of tumor? How may the diagnosis be made?

Early diagnosis is made by the patient complaining of paroxsymal hypertension, excessive sweating, elevated temperatures, frequent headaches, weight loss, recent onset of hypertension with severe retinopathy, elevated basal metabolic rate, and a diabetes like syndrome with an elevated fasting blood sugar. The hypertension in adults is paroxysmal in about 30% of patients. However, 65% of patients show sustained hypertension. The severe attacks are paroxysmal in nature. The symptoms are severe headache, palpitation, profuse sweating, nausea and vomiting, pallor, epigastric or substernal pain, dyspnea, vertigo, apprehension, fear of impending death, and visual difficulties. All these symptoms might not be present in all attacks, but usually two of them are always manifest. The attack may last for a few moments or hours, frequently precipitated by emotional upset, change in position, physical effort, sneezing, urination, or the induction of anesthesia. One has to make a differential diagnosis between pheochromocytoma and renal vascular hypertension, anxiety states, eclampsia, hysteria, thyroid crisis, brain tumors, and recently, monoamine oxidase inhibitors, occasionally shown to produce attacks similar to pheochromocytoma.

The diagnosis is made by measuring urinary catecholamines. Other tests that were used in the past, such as the phentolamine test or histamine test, are of little value today. It is far better to make the diagnosis of pheochromocytoma by measurement of urinary catecholamines and their metabolites. It is important that patients on alphamethyldopa (Aldomet), should have this drug stopped at least 3 weeks prior to collecting urine for analysis. The drug interferes with metanephrine and normetanephrine measurement. Urinary VMA is a less sensitive test and certainly nonspecific for epinephrine or norepinephrine, as tumors other than pheochromocytomas or neuroblastomas can secrete catecholamines and increased secretions of these substances may be seen in the absence of these tumors. Thus, elevated urinary VMA has been seen in ganglioneuromas, ganglioneuroblastomas, retinoblastomas, carotid body tumors, and malignant carcinoid.

Radiology can help greatly in localization of these tumors using arteriography, venography, nephrotomography, sonography, and computerized tomography.

Katz J, Benumof J, Kadis LB: Anesthesia and Uncommon Diseases, 2nd ed, pp 198–199. Philadelphia, WB Saunders, 1981

Manger WM, Gifford RW Jr: Pheochromocytoma, diagnosis and management. NY State J Med 80, No. 2:217–223, 1980

Schwartz SI: Principles of Surgery, 3rd ed, pp 1522–1527. New York, McGraw–Hill, 1979

B. Preoperative Evaluation and Preparation

B.1. Outline an acceptable preparation for these patients prior to anesthesia and surgery.

Of the three blocking agents, dibenzyline, alpha-methyltyrosine and prazosin, we prefer phenoxybenzamine hydrochloride (Dibenzyline). It is a long acting alpha adrenergic blocker that can be used to control hypertension while the patient is being prepared for the surgical procedure. It is given orally, once or twice daily. The initial dose of 20 to 30 mg is increased by 10 to 20 mg per day until the blood pressure has stabilized and there is mild postural hypotension. Usually, a dose of 40 to 100 mg per day is required. Over the years, this type of alpha blocking agent has produced the most stable blood pressure of any other drugs used to prepare these patients.

If cardiac arrhythmias are a prominent feature, propranolol also can be given, in doses of 20 to 40 mg four times daily. In addition to the alpha and beta blockade, it is important that the state of hydration be evaluated because many patients have a decreased intravascular volume. One or two units of blood may be needed to increase the intravascular volume as the Dibenzyline dilates the peripheral vascular bed. The alpha adrenergic blocker should be used up to and including the day of surgery. During the surgical procedure, alpha and beta adrenergic blocking agents are used intravenously as needed to control blood pressure, arrhythmias, and cardiac rate.

Himathongkam T et al: Pheochromocytoma. J Am Med Assoc 230, No. 12:1692, 1974

B.2. How would you manage the drugs for premedication?

Atropine, 0.4 mg, is given to decrease vagal tone. Sedation is given in doses appropriate to age and weight, to have the patient arrive in the operating room relatively free from fear and anxiety. To accomplish this degree of sedation, we choose pentobarbital sodium, in doses of 100 to 300 mg, one hour prior to the start of anesthesia.

Protocol for Preoperative Medication at The New York Hospital

C. Intraoperative Management

C.1. How would you induce this patient?

We choose thiopental sodium, 2.5%, until the patient enters the state of light hypnosis and loses his eyelid reflex. Care must be taken not to use a large bolus dose of thiopenthal sodium for fear that a significant depressor response may be produced. A significant depressor response may set off a hypertensive attack which may require the intravenous administration of phentolamine (Regitine) to control the severe hypertension.

Katz J, Benumof J, Kadis LB: Anesthesia and Uncommon Diseases, 2nd ed, p 201. Philadelphia, WB Saunders, 1981

C.2. During the surgical procedure, what parameters would you monitor?

At present, we are monitoring intraarterial blood pressure, the central venous pressure, the ECG, using a simulated V-5 lead, and a combined esophageal stethoscope with a temperature thermostat included to measure body core temperature. An indwelling bladder catheter will provide a measurement of urinary output throughout the surgical procedure. Pulmonary artery pressure is monitored if the patient has left ventricular dysfunction.

Katz J, Benumof J, Kadis LB: Anesthesia and Uncommon Diseases, 2nd ed, p 201. Philadelphia, WB Saunders, 1981

C.3. Outline an acceptable anesthetic regimen for this patient.

Following the induction with thiopental sodium, an inhalation anesthetic is preferable to multiple intravenous drugs. Regulating the depth of anesthesia with the inhalation anesthetic may be all that is needed to control the systolic hypertension that occurs with surgical manipulation. At the present time, we are using enflurane (Ethrane) as a suitable nonflammable ether. Prior to this, we used methoxyflurane and diethyl ether. All have worked well for maintenance in previous years. We are about to use isoflurane (Forane) as inhalation agent of choice for these patients.

Janeczko GF et al: Enflurane anesthesia for surgical removal of pheochromocytoma. Anesth Analg (Cleve) 56, No. 1:66, 1977

Manger, WM, Gifford RW Jr: Pheochromocytoma, diagnosis and management. NY State J Med 80, No. 2:225, 1980

Pratilas V, Pratila MG: Management of pheochromocytoma. Anesthesiology Review 6, No. 5:46, 1979

C.4. What are the fluid and volume considerations in these patients?

As mentioned in the preoperative preparation, these patients may have a contracted blood volume; therefore, a balanced salt solution should be administered throughout the surgical procedure to ensure an adequate intravascular volume. When the tumor is removed, the vascular bed will suddenly increase in size because it is no longer being constricted by large amounts of sympathomimetic amines. Preoperative use of whole blood and an adequate amount of intravenous balanced salt solution will minimize any sharp fall in blood pressure. Throughout the surgical procedure, urinary output should be maintained at 30–50 cc/hr. However, at the height of the tumor manipulation, when huge amounts of sympathomimetic amines are being secreted into the circulation, there may be a pause in urinary output. Following tumor removal, a significant compensatory diuresis will occur.

Katz J, Benumof J, Kadis LB: Anesthesia and Uncommon Diseases, 2nd ed, p 203. Philadelphia, WB Saunders, 1981

Manger WM, Gifford RW Jr: Pheochromocytoma, diagnosis and management. NY State J Med 80, No. 2: 225, 1980

C.5. When might you use phentolamine, propranolol, or nitroprusside during surgical removal of a pheochromocytoma?

At present, we prefer to rely on phentolamine (Regitine) as a short acting alpha blocking agent which may be made up in a solution for continuous drip administration—50 mg Regitine per 500 cc Ringer's lactate solution. Using phentolamine and depth of inhalation anesthesia, the systolic blood pressure can be maintained below 200 torr. However, occasionally in spite of the use of phentolamine and depth of anesthesia with Ethrane, the systolic blood pressure cannot be adequately controlled below 200 torr. In those situations, nitroprusside should be used to control blood pressure. We do not use nitroprusside as our primary vasodilator because this drug may be more difficult to control than phentolamine. Frequently the patient may be exquisitely sensitive to this agent and overdose, resulting in hypotension, is a distinct possibility.

Katz J, Benumof J, Kadis LB: Anesthesia and Uncommon Diseases, 2nd ed, p 202. Philadelphia, WB Saunders, 1981

C.6. What are the most critical times during the operative removal of these tumors? How is each portion of the operative procedure managed?

Preoperative alpha blockade by the use of phenoxybenzamine is regulated so as not to produce a totally blocked patient, but only a partial block. In the partially blocked patient, early tumor manipulation will produce minor increases in blood pressure which will demonstrate the reactivity of the peripheral vasculature and will guide the anesthesiologist as tumor removal progresses.

When the blood supply of the tumor has been curtailed, the systolic blood pressure should not be allowed to fall below 100 torr. A rapid further fall in blood pressure may produce an acute decrease in cerebral coronary and renal flow, which may damage these structures. Therefore, following complete removal of the tumor, blood pressure is monitored most carefully. If the blood pressure is maintained above 100 torr, nothing is done to support the circulation. However, if the systolic blood pressure does dip below 100 torr, norepinephrine should be started by continuous drip using a concentration of 4.0 mg in 500 ml of Ringer's lactate. The continuous drip should be regulated to control the blood pressure at approximately 120 to 130 torr. The use of the peripheral vasopressor may be necessary only for a brief period of time, although it may be necessary in some instances to continue it for several hours following the surgical procedure. When the circulation is stabilized and the vascular volume approaches the size of the vascular bed, the vasopressor can be discontinued.

Manger WM, Gifford RW Jr: Pheochromocytoma, diagnosis and management. NY State J Med 80, No. 2:224, 1980

D. Postoperative Management

D.1. What is the significance of postsurgical hypotension? How is it treated?

Postsurgical hypotension may be a result of persistent fatigue of the peripheral constrictor mechanism. Once the massive amounts of catecholamines are stopped by removal of the tumor, the vascular bed may not pick up as quickly as one would expect, and norepinephrine may have to be continued into the postsurgical period. Because this is a rather rare phenomenon today, with preparation of the patient with alpha blockers and whole blood, one should be suspicious of continuous postsurgical bleeding if the blood pressure is not quickly maintained without norepinephrine. If the need for norepinephrine persists, the cause of the hypotension may necessitate a prompt return to the operating room.

Manger WM, Gifford RW Jr: Pheochromocytoma, diagnosis and management. NY State J Med 80, No. 2:225, 1980

Schwartz SI: Principles of Surgery, 3rd ed, p 1532. New York, McGraw–Hill, 1979

Pratilas V, Pratila MG: Management of pheochromocytoma. Anesthesiology Review 8, No. 5:48, 1979

D.2. Can weaning from supportive drugs be a postanesthesia problem? How should it be accomplished?

Weaning from supportive drugs is rarely a postanesthesia problem today. However, when any vasopressor drug is used, it should be decreased slowly, and the pressure carefully followed until the patient can support his own circulation. It should be done by a physician who remains with the patient constantly until homeostasis is achieved and the patient is without vasopressor support and maintains a blood pressure within the acceptable normal range.

Gilman AG, Goodman LS, Gilman A: Goodman and Gilman's The Pharmacological Basis of Therapeutics, 6th ed, p 153. New York, Macmillan, 1980

20 Diabetes
Vinod Malhotra

A 45-year-old woman had a known history of diabetes for 30 years. Her diabetes was controlled with regular crystalline insulin 35 units daily. She was scheduled for emergency surgery for tubo-ovarian abscess. Blood glucose was 350 mg%.

A. Medical Disease and Differential Diagnosis

1. What is the incidence of diabetes mellitus in the general population?
2. What are the factors in the etiology of the disease?
3. How do you classify diabetes mellitus?
4. What are the complications of diabetes mellitus?
5. How would you treat the different forms of this illness?
6. How do you adequately monitor the control of the disease?
7. What are some of the factors that alter insulin requirement?
8. What are the principles in management of diabetic ketoacidosis?

B. Preoperative Evaluation and Preparation

1. How would you evaluate this patient preoperatively?
2. How would you prepare this patient for anesthesia and surgery?

C. Intraoperative Management

1. What is the effect of anesthesia and surgery on insulin and glucose metabolism?
2. What anesthetic techniques would you employ?
3. How would you monitor this patient?

4. How would you employ insulin intraoperatively?
5. How would you recognize and treat hypoglycemic shock intraoperatively?

D. Postoperative Management

1. How would you control diabetes in this patient postoperatively?
2. What are the common postoperative complications you expect in a diabetic?

A. Medical Disease and Differential Diagnosis

A.1. What is the incidence of diabetes mellitus in the general population?

In the United States, the incidence of the disease is 5% and it is on the increase. It is currently the third ranking cause of death.

Report of the National Commission on Diabetes of the Congress of The United States, Vol. 1. The Long Range Plan to Combat Diabetes. DHEW publication no. (NIH) 76-1018

A.2. What are the factors in the etiology of the disease?

Three main factors have received widespread recognition in the etiology of the disease and these include genetics, immune response, and viruses. The role of genetic factors in the development of the disorder is undisputed, although the mode of inheritance still remains controversial. Studies on monozygotic twins show a concordance rate for the disease to be less than 50% if the age at onset in the index twin is less than 40 years. The rate approaches 100% if the age at onset is over 40 years in the index twin. In the offspring of congugal diabetic parents, the incidence of the overt disease is 6% to 10%, and that of chemical diabetes 25% to 40% based on glucose tolerance test. In view of such diverse findings, it is reasonable to assume a polygenic transmission further modified by environmental factors.

Histopathological studies, elevated titres of histocompatibility antigens (notably human leukocyte antigen (HLA)), presence of insulin antibodies, and association of juvenile onset diabetes with certain well-known autoimmune diseases like thyroiditis and myasthenia gravis, underline the significance of immune factors in the pathogenesis of this entity. Virus–beta cell interactions have been postulated in the pathogenesis of juvenile diabetes in recent years, with supportive evidence of antiviral antibody titers implicating several common RNA and DNA viruses.

Craighead JE: Current views on the etiology of insulin–dependent diabetes mellitus. N Engl J Med 299:1439–1445, 1978

Ganda OP, Soeldner SS: Genetic, acquired, and related factors in the etiology of diabetes mellitus. Arch Intern Med 137:461–469, 1977

A.3. How do you classify diabetes mellitus?

Although several classifications exist for diabetes mellitus, the best way to classify the disease is to differentiate the two different forms of the clinical entity. Type A, then, is the insulin dependent diabetes. It is more severe, and the onset is usually in the young. A gene–virus interaction and immune disturbance are believed to be the main causative factors.

Type B, on the other hand, is noninsulin dependent, mild, and affects all ages, the incidence increasing with age. The genetic factors probably predominate in the etiology of this form.

Ganda OP, Soeldner SS: Genetic, acquired, and related factors in the etiology of diabetes mellitus. Arch Intern Med 137:461–469, 1977

A.4. What are the complications of diabetes mellitus?

Diabetic retinopathy, neuropathy, nephropathy, and vascular changes are well-known complications of the long-standing disease. In a juvenile diabetic like this patient, however, the common life-threatening complications are mainly due to poor control and include hypoglycemia, hyperglycemia, diabetic ketoacidosis, and coma.

Isselbacher KJ et al: Harrison's Principles of Internal Medicine, 9th ed, pp 1741–1755. New York, McGraw–Hill, 1980

A.5. How would you treat the different forms of this illness?

The type A diabetic, who has the severe form of the disease, is insulin dependent and prone to diabetic ketoacidosis. Two preparations of insulin in common use today include the regular crystalline insulin and the NPH (Neutral Protamine Hagedorn) insulin. The onset and duration of action of these agents by subcutaneous injection are shown in Table 20–1.

The type B patient is a mild diabetic and is usually obese. The rationale for treatment in these patients centers around weight loss and diet control. Weight reduction and diet control together can control the majority of these patients. Those patients not controlled well on this regimen require oral hypoglycemics, or insulin. The University Group Diabetes Program study revealed a higher incidence of cardiovascular

Table 20–1. The onset and duration of action of subcutaneous insulin injection

TYPE	ONSET (HOURS)	PEAK ACTIVITY (HOURS)	DURATION (HOURS)
Regular insulin (Crystalline insulin)	1	2–4	5–7
NPH insulin (Isophane insulin)	2	6–12	24–28

deaths in patients treated with tolbutamide, with no significant difference in efficiency of treatment compared with placebo. Ever since their first report in 1970, this study has been a subject of major controversy regarding the toxicity of oral hypoglycemics. However, both tolbutamide and phenformin have been shown to be inadequate in sustained lowering of blood sugar in treated populations. The question of efficiency of other agents is still open. At present, then, there is no demonstrable role for oral hypoglycemics, except in selected individuals where insulin control poses problems in a maturity onset diabetic. Most maturity onset diabetics can be treated with diet alone, and if that fails to control it adequately, insulin should be added to the regimen.

A study of the effects of hypoglycemic agents on vascular complications with adult-onset diabetes: II, Mortality results University Group Diabetes Program. Diabetes (Suppl) 19:787–830, 1970

A study of the effects of hypoglycemic agents on vascular complications in patients with adult-onset diabetes VI. Supplementary report on nonfatal events in patients treated with tolbutamide, UGDP. Diabetes 25:1129--1153, 1976

Feinstein AR: Clinical biostatistics XXXV, The persistent clinical failures and fallacies of the UGDP study. Clin Pharmacol Ther 19:78–93, 1976

Scott J, Poffenbarger PL: Tolbutamide pharmacogenetics and the UGDP study. JAMA 242:45–48, 1979

A.6. How do you adequately monitor the control of the disease?

Mild diabetics and well-controlled diabetics are usually self monitored by daily urine test for reducing sugars and ketones. In acute management of hyperglycemia, or situations where insulin requirement is altered (as in the above patient secondary to infection), the best control is achieved with regular crystalline insulin and monitored by frequent blood sugars, since the changes in urinary sugar appear after a lag period. A quick bedside method of blood sugar assessment involves the use of Dextrostix.

Isselbacher KJ et al: Harrison's Principles of Internal Medicine, 9th ed, pp 1741–1755. New York, McGraw–Hill, 1980

Jenkins MT: Common and Uncommon Problems in Anesthesiology, Clinical Anesthesia, pp 264–274. Philadelphia, FA Davis, 1968

A.7. What are some of the factors that alter insulin requirement?

Factors commonly known to increase the insulin requirement include a high carbohydrate diet, infection, sepsis, stress, and certain frequently employed drugs, namely, corticosteriods, thyroid preparations, oral contraceptives, and thiazide diuretics. Exercise and alcohol commonly result in decreased requirements, as do certain drugs such as phenylbutazone, dicumarol, and salicylates, which mainly interfere with the pharmacodynamics of oral hypoglycemics.

Gilman AG, Goodman LS, Gilman A: Goodman and Gilman's The Pharmacological Basis of Therapeutics, 6th ed. New York, Macmillan, 1980

Isselbacher KJ et al: Harrison's Principles of Internal Medicine, 9th ed, pp 1741–1755. New York, McGraw–Hill, 1980

Shen SW, Bressler R: Clinical pharmacology of oral antidiabetic agents. N Engl J Med 296, No. 9:493–497, 1977

A.8. What are the principles in management of diabetic ketoacidosis?

Diabetic ketoacidosis is an acute medical emergency characterized by an absolute or relative deficiency of insulin resulting in an accumulation of ketone acids in the blood. The main disturbances are hyperglycemia, glycosuria, intracellular dehydration, acidosis, and electrolyte imbalance. Conventionally, severe ketoacidosis implies levels of ketone acids in the blood generally greater than 7 mMoles/liter, a decrease in serum bicarbonate to less tha 10 mEq/liter or a decrease in pH to less than 7.25. Initial physical examination should be supported with urinalysis, venous blood analysis for glucose, electrolytes, urea nitrogen, complete blood count, and serum ketone estimation. Reagent strips may be used to determine the blood glucose (Dextrostix) and ketones (Ketostix) quickly, and therapy initiated. An arterial blood gas sample should be analyzed to determine acid–base imbalance. The mainstay of treatment includes fluids, insulin, bicarbonate, and potassium.

- Fluids
  Most patients are dehydrated and the loss of water relatively exceeds that of salt. Therefore, a hypotonic saline solution (0.45% sodium chloride) is considered optimal. Five percent glucose should be instituted once the serum glucose falls below 250 mg per 100 ml. A central venous pressure measurement and urine output are good guidelines for fluid therapy.
- Insulin
  All patients in ketoacidosis are in immediate need of insulin. Therefore, a rapid onset, short acting insulin should be employed to attain better control. Conventionally, an initial dose of 100 units of regular crystalline insulin is given—half intravenously and the other half intramuscularly. Half the initial dose is repeated every 2 to 4 hours, monitored by frequent blood glucose and ketone determinations. Another regimen includes administering small doses of regular insulin (10–20 units) intravenously initially and then intramuscularly every hour. Yet another way to give insulin is in a constant intravenous infusion of insulin (10–20 units) using the Harvard pump.
- Bicarbonate
  Sodium bicarbonate should be used to correct severe metabolic acidosis (with pH 7.20) as guided by determinations of arterial blood pH, P_{CO_2} and bicarbonate. Over correction should be avoided.

- Potassium
  Following acidosis, osmotic diuresis, and vomiting, body potassium stores are depleted by 5 to 10 mEq per kilogram of body weight. Serum potassium, although initially normal, usually decreases because the correction of hyperglycemia and acidosis results in movement of potassium from extracellular space to intracellular space. Therefore, potassium should be added to the intravenous infusion 3 to 4 hours after initiating the therapy, provided the renal function is adequate. Frequent laboratory data and clinical findings should dictate the dose and frequency regimen of the treatment. Supportive therapy for associated problems should continue, and over correction should be avoided.

Felig P: Current concepts, diabetic ketoacidosis. N Engl J Med 290:1360–1362, 1974

Isselbacher KJ et al: Harrison's Principles of Internal Medicine, 9th ed, pp 1741–1755. New York, McGraw–Hill, 1980

B. Preoperative Evaluation and Preparation

B.1. How would you evaluate this patient preoperatively?

A complete preoperative evaluation includes a history and physical examination supported by the following laboratory data:
- Chest x-ray
- Electrocardiogram
- Urinalysis for reducing sugar and ketones
- Venous blood estimation of complete blood count, serum electrolytes, urea nitrogen, sugar, and ketones (Serum osmolality if available)
- Arterial blood gas analysis to determine acid-base status
  Of great pertinence is the history of the last intake of meal and the last dose of insulin. Nausea and vomiting in this patient will affect her state of hydration, acid base status, and electrolyte balance significantly.

Alberti KGMM, Thomas DJB: The management of diabetes during surgery. Br J Anaesth 51:693–710, 1979

Jenkins MT: Common and Uncommon Problems in Anesthesiology pp 264–274. Philadelphia, FA Davis, 1968

Rosenbaum, S: Anesthetic management of the diabetic patient. ASA Refresher Courses in Anesthesiology, 9:143–154, 1981

B.2. How would you prepare this patient for anesthesia and surgery?

The preoperative evaluation will determine the preparation of this patient, the principles of which are as follows:
- Hydration
  Poor oral intake secondary to malaise and abdominal pain, concomitant vomiting, if present, and osmotic diuresis due to glycosuria, will make dehydration quite likely in this patient. Any dehydration that is present,

therefore, should be rapidly corrected. Normal or half-normal saline is a preferred intravenous solution because the blood glucose is already elevated in this instance.

- Insulin

Infection and stress are known to increase insulin requirements, which explains hyperglycemia in this patient. Insulin can be given to this patient either in small doses (10 units intramuscularly) every hour or as a continuous infusion using a pump. Hourly blood and urine glucose and acetone measurements should be used to adequately monitor this therapy. Acid–base and electrolyte correction should be carried out as dictated by blood tests. Antibiotics should be instituted once appropriate culture samples are obtained.

Alberti KGMM, Thomas DJB: The Management of Diabetes During Surgery. Br J Anaesth 51:693–710, 1979

Jenkins MT: Common and Uncommon Problems in Anesthesiology, pp 264–274. Philadelphia, FA Davis, 1968

Rosenbaum S: Anesthetic management of the diabetic patient. ASA Refresher Courses in Anesthesiology 9:143–154, 1981

C. Intraoperative Management

C.1. What is the effect of anesthesia and surgery on insulin and glucose metabolism?

Anesthesia alone, in normal man, is unaccompanied by significant change in plasma insulin level during halothane, methoxyflurane, enflurane, thiopental–nitrous oxide, and spinal anesthesia. Glucose levels have been shown to rise significantly during halothane, methoxyflurane, and thiopental–nitrous oxide anesthesia, thereby resulting in a decreased plasma insulin level to blood glucose ratio. The insulin to glucose ratio has been reported to be unchanged during enflurane and spinal anesthesia. The earlier studies were done with ether and cyclopropane, both of which are not in use today, and hence, these results are not clinically significant. Over all, the metabolic effects of modern anesthetics are minor compared with the stress of surgery itself. Muscle relaxants and premedicant drugs in common use today are of little concern to diabetics.

Surgery provides a classical stress situation with catabolic response. The extent of the metabolic response is related to the severity of the operation and other concomitant factors such as sepsis in this patient, and shock, if present. The well recognized hormonal changes include increased catecholamines, ACTH, and cortisol secretions, as well as plasma cyclic–AMP and glucagon levels. Despite unaltered plasma insulin levels, blood glucose levels are known to increase during and after surgery. There is also a phase of relative insulin resistance following surgery. All these changes increase the insulin requirement acutely in a diabetic.

Alberti KGMM, Thomas DJB: The management of diabetes during surgery. Br J Anaesth 51:693–710, 1979

Rosenbaum S: Anesthetic management of the diabetic patient. ASA Refresher Courses in Anesthesiology, 239:1–6, 1980

C.2. What anesthetic techniques would you employ?

A general anesthetic with intubation of the trachea will be a satisfactory choice. There is no significant difference between the commonly employed general anesthetics regarding their effect on the diabetic control. Close monitoring will be necessary to provide cardiovascular stability and adequate control of diabetes.

Alberti KGMM, Thomas DJB: The management of diabetes during surgery. Br J Anaesth 51:693–710, 1979

Rosenbaum S: Anesthetic of the diabetic patient. ASA Refresher Courses in Anesthesiology 239:1–6, 1980

C.3. How would you monitor this patient?

In addition to continuous electrocardiogram, blood pressure, temperature recording, and precordial stethoscope, frequent determinations of blood glucose and urine glucose should be made. The blood glucose can be estimated easily in the operating room with the use of Dextrostix, which will dictate further insulin therapy.

Alberti KGMM, Thomas DJB: The management of diabetes during surgery. Br J Anaesth 51:693–710, 1979

Jenkins MT: Common and Uncommon Problems in Anesthesiology, pp 264–274. FA Davis, 1968

C.4. How would you employ insulin intraoperatively?

A good way to control hyperglycemia intraoperatively is to use a continuous infusion of insulin, starting at 1 unit per hour if the patient required 20 units less of NPH insulin daily, preoperatively. In this patient, a starting rate of 2 units per hour, further dictated by frequent blood and urine glucose estimations, will be an adequate regimen. The use of an infusion pump with a plast syringe affords a 90% recovery of insulin. The keystone to intraoperative diabetes management is the measurement of blood glucose concentration.

Alberti KGMM, Thomas DJB: The management of diabetes during surgery. Br J Anaesth 51:693–710, 1979

Taitelman U, Reece EA, Bessman AN: Insulin in the management of the diabetic surgical patient. JAMA 237: 658–660, 1977

C.5. How would you recognize and treat hypoglycemic shock intraoperatively?

It is virtually impossible to differentiate hypoglycemic shock from other forms of shock intraoperatively, unless supported by low blood glucose concentrations measured concomitantly. Treatment lies in administration of glucose, which may be given as a bolus of 50% glucose followed by a 10% glucose—insulin infusion.

Alberti KGMM, Thomas DJB: The management of diabetes during surgery. Br J Anaesth 51:693–710, 1979

Jenkins MT: Common and Uncommon Problems in Anesthesiology, pp 264–274. Philadelphia, FA Davis, 1968

D. Postoperative Management

D.1. How would you control diabetes in this patient postoperatively?

Infusions of 10% glucose–insulin–potassium, as determined by blood glucose and potassium every 4–6 hours, should be continued. NPH insulin should be replaced by regular insulin in divided doses. An additional 20% of insulin may be given since infection is present. As the patient totally resumes her controlled diet, the original preoperative regimen should be restored.

Alberti KGMM, Thomas DJB: The management of diabetes during surgery. Br J Anaesth 51:693–710, 1979

D.2. What are the common postoperative complications you expect in a diabetic?

In addition to the usual complications, the common problems in a diabetic include poor diabetes control and infection. A higher incidence of cardiovascular and renal problems and autonomic neuropathy, resulting in postural hypotension and urinary retention, may be encountered. The over-all morbidity and mortality is increased.

Alberti KGMM, Thomas DJB: The management of diabetes during surgery. Br J Anaesth 51:693–710, 1979

21 Adrenocortical Tumor
Vinod Malhotra

A 35-year-old man with an adrenocortical tumor was scheduled for left adrenalectomy. Blood pressure, 160/100 torr; pulse, 100/m; blood glucose, 220 mg%.

A. Medical Disease and Differential Diagnosis

1. What is Cushing's syndrome?
2. What are the common causes of Cushing's syndrome?
3. List the major hormonal secretions of the adrenal cortex.
4. What are the other clinical syndromes associated with hyperfunction of the adrenal cortex?
5. What are the clinical features of hyperaldosteronism?
6. What is the treatment of aldosteronism?
7. What are the common indications for adrenalectomy?

B. Preoperative Evaluation and Preparation

1. How would you evaluate this patient preoperatively?
2. What is the screening dexamethasone suppression test?
3. How would you prepare this patient for surgery?

C. Intraoperative Management

1. What anesthetic agents and technique would you employ?
2. What monitors would you use for this procedure?
3. What are the anesthetic considerations in this patient?

D. Postoperative Management

1. What are the possible postoperative complications in this patient?

A. Medical Disease and Differential Diagnosis

A.1. What is Cushing's syndrome?

Cushing's syndrome is a clinical entity resulting from adrenocortical hyperfunction. The signs and symptoms of Cushing's syndrome are related to excess glucocorticoids. The patient presents with increased body weight, truncal obesity with the "buffalo hump" in the interscapular area, "moon" facies, easy fatigability, weakness, hypertension, hirsutism, amenorrhea, easy bruisability, cutaneous striae, personality changes, edema, polyuria, polydypsia, hypokalemia, and impaired glucose tolerance. Abnormally high levels of corticosteroids also result in osteoporosis, peptic ulcers, cataracts, and glaucoma.

Isselbacher KJ, Adams RD, Braunwald E et al: Harrison's Principles of Internal Medicine, 9th ed, pp 1719–1724. New York, McGraw–Hill, 1980

A.2. What are the common causes of Cushing's syndrome?

The most common cause of Cushing's syndrome is iatrogenic, resulting from the administration of corticosteroids. Approximately 40% of the endogenous causes of Cushing's syndrome are ACTH-producing pituitary tumors (more common in women) and another 15% are ACTH-producing nonpituitary tumors such as tumors of the lung, prostate, testis, parotid, or pancreas (more common in men). Nearly 25% of cases are due to adrenal hyperplasia without an ACTH-secreting tumor. Twenty percent of patients with endogenous Cushing's syndrome are due to adrenocortical tumors, about half of which are benign adenomas.

Brown BR: Anesthesia and the Patient with Endocrine Disease. Contemporary Anesthesia Practice, pp 1–9. Philadelphia, FA Davis, 1980

A.3. List the major hormonal secretions of the adrenal cortex.

More than 50 steroids have been isolated from the adrenal cortex. Not all of these are normally secreted or released into the circulation, many of these do not possess any significant biological activity. Based on their physiologic roles, three principle categories of hormone can be described as follows:

- Glucocorticoids. The principle glucocorticoid is cortisol (hydrocortisone) of which 15 to 30 mg are secreted daily. Cortisol exerts its action primarily on glucose metabolism and to a certain extent on protein and lipid metabolism. The effects are generally catabolic with increased release of glucose into the blood. Cortisol possesses antiinflammatory action and is involved in immune and stress responses. Following biotransformation in the liver, it is excreted in the urine. Normal blood levels show diurnal variation with a range of 9 to 24 $\mu g/100$ ml in the morning and 3 to 12 $\mu g/100$ ml in the evening.

- Mineralocorticoids. The principle mineralocorticoid is aldosterone with an average daily secretion of between 50 and 250 μg and a blood level of 15 ng/100 ml on a normal salt intake. Aldosterone promotes the reabsorption of sodium with resultant loss of potassium and hydrogen ions in the distal tubules of the kidney. Secondarily, intravascular fluid volume increases. Aldosterone is biotransformed in the liver and excreted in the urine. Although the glucocorticoids also possess some mineralocorticoid activity, their potency is relatively low (see Table 21–1).
- Androgens. The major androgenic compound is dehydroepiandrosterone (DHEA) secreted at the rate of 15 to 30 mg/day. In the male, it is biotransformed to testosterone and in the female to estrogens. These sex hormones are anabolic in nature and are precursors of 17-keto steroids in the urine. About two thirds of urinary 17-ketosteroids are normally derived from adrenal androgens in the male. In the female, almost all urine 17-ketosteroids are derived from the adrenal gland.

Gilman AG, Goodman LS, Gilman A: The Pharmacologic Basis of Therapeutics, 6th ed, pp 1466–1496. New York, Macmillan, 1980

Glenn F, Peterson RE, Mannix H Jr: Surgery of the Adrenal Gland, pp 13–43. New York, Macmillan, 1968

Isselbacher KJ, Adams RD, Braunwald E et al: Harrison's Principles of Internal Medicine, 9th ed, pp 1711–1736. New York, McGraw–Hill, 1980

A.4. What are the other clinical syndromes associated with hyperfunction of the adrenal cortex?

Besides Cushing's syndrome, there are primary hyperaldosteronism or Conn's syndrome due to hypersecretion of aldosterone and the adrenogenital syndrome, due to hypersecretion of androgenic adrenocortical steroids.

Brown BR: Anesthesia and the Patient with Endocrine Disease. Contemporary Anesthesia Practice, pp 1–9. Philadelphia, FA Davis, 1980

Isselbacher KJ, Adams RD, Braunswald E et al: Harrison's Principles of Internal Medicine, 9th ed, pp 1719–1729. New York, McGraw–Hill, 1980

Table 21–1. Relative properties of major corticosteroids and the commonly employed synthetic analogues

STEROIDS	DAILY SECRETION	PLASMA CONCENTRATION	BIOLOGICAL HALF-LIFE HOURS	POTENCY GLUCOCORTICOID/ MINERALOCORTICOID
Cortisol (hydrocortisone)	15–30 mg	9–24 μg/100 ml (am) 3–12 μg/100 ml (pm)	8–12	1/1
Aldosterone	50–250 μg	1–5 ng/100 ml	2–3	0.3/3000
Prednisone	—	—	12–36	4/0.25
Methylprednisolone	—	—	12–36	5/0.25
Dexamethasone	—	—	> 24	25/±
Fluorohydrocortisone	—	—	—	5/200

A.5. What are the clinical features of hyperaldosteronism?

Primary hyperaldosteronism, described by Conn in 1956, is a rare disease. It may account for less than 1% of known hypertensive patients. The usual etiology is an adrenal adenoma or hyperplasia and more infrequently a carcinoma of the adrenal gland. Secondary hyperaldosteronism results from excessive production of aldosterone secondary to increased renin-angiotension activity. The signs and symptoms are due to the two main features of the disease, namely, diastolic hypertension and hypokalemia. Patients commonly complain of headache, fatigue, muscle weakness, polyuria, and polydypsia. Serum hypernatremia may be seen. Electrocardiographic manifestations of electrolyte disturbance are evident. With the onset of nephropathy, renal function may be impaired. Plasma renin levels are low in primary aldosteronism and high in the secondary form of the disease.

Isselbacher KJ, Adams BD, Braunswald E et al: Harrison's Principles of Internal Medicine, 9th ed, pp 1724–1727. New York, McGraw–Hill, 1980

A.6. What is the treatment of aldosteronism?

Medical treatment is indicated for patients with bilateral hyperplasia. It consists of the administration of the aldosterone antagonist, spironolactone 25 to 100 mg twice a day. Triamterene is a good adjunct therapy for hypokalemia. Surgical intervention is indicated for failed medical therapy and in cases of an adrenal adenoma.

Isselbacher KJ, Adams RD, Braunswald E et al: Harrison's Principles of Internal Medicine, 9th ed, p 1726. New York, McGraw–Hill, 1980

A.7. What are the common indications for adrenalectomy?

The common indications for adrenalectomy are adrenal cortical adenomas and carcinomas, bilateral cortical hyperplasia, pheochromocytoma, and palliation for metastatic breast and prostatic carcinoma.

Brown BR: Anesthesia and Patient with Endocrine Disease. Contemporary Anesthesia Practice, pp 3–4. Philadelphia, FA Davis, 1980

B. Preoperative Evaluation and Preparation

B.1. How would you evaluate this patient preoperatively?

A thorough evaluation of the patient's medical history is necessary. The patient's diabetic status, including efficacy of insulin therapy if indicated, should be evaluated by blood glucose and glucose tolerance tests. Although usually mild, significant hypertension may exist in the patient along with salt retention and increased intravascular and interstitial volume. Look for any evidence of congestive heart failure. Hypokalemia predisposes to arrhythmias. Hypokalemia also causes muscle weakness, which coupled with truncal obesity may compromise respiration in this patient. Therefore, a careful evaluation of electrolyte balance and acid–base status is mandatory. Osteoporotic changes should be searched for as they predispose to compression and spontaneous fractures. Increased gastric acidity is common. Psychological evaluation should also be made. The site and vascularity of the tumor should be assessed preoperatively because a large vascular tumor with local infiltration may result in massive blood loss during surgery.

Brown BR: Anesthesia and Patient with Endocrine Disease. Contemporary Anesthesia Practice, pp 1–9. Philadelphia, FA Davis, 1980

Katz J, Benumof J, Kadis LB: Anesthesia and Uncommon Diseases. Pathophysiologic and Clinical Correlations, pp 191–194. Philadelphia, WB Saunders, 1981

B.2. What is the screening dexamethasone suppression test?

This test usually distinguishes Cushing's syndrome from other diseases with similar clinical pictures in more than 95% of cases. The test consists of oral administration of 1 mg of dexamethasone at bedtime followed by morning blood sampling for cortisol level, which is normally less than 5 $\mu g/100$ ml.

Katz J, Benumof J, Kadis LB: Anesthesia and Uncommon Diseases. Pathophysiologic and Clinical Correlations, p 191. Philadelphia, WB Saunders, 1981

Vandam LD: To Make the Patient Ready for Anesthesia. Medical Care of the Surgical Patient, p 121. Menlo Park, CA, Addison–Wesley, 1980

B.3. How would you prepare this patient for surgery?

The key factor to remember when preparing this patient for surgery is to get him medically stabilized. Hyperglycemia is best controlled with regular insulin given intravenously in repeated doses or as an infusion in small doses. Hypertension may require treatment that usually can be achieved with the use of diuretics. Most diuretics will augment the already existing hypokalemia that should be treated concomitantly. Look for any evidence of congestive failure and treat it properly. Hypokalemic alkalosis predisposes to ventricular arrhythmias and may lead to a compensatory respiratory acidosis. The muscle weakness associated with hypokalemia also may contribute to hypoventilation. Therefore, hypokalemia should be adequately treated and acid–base status stabilized. Use of Cimetidine and antacids is indicated for gastric hyperacidity. Respiratory therapy should begin preoperatively. Because of upper abdominal surgery and possible massive blood transfusion, the pulmonary problems secondary to electrolyte disturbance, volume overload and truncal obesity will be further aggravated postoperatively. The patient, even though scheduled for unilateral adrenalectomy should be treated as addisonian intraoperatively and postoperatively because the normal adrenal tissue is suppressed by high levels of circulating corticosteroids. Preoperative steroids are not indicated unless the patient has been treated with cortisol inhibitors.

Katz J, Benumof J, Kadis LB: Anesthesia and Uncommon Diseases. Pathophysiologic and Clinical Correlation, pp 191–194. Philadelphia, WB Saunders, 1981

Schwartz SJ: Principles of Surgery, p 1502. New York, McGraw–Hill, 1979

C. Intraoperative Management

C.1. What anesthetic agents and technique would you employ?

Anesthesia is induced with thiopental and tracheal intubation facilitated by the use of succinylcholine. Following induction, anesthesia may be maintained with an inhalation agent or with intravenous drugs. The effects of various anesthetic agents on adrenocortical function do not provide any significant advantages or disadvantages. Adequate muscle relaxation is necessary for good exposure of the surgical field. Any of the nondepolarizing muscle relaxants may be employed.

Brown BR: Anesthesia and the Patient with Endocrine Disease. Contemporary Anesthesia Practice, p 6. Philadelphia, FA Davis, 1980

Katz J, Benumof J, Kadis LB: Anesthesia and Uncommon Diseases. Pathophysiologic and Clinical Correlation, p 195. Philadelphia, WB Saunders, 1981

Oyama T: Endocrine responses to anesthetic agents. Br J Anaesth 45:276–281, 1973

C.2. What monitors would you use for this procedure?

For this procedure we usually monitor ECG, blood pressure, urine output, heart and breath sounds using a esophageal stethoscope, temperature, and muscle relaxation with a peripheral nerve stimulator. In the severely ill patient, a radial arterial line and a central venous or pulmonary artery catheter are placed in addition to the usual monitors.

Brown BR: Anesthesia and the Patient with Endocrine Disease. Contemporary Anesthesia Practice, p 6. Philadelphia, FA Davis, 1980

C.3. What are the anesthetic considerations in this patient?

Almost all adrenalectomies at our institution are carried out through a transabdominal approach. The patient is put in the supine position, with moderate flank support on the operative side, which makes it easier for us to position the patient and reduces the risk of complications from moving the patient to other positions for surgery. The lateral decubitus or prone position may have to be employed if the lateral retroperitoneal or the posterior approach is used. In these cases, the complications from the lateral decubitus or the prone position under anesthesia should be carefully avoided. These patients require adequate muscle relaxation to afford access to the adrenal gland. Because the gland lies just beneath the diaphragm, pleura may be easily entered inadvertently. Therefore, controlled positive pressure ventilation is recommended. Massive blood transfusions may be necessary. Proper precautions in transfusion including the use of microfilters and blood warmers should be employed. Following the removal of the affected gland, the patient is essentially an addisonian because the normal tissue is already suppressed. Therefore, steroid therapy must be instituted intraoperatively and continued postoperatively. We administer 100 mg of hydrocortisone intravenously during surgery and repeat the same dose twice on the same day to a total of 300 mg. On the first postoperative day, a total of 300 mg of hydrocortisone is repeated in divided doses. Over the next 5 days, the steroids are tapered gradually to 75 mg/day of intravenous hydrocortisone, or the same dose of cortisone acetate if used intramuscularly or orally. The steroids may be given in equally divided doses or preferably in physiologic replacement schedule of $2/3$ of the daily dose in the morning and $1/3$ in the evening.

Katz J, Benumof J, Kadis LB: Anesthesia and Uncommon Diseases. Pathophysiologic and Clinical Correlation, pp 190–197. Philadelphia, WB Saunders, 1981

Martin JT: Positioning in Anesthesia and Surgery, pp 32–43, 116–141. Philadelphia, WB Saunders, 1978

Schwartz SI: Principles of Surgery, p 1502. New York, McGraw–Hill, 1979

D. Postoperative Management

D.1. *What are the possible postoperative complications in this patient?*

The possible postoperative complications include fluid and electrolyte imbalance, hyperglycemia, hypertension, pneumothorax, wound infection, pulmonary infection and atelectasis, and pancreatitis. Fluid and electrolyte imbalances are common and potassium supplements should be given to maintain normal potassium. Sodium intake should be restricted during steroid therapy. Hyperglycemia and hypertension may need to be treated. Steroid therapy should be continued in the postoperative period to prevent addisonian crisis. Pneumothorax is a potential complication due to the proximity of surgical site to the pleura. Therefore, a chest x-ray should be obtained in the recovery room. Poor wound healing and wound infection are more common. Postoperative pancreatitis due to surgical manipulation during left adrenalectomies is a serious complication. Pulmonary atelectasis and infection are more common especially when lateral decubitus position was used during surgery.

Katz J, Benumof J, Kadis LB: Anesthesia and Uncommon Diseases. Pathophysiologic and Clinical Correlation, p 196. Philadelphia, WB Saunders, 1981

Martin JT: Positioning in Anesthesia and Surgery, pp 138–140. Philadelphia, WB Saunders, 1978

Schwartz SI: Principles of Surgery, p 1503. New York, McGraw–Hill, 1979

Section Six
The Genitourinary System

22 Transurethral Resection of the Prostate

Joseph F. Artusio, Jr.

A 73-year-old man suffers from benign prostatic hyperplasia. A transurethral resection is planned. Seven months ago he suffered a myocardial infarction followed by congestive heart failure from which he recovered uneventfully. Blood pressure 150/80, pulse 88, weight 167 lbs.

A. Medical Disease and Differential Diagnosis

1. What is benign prostatic hyperplasia?
2. How would you evaluate this patient's cardiac disease? How would you determine this patient's physical status and risk for transurethral resection of the prostate?
3. Would you recommend that surgery be postponed for an extended period of time? If so, why?
4. Does the present ECG help you to make this decision?
5. What tests are needed to determine the renal status of this patient? What does each test measure and what are the normal values for each one?

B. Preoperative Evaluation and Preparation

1. What drugs would be used chronically by this patient? Which would you discontinue prior to surgery and which would you continue?
2. Some chronically used drugs are affected by the level of serum potassium. Which are they? Would the level of potassium be suspect in this patient? Why?

C. Intraoperative Management

1. What anesthetic regimen could be chosen for this patient? Why? Would you intubate this patient?

2. What intraoperative fluids would you use?
3. How may the position of this patient on the operating table affect the parameters you are measuring?
4. What is water intoxication? How does it occur? What is the significance of the fluids used to irrigate the urinary bladder?
5. How is the diagnosis of dilutional hyponatremia made? What is a significantly low serum sodium? What central nervous system effects may be observed during anesthesia?
6. How would you treat hyponatremia?
7. Does intraoperative perforation of the bladder produce any change in the monitored parameters? Why?
8. What are the causes of hypotension during TURP?
9. What are the signs of an intraoperative myocardial infarction?

D. Postoperative Management

1. What are the signs and symptoms of postoperative hyponatremia?
2: If this patient sustains a myocardial infarction postoperatively, when is it most likely to be recognized?
3. Are there any clotting defects more likely to occur following TURP?

A. Medical Disease and Differential Diagnosis

A.1. What is benign prostatic hyperplasia?

Benign prostatic hyperplasia is a tumor that originates from the periurethral tissues. Adenoleiomyofibromatosis produces symptoms of mechanical obstruction. The onset of obstruction is insidious. Nocturia is frequent and eventually, symptoms related to residual urine are present. Normally, a person voids 20 ml per second; in patients with prostatic obstruction the voiding rate is less than 5 ml per second. Acute retention of urine is the ultimate consequence of detrusor decompensation. Eventually, prostatic hyperplasia produces thickening of bladder wall, formation of vesical diverticula, ureteral dilatation, and hydronephrosis.

Schwartz, S: Principles of Surgery, p 1698. New York, McGraw–Hill, 1979

A.2. How would you evaluate this patient's cardiac disease? How would you determine this patient's physical status and risk for transurethral resection of the prostate?

The patient's cardiac disease may be evaluated by a careful history of his ability to perform simple exercises such as walking, or climbing one flight of stairs. An increase in heart rate above 140 beats/min, cardiac arrhythmia, the development of precordial pain, severe dyspnea, or extreme fatigue indicate a lack of ability to compensate for mild stress. The physical status of the patient may be determined by evaluating the effect of mild exercise and reviewing the patient's history, physical examination, and laboratory data. Using the ASA classification, each patient can be placed in a class I through V. If Goldman's "Multifactorial Index of Cardiac Risks in Noncardiac Surgical Procedures" is used, the cardiac risk index score can be obtained and the patient classified as follows: Class I, 0–5 points; Class II, 6–12 points; Class III, 13–25 points; Class IV, 26 points or more. The operative risk takes into account the physical status, but also considers the skill of the surgeon, the skill of the anesthesiologist, and the site and duration of the procedure. All these factors must be considered in determining operative risk.

Goldman L, Caldera DL, Nussbaum SR et al: Multifactorial index of cardiac risk in noncardiac surgical procedures. N Eng J Med 297:845–850, 1977

Saklad M: Grading patients for surgical procedures. Anesthesiology 2:281–284, 1941

A.3. Would you recommend that surgery be postponed for an extended period of time? If so, why?

This man suffered a documented myocardial infarction 7 months prior to the date of planned surgery. All studies agree that the incidence of reinfarction and morbidity are much higher if surgery is performed during the first 6 months following a myocardial infarction. Although 7 months have elapsed since this patient's infarction, there is still a significant incidence of reinfarction and morbidity until 2 years have elapsed between the documented infarction and the surgical procedure. It is obvious that surgery cannot be delayed that long, but if the prostatic symptoms are not too severe, and urinary back pressure has not significantly decreased urinary function, it is recommended that at least 6 months to a year elapse between the myocardial infarction and the surgical procedure. Under these circumstances, the risk of reinfarction is only 4% to 5%.

Knapp RB, Topkins MJ, Artusio JF Jr: The cerebrovascular accident and coronary occlusions in anesthesia. JAMA 182:332–334, 1962

Tarhan S et al: Myocardial infarction after general anesthesia. JAMA 200:1451–1454, 1972

Topkins MJ, Artusio JF Jr: Myocardial infarction and surgery, a five year study. Anesth Analg (Cleve) 43:716–720, 1964

A.4. Does the present ECG help you make this decision?

No. The present ECG does not help in this decision, since Q waves and T wave inversion or ST depression may be present for many months.

Braunwald E: Heart Disease, p 1333. Philadelphia, WB Saunders, 1980

A.5. What tests are needed to determine the renal status of this patient? What does each test measure and what are the normal values for each one?

The blood level of urea nitrogen and creatinine are helpful when determining the renal status of the patient. The level of creatinine is more reliable than BUN, as it is affected by diet and liver disease. If both the blood urea nitrogen and the blood creatinine are within normal limits (BUN 10–20 mg/100 ml, creatinine 0.6–1.3 mg/100 ml), it is sufficient evidence that renal status has not been significantly impaired. However, if the BUN and creatinine both are elevated, a creatinine clearance test is to be recommended. The creatinine clearance test is accomplished by 24 hr urine collection. The normal value for creatinine clearance is 95 to 140 ml/min.

Harries JD: Evaluation of renal function. ASA Refresher Courses in Anesthesiology: 4:43–44, 1976

B. Preoperative Evaluation and Preparation

B.1. What drugs would be used chronically by this patient? Which would you discontinue prior to surgery and which would you continue?

Digitalis, propranolol, furosemide, and nitroglycerine are the drugs most likely to be used chronically by this patient. All these drugs may be continued to the day scheduled for surgery. Some physicians recommend that the daily dose of digitalis be omitted on the morning of surgery to ensure against digitalis toxicity. It is also recommended that the diuretic, furosemide, be omitted on the day of surgery. Propranolol (Inderal) or clonidine should not be stopped because a severe withdrawal reaction can occur, which may result in hypertension, tachycardia, and arrhythmia.

Dripps RD et al: Introduction to Anesthesia. The Principles of Safe Practice, 5th ed, pp 28–29. Philadelphia, WB Saunders, 1977

B.2. Some chronically used drugs are affected by the level of serum potassium. Which are they? Would the level of potassium be suspect in this patient? Why?

Digitalis is the classic example where a pharmacologic effect is significantly affected by the level of serum potassium. If the serum potassium level is high, the intensity of the digitalis effect is decreased. If the potassium level is lower than normal, the digitalis action is enhanced and digitalis toxicity may result. The critical level of potassium on the high side is 7.0 mEq/L; on the low side, 2.5 mEq/L. Digitalis toxicity results in nausea, vomiting, ventricular arrhythmia, A.V. block, and ventricular fibrillation. The patient's potassium level might be low from diuretic therapy for congestive heart failure.

Gilman AG, Goodman LS, Gilman A: Goodman and Gilman's Basis of Therapeutics, 6th ed, p 755. New York, Macmillan, 1980

C. Intraoperative Management

C.1. What anesthetic regimen could be chosen for this patient? Why? Would you intubate this patient?

Due to the location of the planned surgery (TURP), general or regional anesthesia are definite considerations as anesthetic techniques of choice. The case to support the choice of subarachnoid or epidural analgesia includes the following:

- Minimal disturbance to respiration when the level of analgesia is at T_9
- Analgesia to pin prick to T_9 produces sufficient sympathetic blockade to produce vasodilatation in the lower extremities. This results in an increase in the peripheral vascular bed and permits an increase in vascular volume without increasing venous return to the right heart.

The case that is made against using regional anesthesia highlights the potential danger of an inadvertently high spinal anesthesia. This results in total sympathetic blockade, thereby producing a sharp fall in blood pressure. Even a relatively brief fall in cardiac output, which decreases coronary perfusion, may result in a hypoxic insult to this myocardium that already has a compromised coronary circulation.

A general anesthetic provides a state free from the anxiety which is frequently encountered during a regional anesthetic. A nonflammable inhalation anesthetic provides the anesthesiologist with easy control of the depth of anesthesia, which can be regulated moment to moment during the changing sensory input associated with TURP. Because the rate pressure product is a good guide to use when estimating the oxygen demands of the myocardium, inhalation anesthesia can be used to control the systolic blood pressure and heart rate.

Inhalation anesthesia also produces a controllable peripheral dilatation that will increase the vascular bed and act as a buffer to prevent heart failure from fluid overload. However, if the anesthesiologist attempts to dilate the peripheral vascular bed by general anesthesia, he must be aware that simultaneous myocardial depression will occur. If general anesthesia is chosen for this patient, we do not favor a narcotic or neurolept technique because sensory blockade may be inadequate and may result in hypertension and tachycardia. An increase in heart rate and systolic blood pressure produces an increased oxygen demand by myocardial muscle, which cannot be met by this compromised coronary circulation.

The anesthesiologist should decide whether or not to intubate this patient. The ease of airway management in this patient, the anesthesiologist's own familiarity with general anesthesia by mask, will enter into this decision. In general, however, we recommend intubation to ensure a patent and unobstructed airway. The endotracheal tube also allows the anesthesiologist more freedom to care for fluid replacement. In addition, the endotracheal tube, if properly placed and attended, helps to prevent gastric aspiration into the tracheobronchial tree and gastric inflation during assisted or controlled respiration.

C.2. What intraoperative fluids would you use?

The volume of fluids necessary during the surgical procedure will be determined primarily by the state of the patient's fluid balance prior to surgery. During the operation, particularly in this patient with a previous myocardial infarction, intravenous fluids should be kept to a minimum. Even when the surgeon is careful to remove the prostate without cutting close to the capsule or actually perforating the capsule, it is impossible not to open large venous sinuses. As the hydrostatic pressure of the irrigation fluids entering the bladder is higher than the venous pressure, isotonic glycerine solution enters the circulation. This additional fluid constitutes a water load for the patient. A dilutional effect will occur and will decrease electrolyte concentration. Serum sodium may be lowered significantly. To prevent this, any intravenous fluids administered to the patient should contain sodium, but over zealous administration of sodium may hold the fluid in the vascular space and precipitate cardiac failure. Serial determinations of serum sodium will serve as a guide for intelligent administration.

Katz J, Benumof J, Kadis LB: Anesthesia and Uncommon Diseases: Pathophysiologic and Clinical Correlations, 2nd ed, pp 431–432. Philadelphia, WB Saunders, 1981

C.3. How may the position of this patient on the operating table affect the parameters you are measuring?

In order to accomplish this surgical procedure, the patient is placed in the dorsal lithotomy position. The elevation of the legs effectively adds a 600 ml fluid load to the central circulation as the lower extremities are drained of blood. This additional fluid load occurs under spinal, epidural, and general anesthesia, and the extra volume in a smaller vascular space may be sufficient to produce an inordinate circulatory load in this patient with a previously damaged myocardium. Cardiac failure may ensue. A central venous pressure monitor will aid in determining the effect of position on the right side of the heart. To help minimize this volume effect the head and torso of the patient can be elevated to decrease the full impact of the added venous return.

Glenn F et al: Surgery in the Aged, p 65. New York, McGraw–Hill, 1960

C.4. What is water intoxication? How does it occur? What is the significance of the fluids used to irrigate the urinary bladder?

Although we have alluded to the problem in a previous question, water intoxication is caused by the entrance of the irrigating solution into venous sinuses of the resected prostatic bed. The hydrostatic pressure of the irrigating solution is greater than the venous pressure and isotonic glycerine solution enters the venous side of the circulation and expands the intravascular volume. The irrigating fluid, being devoid of electrolytes, dilutes the serum and can produce rather severe electrolyte disturbance. The quantity of water that enters the circulation is a function of how many venous sinuses are open and the total time of prostatic resection. Although this isotonic solution (5% glycerine) does not change the tonicity of the blood, it does dilute the blood electrolytes. The glycerine itself has little or no physiological effect, and is used because its refractive index allows good vision for prostatic resection. In the early days of prostatic resection, plain water was used as the irrigating fluid. Because it was hypotonic when it entered the circulation, it produced significant hemolysis.

Katz J, Benumof J, Kadis LB: Anesthesia and Uncommon Diseases: Pathophysiologic and Clinical Correlations, 2nd ed, p 109. Philadelphia, WB Saunders, 1981

Marx GF, Orkin LR: Complications associated with transurethral surgery. Anesthesiology 23:802–813, 1962

C.5. How is the diagnosis of dilutional hyponatremia made? What is a significant low serum sodium? What central nervous system effects may be observed during anesthesia?

It may be difficult to determine the prodromal stage of hyponatremia during the surgical procedure, particularly if the surgery is being done under general anesthesia. The only sign of impending difficulty may be a rising venous pressure, indicating that a significant amount of fluid is entering the circulation. If the TURP is done under spinal or epidural anesthesia, irritability, restlessness, and confusion of the patient may be an early symptom of dilutional hyponatremia. Aasheim outlines some of the signs of dilutional hyponatremia at various levels of serum sodium.

- With regional anesthesia, restlessness is an early symptom and may be associated with irritability and confusion. A serum sodium of 120 mEq/L appears to be borderline between mild and severe reactions.
- Hypotension and tachycardia
- ECG changes characterized by widening of the QRS complex and ST segment elevation when serum sodium is 102 mEq/L (approx)
- Seizures occur at serum sodium of 102 mEq/L (approx)
- Ventricular tachycardia or fibrillation may occur at serum sodium of 100 mEq/L or less.

Aasheim GM: Hyponatremia during transurethral surgery. Can Anaesth Soc J 20:274–280, 1973

C.6. How would you treat hyponatremia?

Early detection leads to the most successful treatment. When the diagnosis is made by symptoms and confirmed by a low serum sodium level, the procedure should be terminated and anesthesia discontinued. A prompt diuresis usually ensues. Diuretics may be used to decrease the water load and sodium given until serum sodium determinations show a return toward the normal serum sodium level of 140 mEq/L.

Aasheim GM: Hyponatremia during transurethral surgery. Can Anaesth Soc J 20:274–280, 1973

C.7. Does intraoperative perforation of the bladder produce any change in the monitored parameters? Why?

Perforation of the urinary bladder may go unnoticed under general anesthesia. However, an increase in blood pressure and tachycardia are usually seen. A sudden fall in blood pressure may occur. Occasionally, suprapubic fullness and abdominal wall spasm may be observed.

The patient under regional anesthesia may complain of abdominal and shoulder pain from diaphragmatic irritation.

Marx GF, Orkin LR: Complications associated with transurethral surgery. Anesthesiology 23:802–813, 1962

C.8. What are the causes of hypotension during TURP?

- Deep general anesthesia or high spinal or epidural anesthesia
- Inadequate blood volume due to the following:
  - Use of diuretics preoperatively
  - Bleeding. Obvious or occult DIC or platelet consumption
- Fluid overload, if cardiac failure ensues
- Bladder perforation may cause hypotension, but usually there is an increase in blood pressure
- Sepsis
- Intraoperative myocardial infarction

Marx GF, Orkin LR: Complications associated with transurethral surgery. Anesthesiology 23:802–813, 1962

C.9. What are the signs of an intraoperative myocardial infarction?

An intraoperative myocardial infarction may be totally silent or may be called to the attention of the anesthesiologist by a sudden fall in blood pressure. The sudden fall in blood pressure may be accompanied by tachycardia which is indistinguishable from the hypovolemic hypotension resulting from acute blood loss.

The electrocardiogram is a good monitor of the adequacy of the coronary circulation. By recording a simulated V-5 lead, one can observe for J point depression and ST segment changes. The depression of ST segments from base-lines (depressed J point) with up sloping of ST segments suggests ischemia. J point depression with down sloping of ST segments reflects definite ischemia. When the ischemia becomes subendocardial it is manifested by inverted T waves. This may be the only thing seen during the surgical procedure. ST-segment elevations of greater than 1.0 mm are considered significant signs of severe transmural myocardial ischemia. Only the appearance of Q waves more than 0.03 seconds in width is diagnostic of definite myocardial infarction. However, the Q waves usually appear postoperatively instead of intraoperatively. No change in blood pressure may be apparent, but in the third to the seventh postoperative day, a reinfarction picture may become quite obvious. Postoperative measurements of the myocardial isoenzymes of creatine phosphokinase (CPK–MB) may confirm the diagnosis. Although this patient was not monitored by a pulmonary artery balloon tip catheter, it would have allowed measurements of the magnitude and shape of the pulmonary capillary wedge pressure. When the pulmonary pressure rises coronary perfusion pressue and thus the oxygen supply may fall significantly. In addition, high pulmonary wedge pressure signifies the distended heart with increased oxygen demand. Large "A" waves in the pulmonary capillary wedge pressure wave form indicate an uncompliant left ventricle. Large V waves indicate mitral regurgitation from ventricular dysfunction. These are the signs of impending or existing ischemia. Diuretic therapy under these conditions is vitally important to decrease the distension of the heart and decrease the oxygen demand.

Kaplan JA: Cardiac Anesthesia, pp 151–155. New York, Grune & Stratton, 1979

D. Postoperative Management

D.1. What are the signs and symptoms of postoperative hyponatremia?

Occasionally, hyponatremia is not suspected until the patient arrives in the recovery room, particularly if the surgery has been done under general anesthesia. Unlike the usual emergence from general anesthesia, the patient may emerge confused and may even mimic the effects of an intraoperative cerebrovascular accident.

Aasheim GM: Hyponatremia during transurethral surgery. Can Anaesth Soc J 20:274–280, 1973

D.2. If this patient sustains a myocardial infarction postoperatively, when is it most likely to be recognized?

The recognition of a postoperative myocardial infarction occurs most frequently in the first 3 postoperative days. It may be recognized as late as the 21st postoperative day or as early as the same day of operation.

Miller R et al: Anesthesia, surgery and myocardial infarction: A review. Anesthesiology Review 6, No. 1:14–20, 1979

D.3. Are there any clotting defects more likely to occur following TURP?

Very few clotting defects occur following TURP because all of the irrigating fluid that is used today is isotonic. However, if a large amount of bank blood is used, a dilutional thrombocytopenia is the most frequent finding. Rarely a consumption coagulopathy such as primary fibrinolysis occurs.

Marx GF, Orkin LR: Complications associated with transurethral surgery. Anesthesiology 23:802–813, 1962

23 Kidney Transplant
Fun-Sun F. Yao

A 35-year-old man with a long-standing history of chronic glomerulonephritis had end-stage renal disease (ESRD). He had been on hemodialysis for 3 years. He was scheduled for emergency renal transplantation using a cadaver kidney.

A. Medical Disease and Differential Diagnosis

1. What are the common etiologies of chronic renal failure?
2. What are the common problems related to ESRD?
3. What hemoglobin level would you expect to find in this patient? Why?
4. What is the oxygen carrying capacity? How can you improve it?
5. How do uremic patients compensate for anemia? Are there any changes in 2,3-DPG levels?
6. When are you going to transfuse the patient? What kind of blood would you use? Why?
7. What kind of bleeding disorder would you expect?
8. Do these patients have electrolyte imbalances? Discuss Na, K, Mg, Ca, P, and CO_2 content.
9. How would you treat the hyperkalemia?
10. When would you correct the metabolic acidosis? What are the dangers of overzealous correction?
11. Discuss the cardiovascular disorders of ESRD and their treatment.
12. What are the problems related to chronic hemodialysis?

B. Preoperative Evaluation and Preparation

1. What medication might the patient have been receiving? What steroid preparation would you order?

2. What preoperative work-up would you order?
3. What are the normal values of BUN, serum creatinine, and creatinine clearance?
4. How would you differentiate prerenal, renal, and postrenal oliguria?

C. Intraoperative Management

1. What premedication would you choose? Why?
2. What anesthesia equipment and monitors would you use? Why?
3. How would you conduct the anesthesia induction?
4. Is succinylcholine dangerous for this patient?
5. What anesthetic agents would you use for maintenance? Discuss the advantages and disadvantages of inhalation and intravenous agents.
6. What percentage of the halogenated inhalation anesthetics are metabolized in the body? What concentrations of inorganic fluoride would you consider nephrotoxic?
7. Would you consider using regional anesthesia? Why?
8. What muscle relaxants would you choose? Discuss the excretion of d-tubocurarine, pancuronium, and gallamine.
9. How would you handle intraoperative fluid therapy?
10. At the end of surgery, the patient is apneic. What are you going to do?
11. How much neostigmine would you use? Are there any limits? Why?
12. What are the other unusual situations that cause prolonged neuromuscular blockade?
13. What is apneic oxygenation? Who did the pioneer study?

D. Postoperative Management

1. What are the early postoperative complications?
2. How would you make the diagnosis of rejection?

A. Medical Disease and Differential Diagnosis

A.1. What are the common etiologies of chronic renal failure?

The common causes of chronic renal failure are glomerulonephritis, pyelonephritis, polycystic kidney, and some systemic diseases such as diabetes mellitus, malignant hypertension, lupus erythematosus, vasculitis, Wegener's granulomatosis, and congenital anomalies. Generally, the particular cause of chronic renal failure has little effect on the decisions of anesthesiologists or surgeons.

Isselbacher KJ, Adams RD, Braunwald E et al: Harrison's Principles of Internal Medicine, 9th ed, pp 1299–1307. New York, McGraw–Hill, 1980

A.2. What are the common problems related to end-stage renal disease?

The common problems are the following:
- Anemia
- Coagulopathies
- Electrolyte imbalance and acidosis
- Hypertension
- Treatment with steroids and immunosuppressants
- Psychological factors
- Chronic hemodialysis

Zauder HL: Anesthesia for patients who have terminal renal disease. ASA Refresher Courses in Anesthesiology 4:163–173, 1976

A.3. What hemoglobin level would you expect to find in this patient? Why?

It is not uncommon for uremic patients to have hemoglobin concentrations of 5 to 7 g/100 ml, corresponding to hematocrits of 15% to 25%. Erythropoiesis is depressed in ESRD, due both to the effects of retained toxins on bone marrow and to diminished biosynthesis of erythropoietin by the diseased kidney.

Isselbacher KJ et al: Harrison's Principles of Internal Medicine, 9th ed, pp 1299–1307. New York, McGraw–Hill, 1980

A.4. What is the oxygen carrying capacity? How can you improve it?

The oxygen carrying capacity is equivalent to the oxygen content, which consists of the amount of oxygen carried by hemoglobin and dissolved oxygen in plasma. O_2 content (ml/100ml blood) = 1.34 × Hb × O_2 saturation + 0.0031 × PaO_2. Normal oxygen content is 20.3 ml/100 ml blood. Dissolved oxygen, 0.3 ml/100 ml blood, normally is only 1.5% of the total oxygen content, but in severely anemic patients with a hemoglobin of 5 g%, the dissolved oxygen is 4.5% of the total oxygen content in room air. If the patient breathes 100% oxygen, the PaO_2 is normally over 600 torr. The dissolved oxygen will be 1.86 ml/100 ml blood, which is 21.7% of the total oxygen content. This is why a high inspired oxygen concentration during anesthesia can significantly increase the oxygen carrying capacity. We can improve the oxygen carrying capacity by increasing hemoglobin, oxygen saturation, and oxygen tension.

Shapiro BA, Harrison RA, Walton JR: Clinical Application of Blood Gases, 2nd ed, p 83. Chicago, Year Book Medical Publishers, 1977

A.5. How do uremic patients compensate for anemia? Are there any changes in 2,3-DPG levels?

The oxygen carrying capacity is decreased to less than half normal. This is tolerated because of increased cardiac output. Although the 2,3-DPG is significantly higher in patients with renal disease than in normal subjects, it is below that expected for the degree of anemia present.

Zauder HL: Anesthesia for patients who have terminal renal disease. ASA Refresher Courses in Anesthesiology 4:163–173, 1976

A.6. When are you going to transfuse the patient? What kind of blood would you use? Why?

Well controlled uremic patients usually tolerate hematocrits of 15% to 25% very well. Preoperative transfusion is usually not indicated. However, recent information demonstrated an association between recipients having received pretransplantation blood transfusions and an improved allograft survival. Patients with no blood transfusions have a particularly poor prognosis. The reasons for this association are unknown. We agree that transfusions are not contraindicated in dialysis or potential transplant patients and that blood should be administered as necessary, such as for hypotension from blood loss or a hematocrit below 15%. When indicated, packed, washed red cells (leukocyte-poor blood) are transfused, because the introduction of leukocytic antigens may induce production of additional antibodies, predisposing to rejection of a subsequently implanted kidney.

Cuttmann RD: Renal Transplantation. N Engl J Med 301:975–982, 1038–1048, 1979

A.7. What kind of bleeding disorder would you expect?

Although the platelet count is often low, the primary effect is platelet dysfunction. Prolonged bleeding time, decreased platelet adhesiveness, and abnormal prothrombin consumption and thromboplastin generation are the clinical manifestations of platelet dysfunction. Increased plasma levels of guanidinosuccinic acid cause a decline in platelet factor 3 availability, thereby inhibiting secondary platelet aggregation. Hemodialysis effectively eliminates the offending compounds and usually restores adequate platelet function.

Isselbacher KJ et al: Harrison's Principles of Internal Medicine, 9th ed, pp 1299–1307. New York, McGraw-Hill, 1980

A.8. Do these patients have electrolyte imbalances? Discuss Na, K, Mg, Ca, P, and CO_2 content.

Hyponatremia is usually found in uremic patients and is due to urinary loss, salt restriction, vomiting, and diarrhea. Serum potassium may rise to dangerous levels when oliguria supervenes and urinary output falls below 500 to 1000 ml daily in patients with renal decompensation. Hypermagnesemia is not uncommon, although this is usually controlled by dialysis. Hypermagnesemia may enhance the effects of neuromuscular blocking agents. Phosphate is excreted by glomerular filtration. As the glomerular filtration rate diminishes, phosphate is retained, thereby depressing the serum calcium level. Meanwhile, absorption of calcium from the gastrointestinal tract is impaired. Both protein bond and ionized calcium are reduced in uremic patients. Moderate metabolic acidosis is frequently present because the kidneys are unable to excrete hydrogen ions.

Isselbacher KJ et al: Harrison's Principles of Internal Medicine, 9th ed, Chap. 276. New York, McGraw–Hill, 1980

A.9. How would you treat the hyperkalemia?

No patient should be anesthetized who has a serum K^+ in excess of 5.5 mEq/L. Hyperkalemia should be controlled by dialysis prior to operation. Serial electrolyte determinations should be taken during the operative procedure. Should a significant increase in potassium occur, 50 ml of 50% glucose and 50 mEq $NaHCO_3$ may be given to a 70 kg patient to shift extracellular potassium intracellularly. One half to 1.0 g of calcium gluconate or calcium chloride may be given to counteract the effect of hyperkalemia on the myocardial conduction system. One unit of insulin for every 2 to 5 g glucose should be given for a diabetic patient. If possible, patients should undergo preoperative dialysis 12–24 hours before anesthesia and surgery.

Vandam LD: To make the patient ready for anesthesia, pp 97–99. Menlo Park, CA, Addison–Wesley Publishing Co, 1980

A.10. When would you correct the metabolic acidosis? What are the dangers of overzealous correction?

Moderate metabolic acidosis (HCO_3^- of 10–20 mEq/L) is frequently seen in uremia and may not require correction. More severe acidosis (pH below 7.20) reflects a need for repeated dialysis. If dialysis is not possible because of the emergency nature of the surgical procedure, sodium bicarbonate therapy is indicated. We tend to correct the extracellular base deficit only. HCO_3^- required = 0.2 × body weight (kg) × base deficit. Only half of the calculated HCO_3^- is given. Repeated HCO_3^- analyses are critical to titrate the amount of HCO_3^- needed for each patient. Overzealous use of $NaHCO_3$ may cause volume overload, precipitation of tetany in uremic patients with preexisting hypocalcemia, and overshoot alkalosis.

Vandam LD: To make the patient ready for anesthesia, Chapter 4. Menlo Park, CA, Addison–Wesley Publishing Co, 1980

A.11. Discuss the cardiovascular disorders of ESRD and their treatment.

Hypertension is almost always present at some stage of chronic renal failure. In the majority of patients, hypertension is the result of fluid overload. Adequate dialysis, sodium depletion, and fluid restriction usually control hypertension in this group. In a few patients, plasma renin levels are very high and potent antihypertensive drugs such as methyldopa, propranolol, hydralazine, or guanethidine may be needed. Congestive heart failure, pulmonary edema, pericarditis, and pericardial effusion may exist in uremic patients.

Isselbacher KJ et al: Harrison's Principles of Internal Medicine, 9th ed, Chapter 276. New York, McGraw–Hill, 1980

A.12. What are the problems related to chronic hemodialysis?

Hepatitis B may be found in 19% to 50% of patients. Plasma cholinesterase levels were significantly depressed when the relatively crude cellophane membranes were used. The newer types of membranes now in use apparently cause less decrease in pseudocholinesterase levels. Prolonged apnea due to reduced pseudocholinesterase titers has not been any more prevalent in patients with ESRD than in the general population.

Desmond JW, Gordon RA: The effect of hemodialysis on blood volume and plasma cholinesterase levels. Can Anesth Soc J 16:292–301, 1969

Lutterman RD: Renal transplantation. N Engl J Med 301:1038–1048, 1979

B. Preoperative Evaluation and Preparation

B.1. What medication might the patient have been receiving? What steroid preparation would you order?

Transplant recipients might have been receiving steroids or immunosuppressants. Steroids should be given to prevent rejection and possible adrenal insufficiency secondary to chronic administration of steroids. The usual preoperative preparation is hydrocortisone phosphate 100 mg IV at 10 p.m. the night before surgery, 6 a.m. the morning of surgery, and before the induction of anesthesia. If emergency surgery is required, we usually give 300 mg hydrocortisone phosphate or 100 mg methylprednisolone (Solu-Medrol) before the induction of anesthesia. It is recommended that the total dose of hydrocortisone on the day of operation should be approximately 300 mg/24 hr. Thereafter, the total dose is reduced approximately 20% per day until replacement levels are reached.

Vandam LD: To make the patient ready for anesthesia, p 125. Menlo Park, CA, Addison–Wesley Publishing Co, 1980

B.2. What preoperative work-up would you order?

In addition to the routine systemic tests such as ECG, chest radiograph, blood counts, urinalysis, electrolytes, blood sugar, BUN, creatinine, platelet count, prothrombin time, partial thrombin time, SGOT, SGPT, bilirubin, albumin, and globulin, we would like to have arterial blood gases to determine the acid–base balance.

B.3. What are the normal values of BUN, serum creatinine, and creatinine clearance?

Normal BUN is 10 to 20 mg/100 ml. Normal serum creatinine is 0.6 to 1.3 mg/100 ml. Normal values for creatinine clearance are 85 to 125 ml/min for women and 95 to 140 ml/min for men (average 120 ml/min).

Vandam LD: To make the patient ready for anesthesia. In Renal System, pp 64–111. Menlo Park CA, Addison–Wesley Publishing Co, 1980

B.4. How would you differentiate prerenal, renal, and postrenal oliguria?

The diagnosis of postrenal obstruction is characteristically established by complete anuria, as opposed to the oliguria found in patients with hypovolemic and acute tubular necrosis. It must be emphasized that all collection tubing should be checked to be sure it is properly connected, patent, and not kinked.

Careful examination of urine sediment is of major importance in determining the cause of oliguria. The presence of renal tubular cells, casts, and many pigmented granular casts is strong evidence of acute tubular necrosis. A normal sediment suggests a diagnosis of hypovolemic prerenal failure. In prerenal hypovolemic oliguria, there is a decrease in glomerular filtration and an increase in water, sodium, and urea reabsorption, resulting in concentration of nonresorbable solute. Usually urine sodium is less than 20 mEq/L; urine:plasma creatinine is greater than 30; BUN:serum creatinine is greater than 20. The response to mannitol is brisk when blood pressure and hydration are adequate. In renal failure, the nephrons that continue to function do so in a state of osmotic diuresis. Creatinine is not concentrated in urine. BUN and serum creatinine are both increased and their ratio is normal, 10 to 1, because the urea reabsorption is not potentiated. Mannitol is uniformly ineffective in promoting diuresis (Table 23–1).

Bastron RD: Pathophysiology of acute renal failure. ASA Refresher Courses in Anesthesiology 8:1–12, 1980

Harries JD: Evaluation of renal function. ASA Refresher Courses in Anesthesiology 4:39–50, 1976

Table 23–1. Differentiation of prerenal and renal failure

	PRERENAL	RENAL
Urinary sediment	Normal	Tubular cells, casts
Urinary specific gravity	>1.014	1.005–1.014
Urinary osmolality (mOsm/kg)	> 400	< 350
Urinary Na (mEq/L)	< 20	> 20
Urine: plasma creatinine ratio	> 30	< 20
BUN: serum creatinine ratio	> 20	< 20
Mannitol response	Brisk	None

C. Intraoperative Management

C.1. What premedication would you choose? Why?

Numerous combinations of sedatives, tranquilizers, and narcotics, with or without vagolytic agents, have been used satisfactorily. We usually give pentobarbitol (Nembutol) 100 mg and atropine 0.4 mg intramuscularly one hour prior to surgery for a 70 kg patient. Pentobarbitol will achieve adequate sedation without significant respiratory and circulatory depression. Atropine is to prevent a vagal reflex from tracheal intubation.

C.2. What anesthesia equipment and monitors would you use? Why?

Because of a high incidence of serum hepatitis from chronic hemodialysis and low resistance to infection from steroid and immunosuppresant therapy, a sterile disposable anesthetic circuit, endotracheal tube, and laryngoscope are used to prevent cross infection from patient to patient. The anesthesiologist is required to use gloves and gown to protect the patient and himself. We routinely monitor blood pressure, use a precordial or esophageal stethoscope, monitor rectal or esophageal temperature, and record electrocardiography and central venous pressure. Electrolytes, blood gases, and hematocrit are determined when necessary. Sudden increase in body temperature is an important sign of superacute rejection of the transplanted kidney. Unless there is evidence of left ventricular failure, we do not recommend pulmonary wedge pressure monitoring. Simple central venous pressure monitoring is usually enough to guide the fluid therapy.

C.3. How would you conduct the anesthesia induction?

Anesthesia is usually induced with an ultra-short-acting barbiturate, such as thiopental 250 mg for a 70 kg patient. Succinylcholine is used to facilitate endotracheal intubation.

C.4. Is succinylcholine dangerous for this patient?

When serum potassium is within the normal range, 3.5–5.0 mEq/L, a regular clinical dose of succinylcholine may be used without difficulty. Potassium flux after administration of succinylcholine in patients with renal failure does not differ from that seen in patients with normal renal function. The mean maximal increase in serum potassium was 0.5 mEq/L. When serum potassium is close to or above 5.5 mEq/L, we try to avoid succinylcholine. The pseudocholinesterase levels were significantly depressed when the relatively crude cellophane membranes were used for hemodialysis, but the newer types of membranes now in use cause less decrease in pseudocholinesterase. Prolonged apnea due to reduced pseudocholinesterase has not been any more prevalent than in the general population.

Desmond JW, Gordon RA: The effect of hemodialysis on blood volume and plasma cholinesterase levels. Can Anesth Soc J 16:292–301, 1969

Koide M, Ward BE: Serum potassium concentration after succinylcholine in patients with renal failure. Anesthesiology 36:142–145, 1972

C.5. What anesthetic agents would you use for maintenance? Discuss the advantages and disadvantages of inhalation and intravenous agents.

We use N_2O-O_2 with neuroleptic agents (fentanyl–droperidol) when the anemia is not severe enough to seriously impair the oxygen carrying capacity. Narcotic agents do not depress cardiac and renal function, whereas most potent inhalation agents do. More muscle relaxants may be needed since narcotic agents offer no muscle relaxation. Using a narcotic technique, a high concentration of N_2O is needed to keep the patient unconscious. Therefore, very high concentrations of oxygen cannot be given to improve oxygen carrying capacity by increasing the dissolved oxygen. However, blood transfusion is not contraindicated in transplant patients, and oxygen carrying capacity can be most effectively improved by transfusion of packed red cells. Halothane–oxygen sequence has also been used successfully. The very high concentration of oxygen increases oxygen carrying capacity significantly in those patients with severe anemia. Inhalation agents provide a steady depth of anesthesia, but halothane depresses the cardiovascular system and may cause hepatic dysfunction. We rarely use halothane because of a high incidence of serum hepatitis in those patients under chronic hemodialysis. Enflurane is avoided for renal transplantation, even though the biotransformation of enflurane with liberation of inorganic fluoride is low. Postoperative transplant renal failure has been reported with the use of enflurane.

Methoxyflurane is contraindicated because of a high concentration of free fluoride from biotransformation. For surgery other than renal transplantation, methoxyflurane is a good choice for the anephric patient because the target organ of nephrotoxicity is absent. Isoflurane has very little biotransformation (only 0.2%). This is a relatively new agent and it may become the ideal agent for this kind of patient. Ether and cyclopropane are explosive and have been virtually abandoned.

Zauder HL: Anesthesia for patients who have terminal renal disease. ASA Refresher Courses in Anesthesiology 4:163–173, 1976

C.6. What percentage of the halogenated inhalation anesthetics are metabolized in the body? What concentrations of inorganic fluoride would you consider nephrotoxic?

Isoflurane, 0.2%; enflurane, 2%; halothane, 12%–20%; and methoxyflurane, 20% to 40% are metabolized in the body (rule of 2). When serum inorganic fluoride reaches 50 to 80 μMol/L, subclinical renal toxicity (laboratory abnormalities) occurs. Clinical nephotoxicity usually becomes apparent when serum fluoride is over 80 μMol/L. The high output renal failure is dose-related and characterized by vasopressin–resistant polyuria, hypernatremia, serum hyperosmolarity, increased serum urea nitrogen, and inorganic fluoride concentration.

Cohen EN: Metabolism of the volatile anesthetics. ASA Refresher Courses in Anesthesiology 5:21–32, 1977

Mazze RI: Renal toxicity of anesthetics. ASA Refresher Courses in Anesthesiology 1:85–99, 1973

C.7. Would you consider using regional anesthesia? Why?

Because of possible uremic neuropathy and coagulopathy, epidural or spinal anesthesia is not recommended at Cornell Medical Center. Regional anesthesia has been used successfully for transplantation.

Zauder HL: Anesthesia for patients who have terminal renal disease. ASA Refresher Courses in Anesthesiology 4:163–173, 1976

C.8. What muscle relaxants would you choose? Discuss the excretion of d-tubocurarine, pancuronium, and gallamine.

We prefer to use d-tubocurarine. Both d-tubocurarine and pancuronium have been used widely in the presence of renal failure. Both drugs are eliminated in large part by glomerular filtration and to a lesser extent by biotransformation and biliary excretion. The elimination of both drugs is reduced in renal failure, so the duration of blockade is prolonged. The elimination half-life of pancuronium is prolonged by more than 95%, compared with 43% for d-tubocurarine. This difference has been attributed to a greater capacity for biliary excretion of d-tubocurarine in the presence of renal failure, but this has not been proven. We try to use muscle relaxants as little as possible. The use of a peripheral nerve stimulator is recommended to adjust drug dosage to clinical needs, to assist in avoiding overdose, and to help in evaluating reversal of neuromuscular blockade. Both decamethonium and gallamine are almost quantitatively excreted by the kidney. Their use in aphrenic patients is contraindicated.

Ham J: Factors affecting administration of nondepolarizing neuromuscular blocking agents. ASA Refresher Courses in Anesthesiology 8:61–78, 1980

Miller RD: Reversal of neuromuscular blockade. ASA Refresher Courses in Anesthesiology 5:125–136, 1977

C.9. How would you handle intraoperative therapy?

Central venous pressure monitoring is routinely used to guide fluid therapy. Fluid restriction is essential, but volumes used should be sufficient to replace insensible water loss. Balanced salt solutions are used to replace the estimated volume of sequestered fluid, while 5% dextrose in water is used to replace water loss. Buffy coat poor packed red cells may be transfused to replace blood loss. Hemodialysis can be used effectively to remove excess fluid postoperatively.

Zauder HL: Anesthesia for patients who have terminal renal disease. ASA Refresher Courses in Anesthesiology 4:163–173, 1976

C.10. At the end of surgery, the patient is apneic. What are you going to do?

The possible causes of apnea must be identified and specific treatment established accordingly. Apnea may result from central depression or peripheral neuromuscular blockade. The respiratory center may be depressed by hypocarbia and anesthetics, including both inhalational and intravenous agents such as narcotics and barbiturates. Peripheral blockade is usually the result of residual muscular relaxants. Hypocarbia can be corrected by hypoventilation with high inspired oxygen concentration to prevent hypoxia. When respiration is depressed by narcotics, the pupils are usually miotic. Naloxone in 0.1 mg increments may be titrated to reverse narcotic depression. Potent inhalation agents should be terminated to decrease respiratory depression.

Neuromuscular blockade can be evaluated with a peripheral nerve stimulator. Nondepolarizing blockade is characterized by fade from single twitch stimulations and tetanic stimulation and by posttetanic facilitation. Neostigmine or pyridostigmine may be given with atropine to reverse the blockade. Normally, neostigmine and atropine can be administered concomitantly because the vagolitic effects of atropine precede the cardiac muscarinic effects of neostigmine by 1 to 2 minutes. However, in cardiac patients or in patients with electrolyte or acid–base imbalance, we recommend careful titration of atropine in 0.1 to 0.2 mg increments and neostigmine in 0.25 to 0.5 mg increments in separate syringes, to keep the heart rate change within 10% to 15% of its control value. Cardiac response to atropine and neostigmine may be unpredictable in patients with irritable hearts or electrolyte imbalance. Sinus arrest and severe tachycardia have been experienced by those patients after concomitant administration of atropine and neostigmine.

Miller RD: Anesthesia, pp 1345–1347. New York, Churchill–Livingstone, 1981

C.11. How much neostigmine would you use? Are there any limits? Why?

The dose of neostigmine depends on the intensity of the neuromuscular blockade, which is determined by the total amount of muscle relaxant given, the frequency of administration, and the time of the last dose. Usually 1.5–3.0 mg of neostigmine will antagonize most nondepolarizing blocks in the average adult patients. If the blockade is not reversed adequately, a total dose of up to 5 mg may be given. Larger doses of neostigmine may reinforce the neuromuscular blockade by causing its own nondepolarizing blockade. Other unusual situations have to be studied.

Miller RD: Reversal of neuromuscular blockade. ASA Refresher Courses in Anesthesiology 5:125–136, 1977

C.12. What are the other unusual situations that cause prolonged neuromuscular blockade?

- Electrolyte imbalance
  - Hypokalemia and hypernatremia may increase the transmembrane potential and postjunctional membrane threshold for depolarization, and thus increase the action of a nondepolarizing muscle relaxant. However, the increase of transmembrane potentials also increases release of neurotransmitter from the nerve terminal, and decreases the action of a nondepolarizing relaxant. Clinically, the net effect is unpredictable.
  - Hypermagnesemia enhances the action of a nondepolarizing relaxant by decreasing the release of acetylcholine from the nerve terminal and reducing the sensitivity of the postjunctional membrane to acetylcholine.
  - Calcium has various effects at the neuromuscular junction. It enhances the release of acetylcholine from the nerve terminal, decreases the sensitivity of the postjunctional membrane to acetylcholine, and enhances excitation–contraction coupling in the muscle. Calcium appears to be effective in antagonizing neuromuscular blockade associated with muscle relaxants, magnesium, and antibiotics.
- Acid–base imbalance
  - Respiratory acidosis enhances the nondepolarizing relaxants.
  - The effects of respiratory alkalosis, metabolic alkalosis, and metabolic acidosis are inconsistent.
- Drug interactions
  - Antibiotics. Certain antibiotics, alone or in combination with nondepolarizing relaxants, cause apnea by neuromuscular blockade. The aminoglycosides (neomycin, gentamycin, kanamycin, and streptomycin), as well as tetracycline, decrease acetylcholine release by blocking the influx of calcium ions necessary for transmitter release. Penicillin V, erythromycin, clindamycin, polymyxin, and tetracycline produce partial paralysis by directly decreasing muscle contractility. Paromomycin, viomycin, colistin, lincomycin, amikacin, and netilmicin also produce neuromuscular blockade.
  - Local anesthetics. Both the ester and amide types of local anesthetics enhance the effects of d-tubocurarine. In addition, local anesthetics directly depress the respiratory center.
  - Antiarrhythmic agents. Lidocaine, procainamide, and quinidine enhance the effects of d-tubocurarine.

- Furosemide (Lasix) enhances d-tubocurarine by inhibiting the cyclic AMP system and reducing neurotransmitter output.
- Ketamine enhances the effects of d-tubocurarine, but not pancuronium.
- The hypotensive agents trimethaphan, pentolinium, nitroglycerin, and nitroprusside enhances d-tubocurarine in very high doses, but not in clinical doses.
- Hypothermia. Hypothermia reduces serum clearances as well as renal and biliary excretion of both d-tubocurarine and pancuronium. The metabolism of pancuronium to less active metabolites is reduced. The neuromuscular effects of relaxants are prolonged. Hypothermia may have a direct mechanical effect on the muscle, slowing contraction and relaxation and thus enhancing the blockade.
- Atypical pseudocholinesterase causing prolonged apnea after administration of succinylcholine.

Ham J: Factors affecting administration of nondepolarizing neuromuscular blocking agents. ASA Refresher Courses in Anesthesiology 8:61–78, 1980

Sokoll MD, Gergis SD: Antibiotics and neuromuscular function. Anesthesiology 55:148–159, 1981

C.13. What is apneic oxygenation? Who did the pioneer study?

Draper and Whitehead conducted the pioneer study in 1944. Apneic oxygenation is actually caused by mass movement oxygenation. When the lungs are completely denitrogenized with oxygen and the airway is connected to an oxygen source, continuous oxygenation takes place by mass movement. Normally, every minute, 250 ml of oxygen are removed from the alveoli for metabolism and 200 ml of CO_2 are produced and eliminated from the lungs. When a person is apneic, only 10% of CO_2 accumulates in the alveoli, and 90% of CO_2 stays in the blood as bicarbonate. Consequently, 250 ml of oxygen are removed from the lungs and 20 ml of CO_2 accumulates in the lungs, creating a 230 ml vacuum effect and sucking in oxygen. Carbon dioxide tension continues to rise because there is no elimination during apnea. The total pressure in the alveoli is constant, so the fall in PO_2 equals the rise in PCO_2, ranging from 3 to 6 torr per minute.

Nann JF: Applied Respiratory Physiology, 2nd ed, pp 358–359. London, Butterworth & Co, 1977

D. Postoperative Management

D.1. What are the early postoperative complications?

The early complications are acute renal failure, renal artery occlusion, hyperacute rejection, graft rupture, urinary fistula, wound infection, and lymphoceles.

Guttmann RD: Renal transplantation. N Engl J Med 301:1038–1048, 1979

D.2. *How would you make the diagnosis of rejection?*

The signs of rejection are fever, decreased urine output, and increased serum creatinine. Often there is renal enlargement and tenderness. Unfortunately, without renal biopsy, rejection cannot be distinguished from acute pyelonephritis or recurrent glomerulopathy.

Guttmann RD: Renal transplantation. N Engl J Med 301:1038–1048, 1979

24 Placenta Praevia
Michael Tjeuw

A 34-year-old woman at 34 weeks of gestation required emergency cesarean section for massive painless vaginal bleeding. Blood pressure was 80/50 torr and pulse 120/m. Hemoglobin was 8 gm% and hematocrit 24%. She weighed 55 kg.

A. Medical Disease and Differential Diagnosis

1. What are the major causes of third trimester hemorrhage in a pregnant woman?
2. What is the definition of placenta praevia? Outline the classification of placenta praevia. What is the incidence of placenta praevia?
3. How would you make the diagnosis of placenta praevia?
4. What is the etiology of placenta praevia?
5. What maternal physiological changes occur during pregnancy? Discuss respiratory, circulatory, acid–base and other changes.
6. What factors affect the uteroplacental circulation?
7. Is there autoregulation in the uterus?
8. What is the placental barrier?
9. How does the placenta transfer nutrients to the fetus?
10. What factors affect the diffusion of drugs across the placenta?
11. How is maternal hypotension reflected in the fetus?
12. What methods are available for accurate assessment of the fetal condition?
13. What studies are available for assessment of fetal maturity and placental function?
14. What does the lecithin: sphingomyelin ratio study tell you? Is it a reliable test to assess fetal maturity?
15. What does the amniotic creatinine content tell you?

Placenta Praevia · 287

B. Preoperative Evaluation and Preparation

1. Is this patient in shock?
2. How do you classify shock?
3. Discuss the resuscitative management of hypovolemic shock.
4. What is the mechanism of the supine hypotensive syndrome in pregnancy? Discuss its management.
5. The patient is scheduled for an emergency cesarean section. Would you premedicate this patient? What premedicants would you use and why?

C. Intraoperative Management

1. What is the anesthetic technique you plan to use for emergency cesarean section?
2. What intravenous induction agents would you use?
3. Thiopental sodium crosses the placenta rapidly, and it is not possible to deliver the fetus before the drug is transferred to the fetus. Why is the neonate not affected when 4 mg/kg of thiopental sodium is given to the mother?
4. Describe the technique of general anesthesia for emergency cesarean section.
5. Discuss the effects of muscle relaxants on the fetus (succinylcholine, d-tubocurarine, gallamine, and pancuronium).
6. Would you hyperventilate the patient before the fetus is delivered? Why?
7. Discuss the Apgar scoring system for evaluation of the newborn.
8. If the Apgar score of the newborn is less than 3, how would you manage the newborn?
9. How would you administer drug therapy to the newborn in the initial resuscitation?
10. How do you perform closed chest cardiac massage in the newborn?
11. What factors stimulate the respiratory center of the newborn to initiate the onset of rhythmic breathing?
12. What is the inspiratory volume of the first breath in the newborn?
13. How much inspiratory pressure is required to expand the airless, collapsed lung after delivery of the newborn?
14. Discuss the mechanism of thermoregulation in the newborn.

D. Postoperative Management

1. When would you extubate the patient?
2. This patient was not breathing adequately at the end of surgery. What are the possible causes?

288 · Anesthesiology

A. Medical Disease and Differential Diagnosis

A.1. What are the major causes of third trimester hemorrhage in a pregnant woman?

The major causes are placenta praevia and abruptio placenta.

Shnider SM, Levinson G: Anesthesia for Obstetrics, p 243. Baltimore, Williams & Wilkins, 1979

A.2. What is the definition of placenta praevia? Outline the classification of placenta praevia. What is the incidence of placenta praevia?

In placenta praevia, the placenta is located over or very near the internal cervical os, instead of being implanted in the body of the uterus well away from the internal cervical os. Placenta praevia is classified into the following four types:

- Total placenta praevia—the internal os is totally covered by placenta
- Partial placenta praevia—the internal os is partially covered by placenta
- Marginal placenta praevia—the edge of the placenta is at the margin of the cervical os
- Low-lying placenta—the region of the internal os is encroached upon by the placenta, so that the placenta edge may be palpated by the examining finger when introduced through the cervix

The incidence of placenta praevia varies from 0.1% to 1.0%. It is highest in the multigravida, and the association is actually with age rather than parity. If a patient has a placenta praevia in one pregnancy, the chance of recurrence is 12 times that for the normal parturient.

Shnider SM, Levinson G: Anesthesia for Obstetrics, p 243. Baltimore, Williams & Wilkins, 1979

A.3. How would you make the diagnosis of placenta praevia?

One should always suspect placenta praevia in women with uterine bleeding during the latter half of pregnancy. The diagnosis can rarely be established by clinical examination unless a finger is passed through the cervix and the placenta is palpated. This procedure is never permissible unless the woman is in an operating room with all preparations for immediate cesarean section.

Other methods of localizing the placenta include the following:

- Sonography—this method is safest, simplest, and most precise during the third trimester. It can locate the placenta with an accuracy of 95%.
- Isotopes and roentgenography—this includes soft tissue x-rays, intra-

venous injection of radioactive isotopes, contrast material injection into the amniotic sac, and retrograde arteriography. The most innocuous of these procedures is soft tissue x-rays, but it is the least accurate, giving a correct diagnosis in less than 85% of cases.

Albright G: Anesthesia in Obstetrics, pp 418–419. Menlo Park, CA, Addison–Wesley, 1978

A.4. What is the etiology of placenta praevia?

One factor in the development of placenta praevia is defective vascularization of the decidua, the possible result of inflammatory or atrophic changes. Multiparity and advancing age appear to have higher incidence of placenta praevia. Another factor is a large placenta that spreads over a large area of the uterus and approaches the region of the internal os, completely or partially overlapping it.

Albright G: Anesthesia in Obstetrics, p 417. Menlo Park, CA, Addison–Wesley, 1978

A.5. What maternal physiological changes occur during pregnancy? Discuss respiratory, circulatory, acid–base and other changes.

Respiration

Pregnancy produces significant changes in the respiratory system. In the majority of pregnant women, capillary engorgement takes place throughout the respiratory tract; the nasopharynx, larynx, trachea, and bronchi become swollen and red. Lung volumes do not change until the fifth month of gestation, after which there is a progressive decrease in expiratory reserve volume (ERV), residual volume (RV), and functional residual capacity (FRC). At term, ERV is about 150 ml less, and RV 200 ml less than in the nonpregnant state. Consequently, FRC is about 350 ml or 20% lower than in the nonpregnant state. These changes are accentuated by the recumbent position, obesity, and mitral valve disease. The inspiratory capacity (IC) increases concomitantly, with the result that total lung capacity (TLC) remains unchanged, or just slightly decreases. Vital capacity (VC) remains unchanged but total pulmonary resistance is significantly lower during pregnancy, due to a decrease in airway resistance. The pregnant patient tends to hyperventilate. At term, respiratory rate increases by 10% to 15%, and the tidal volume increases by 40%. Thus, the minute volume increases by 50% above normal. Since dead space remains normal, alveolar ventilation is about 60% to 70% above normal at term. Recent data show that almost maximum hyperventilation occurs as early as the second or third month of gestation. The changes in lung volumes and ventilation lead to a reduction of arterial and alveolar carbon dioxide, which averages 32 torr at term, and an increase in PaO_2 to about 105 torr.

Circulation

The cardiovascular system undergoes multiple changes. Blood volume increases early, reaching a peak at approximately 32 to 34 weeks of gestation. At term, the increase in blood volume is approximately 25%, with a 10% increase in red cell mass, and 30% to 40% expansion of plasma volume. These disproportionate changes in blood components result in the so called physiologic anemia of pregnancy.

Cardiac output increases progressively during pregnancy, reaching a maximum of 30% to 50% above normal at 28 to 32 weeks of gestation and then falls towards normal during the 36th to 40th week. During the last few weeks of gestation, the cardiac output in the supine position may fall below nonpregnant levels, due to compression of the vena cava by the gravid uterus, decreasing venous return to the heart. The heart rate increases progressively until the last trimester when it is 10 beats/minute above nonpregnant levels. Arterial blood pressure decreases slightly during pregnancy because of a decrease in peripheral resistance that more than offsets the increase in cardiac output. The diastolic pressure decreases more than the systolic, therefore, the pulse pressure is increased.

The venous blood pressure is normal throughout the body except in the lower portion, where it increases as pregnancy advances, owing to venous obstruction secondary to pressure exerted by the enlarged uterus on the inferior vena cava and the pelvic veins. In 5% to 10% of patients, the obstruction is so great that they develop the supine hypotension syndrome. Other changes include louder heart sounds with an accentuated first apical and second pulmonic sound, and a faint systolic murmur. ECG changes include large Q wave and an inverted T wave in leads III, V_1, V_2, and occasional S-T segment depression and flattening of the T wave. All these ECG changes disappear during the puerperium.

Acid–base Balance

The total base decreases in pregnant women from the normal nonpregnant level. This is reflected in the decrease of plasma sodium, potassium, calcium, and magnesium. The plasma bicarbonate decreases from an average of 25 mEq/L to 21 mEq/L. $PaCO_2$ decreases to about 32 torr; and the plasma buffer base (which includes the bicarbonate, the protein, and the hemoglobin) decreases from a normal value of 47 mEq/L to 42 mEq/L. In most patients, the *p*H remains unchanged at 7.40; however, in some women mild metabolic acidosis is present.

Gastrointestinal Tract

Pregnancy is assoicated with a decrease of gastric and intestinal motility and a slight delay in gastric emptying time. These changes are exaggerated by sedatives and general anesthetics. The cardioesophageal sphincter tends to dilate; thus, the pregnant woman is prone to gastroesophageal refulx.

Renal Function

During pregnancy, there is a gradual dilatation of the renal pelvis, calyces, and ureters. There is an increase in the glomerular filtration rate. The rate of urine formation is increased because of the increased load of excretory products.

Endocrine System

Estrogen, progesterone, and chorionic gonadotropin are produced by the corpus luteum and placenta. There is hyperplasia of the thyroid and parathyroid glands, marked hypertrophy of the pituitary gland, and enlargement of the adrenal glands.

Metabolism

There is a progressive increase in the basal metabolic rate, oxygen consumption, and retention of water, protein, and minerals.

Bonica J: Principles and Practice of Obstetric Analgesia and Anesthesia, pp 1–25. Philadelphia, FA Davis, 1972

A.6. What factors affect the uteroplacental circulation?

Factors that affect the uteroplacental circulation are as follows:

- Blood pressure. Ewe experiments have shown that the uterus depends on the perfusion pressure of the uterine arteries for its blood flow.
- Uterine contraction. Both spontaneous and oxytocin induced uterine contractions reduce uterine artery blood flow in pregnant ewes.

Marx GF, Bassell GM: Obstetric Analgesia and Anesthesia, p 57. New York, Elsevier–Dutton, 1980

A.7. Is there autoregulation in the uterus?

No. The uterus has no autoregulation.

Marx GF, Bassell GM: Obstetric Analgesia and Anesthesia, p 57. New York, Elsevier–Dutton, 1980

A.8. What is the placental barrier?

The placental barrier or membrane has been defined by Wisloski as those tissues of the developing embryo that are in contact with maternal fluids or tissues at any stage of gestation, which mediate the transfer of substances to and from the fetus.

Bonica J: Principles and Practice of Obstetric Analgesia and Anesthesia, p 124. Philadelphia, FA Davis, 1972

A.9. How does the placenta transfer nutrients to the fetus?

The placenta transfers nutrients to the fetus by means of diffusion, active transport, and special process, such as pinocytosis.

Bonica J: Principles and Practice of Obstetric Analgesia and Anesthesia, p 125. Philadelphia, FA Davis, 1972

A.10. What factors affect the diffusion of drugs across the placenta?

The factors affecting the diffusion of drugs across the placenta are simple diffusion and facilitated diffusion (carrier system). The mechanism of transfer of commonly used drugs appears to be that of simple diffusion from an area of high concentration to one of low concentration following the Fick equation:

$$Q/t = K \frac{A\,(Cm - Cf)}{D}$$

Q/t = the amount of diffused substance per unit time
K = the diffusion constant of a given substance
A = the surface area available for diffusion
Cm = maternal concentration
Cf = fetal concentration
D = thickness of the membrane

In normal pregnancy, the most important factors in the Fick equation are the maternal–fetal concentration gradient and the diffusion constant of a given drug. The former is primarily affected by circulatory factors on both sides of the placenta. Anesthetic techniques and agents may influence placental transfer in a number of ways, both directly and indirectly. For example, by altering maternal cardiovascular dynamics with spinal anesthesia, placental blood flow may be decreased and the delivery of drug to the fetus reduced. A second important element is the nature of the drug itself. Included in the diffusion constant are considerations of lipid solubility, protein binding, degree of ionization, and molecular weight.

Alper MH: What drugs cross the placenta and what happens to them in the fetus. ASA Refresher Courses in Anesthesiology 4:5, 1976

A.11. How is maternal hypotension reflected in the fetus?

Maternal hypotension may be reflected in the fetus as fetal distress, which is characterized by tachybradycardia, fetal acidosis, and the presence of meconium in the amniotic fluid.

Cohen H: Fetal and infant evaluation during labor and delivery. ASA Refresher Courses in Anesthesiology 7:71–86, 1979

A.12. What methods are available for accurate assessment of the fetal condition?

The methods currently available for accurate assessment of the fetal conditions are as follows:

- Continuous monitoring of the fetal heart rate (FHR) by direct and indirect fetal electrocardiography, phonocardiography, and ultrasonography
- Measurement of uterine activity by direct and indirect techniques

Placenta Praevia · 293

- Electroencephalography studies of fetal brain wave patterns
- Acid–base and blood gas determinations through capillary blood sampling
- Amnioscopy, to observe the color and clarity of amniotic fluid
- Amniocentesis, to obtain amniotic fluid for assessment of cell maturity, measurement of bilirubin, creatinine, phospholipids (lecithin and sphingomyelin), and chromosomal abnormalities

Cohen H: Fetal and infant evaluation during labor and delivery. ASA Refresher Courses in Anesthesiology 7:71–86, 1979

A.13. What studies are available for assessment of fetal maturity and placental function?

- Maternal urinary and plasma estriol concentration (E3)
- Maternal plasma levels of human placental lactogen (HPL)
- The oxytocin challenge or stress test (OCT) or contraction stress test (CST)
- The fetal nonstress test (NST)

Cohen H: Fetal and infant evaluation during labor and delivery. ASA Refresher Courses in Anesthesiology 7:71–86, 1979

A.14. What does the lecithin: sphingomyelin ratio study tell you? Is it a reliable test to assess fetal maturity?

This study is the most reliable method for antepartum assessment of maturity of the fetal lung. Gluck found that the concentrations of lecithin (L) and sphingomyelin (S) are equal prior to the 35th week of gestation, following which the lecithin rises to 4 times that of sphingomyelin. The values of the L/S ratio proved to be accurately predictive of lung maturity. Lecithin is the major component of pulmonary surfactant. When the L/S ratio exceeds 2.0, it is unlikely that the newborn will develop respiratory distress syndrome.

Cohen H: Fetal and infant evaluation during labor and delivery. ASA Refresher Courses in Anesthesiology 7:71–86, 1979

Gluck L et al: The interpretation and significance of the L/S ratio in amniotic fluid. Am J Obstet Gynecol 120:142–155, 1974

A.15. What does the amniotic creatinine content tell you?

The amniotic creatinine measurement is the second most reliable method of determining fetal maturity. It reflects the growth of the fetal muscle mass and the development of renal function. A concentration of greater than 1.8 to 2.0 mg/100 ml indicates that the fetus is more than 36 weeks of gestational age and weighs more than 2500 grams.

O'Leary JA et al: Amniotic fluid fetal maturity score. Obstet Gynecol 38:375–378, 1971

B. Preoperative Evaluation and Preparation

B.1. Is this patient in shock?

Her blood pressure was 80/50 torr and pulse rate was 120/m. She could probably be in hypovolemic shock. She is hypotensive and tachycardiac. There is not enough evidence from the history presented here to determine whether she was in shock or not because shock is by definition "inadequate tissue perfusion," and is characterized by a syndrome of pale, mottled, cool skin, tachycardia, and hypotension. If there is a history of cardiac problems, congestive heart failure has to be considered as well. Central venous pressure or pulmonary capillary wedge pressure may confirm the diagnosis.

Schwartz S et al: Principles of Surgery, 3rd ed, p 135. New York, McGraw–Hill, 1979

B.2. How do you classify shock?

For purposes of a working clinical classification, the etiologic classification offered by Blalock in 1934 is still a useful and functional one. Blalock suggested the following four categories:

- Hematogenic (hemorrhagic–hypovolemic) shock
- Neurogenic shock
- Vasogenic septic shock
- Cardiogenic shock

Schwartz S et al: Principles of Surgery, 3rd ed, p 135. New York, McGraw–Hill, 1979

B.3. Discuss the resuscitative management of hypovolemic shock.

Hypovolemic shock results from reduction of the blood volume below a critical level. There is inadequate blood flow to tissues to meet their respiratory and metabolic demands. The management of hypovolemic shock consists of intravenous fluid administration. Therefore, it is essential to have adequate routes for volume replacement. A minimum of two large-bore (16-gauge or 14-gauge) intravenous catheters and a central venous line should be placed. The best rule to follow when administering fluid to a hypovolemic patient is to replace losses as specifically as possible. This patient is most likely to be in hemorrhagic shock. The ideal replacement solution is obviously type-specific, cross-matched whole blood. In most instances a minimum of 30 to 45 minutes is required for typing and cross-matching. In the meantime, crystalloids or colloids can be administered. In desperate cases, O-negative blood may be given until blood typing can be completed.

Schwartz S et al: Principles of Surgery, 3rd ed, pp 163–169. New York, McGraw–Hill, 1979

B.4. What is the mechanism of the supine hypotension syndrome in pregnancy? Discuss its management.

During late pregnancy, the enlarged uterus compresses both the inferior vena cava and the lower aorta whenever the gravida lies flat on her back. Obstruction of the inferior vena cava leads to reduced venous return to the heart and, consequently, a diminished cardiac stroke volume. Most women are capable of compensating for the resultant decrease in stroke volume by increasing peripheral vascular resistance and heart rate so that arterial pressure remains unaffected. However, significant falls in blood pressure or supine hypotension will occur when vasoconstriction is rendered impossible by the sympathetic blockade of high regional analgesia or the vasodilating action of drugs or inhalation agents. Therefore, "supine hypotension" or "postural shock of pregnancy" occurs predominantly in anesthetized gravidae.

Compression of the lower aorta and its branches by the gravid uterus in the supine position occurs as well. During uterine contractions, the degree of displacement is intensified. Therefore, renal and uteroplacental blood flow may be impaired. Fetal arrhythmia, suggestive of uteroplacental insufficiency, can be alleviated by turning the mother from the supine to a lateral position. The management of "supine hypotension" is simple. In most cases, displacement of the uterus to the left can alleviate both the caval and aortic compression. This may be accomplished manually by elevation of the right hip combined with left–down tilt of the table or by self-supporting mechanical devices.

Marx GF, Gassell GM: Obstetric Analgesia and Anesthesia, pp 27–30. New York, Elsevier–Dutton, 1980

B.5. The patient is scheduled for an emergency cesarean section. Would you premedicate this patient? What premedicants would you use, and why?

Yes, I would premedicate this patient with milk of magnesia, 30 ml by mouth. All parturients should receive oral antacid therapy every 2 hours during labor. Women scheduled to have elective cesarean section should be given one dose ½ hour before anesthesia induction. In emergency situation, where insufficient time is available to achieve the full buffering effect of the usual antacid (mixture of $Al(OH)_3$ and $Mg(OH)_2$), it has been shown that a single oral dose of milk of magnesia (30 ml) or sodium citrate (15 ml) requires only 10 minutes to buffer gastric acid to a pH value of more than 2.5.

Premedication with narcotics or ataractics is *not* indicated before cesarean section because the neonatal depressant effects outweigh any possible maternal benefits. Anticholinergic derivatives may be given intravenously immediately before induction if necessary.

Marx GF, Bassell GM: Obstetric Analgesia and Anesthesia, p 285. New York, Elsevier–Dutton, 1980

C. Intraoperative Management

C.1. What is the anesthetic technique you plan to use for emergency cesarean section?

Conduction analgesia is not a good choice for a real emergency cesarean section. General anesthesia is the choice.

C.2. What intravenous induction agents would you use?

The commonly used agent is a thiobarbiturate, usually thiopental sodium. A single dose of 4 mg/kg does not significantly affect the fetal outcome as measured by Apgar score.

Ketamine has been advocated for induction of anesthesia, especially with the presence of unstable maternal hemodynamics associated with blood loss. With doses as high as 1 mg/kg, no deleterious effect was found in the newborn. It has been reported that levels of ketamine in cord blood exceeded those in maternal blood within 97 seconds of injection, with maximal levels at 125 seconds. The place of ketamine in obstetrics remains unsettled.

Stovner and Vangen compared diazepam, 20 mg, with thiopental sodium, 200 mg, and found no difference in neonatal conditions as measured by Apgar scores. However, diazepam has been associated with neonatal hypotonia and increased susceptibility to cold stress.

<small>Datta S, Alper MH: Anesthesia for cesarean section. Anesthesiology 53:142–160, 1980</small>

<small>Ellington A, Haram R, Sagen N et al: Transplacental passage of ketamine after intravenous administration. Acta Anaesthesiol Scand 21:41–44, 1977</small>

<small>Peltz B, Sinclair DM: Induction agents for caesarian section. Anaesthesia 28:37–42, 1973</small>

<small>Stovner J, Vangem O: Diazepam compared to thiopentone as induction agent for caesarian sections. Acta Anaesthesiol Scand 18:264–269, 1974</small>

C.3. Thiopental sodium crosses the placenta rapidly and it is not possible to deliver the fetus before the drug is transferred to the fetus. Why is the neonate not affected when 4 mg/kg of thiopental sodium is given to the mother?

After a single maternal intravenous dose, the drug can be detected in umbilical venous blood within 30 seconds. It reaches its peak concentration in umbilical venous blood in 1 minute and in umbilical arterial blood in 2 to 3 minutes. After 4 mg/kg of thiopental sodium is given, the fetal brain concentration is not high. Umbilical arterial levels of thiopental are much lower than umbilical venous levels. This may be due to the fact that blood from the placenta first passes through the liver, so most of thiopental is either cleared by the liver or diluted by blood from the lower extremities and viscera. Other reasons are swift decline of the drug's concentration in maternal blood, and nonhomogeneous distribution in the intervillous space. *Note*, after large doses of thiopental sodium (8 mg/kg), neonates are delivered depressed.

Shnider SM, Levinson G: Anesthesia for Obstetrics, pp 263–264. Baltimore, Williams & Wilkins, 1979

C.4. *Describe the technique of general anesthesia for emergency cesarean section.*

The patient is placed on the operating table with head slightly elevated and pelvis tilted to the left by a wedge under the right hip. The abdomen is surgically prepared and draped. Blood pressure and ECG are monitored. After preoxygenation for 5 minutes, and precurarization with 3 to 6 mg of d-tubocurarine, anesthesia is rapidly induced with thiopental (4 mg/kg of pregnant body weight) and succinylcholine (1–1.5 mg/kg of pregnant body weight). Cricoid pressure (Sellick's maneuver) is applied during intubation with a cuffed endotracheal tube. Anesthesia is maintained with nitrous oxide/oxygen and a succinylcholine infusion to provide adequate muscle relaxation. Halothane, 0.5%, or enflurane, 1.0%, may be added to prevent maternal awareness and recall. After delivery of the baby and clamping of the umbilical cord, narcotics or other adjuvants are administered as needed to maintain anesthesia. At the end of the procedure, during extubation, extreme care must be taken to avoid aspiration.

Ostheimer GW: Physiologic changes in the paturient. Anesthesiology Review 6, No. 2:17–21, 1979

C.5. *Discuss the effects of muscle relaxants on the fetus (succinylcholine, d-tubocurarine, gallamine, and pancuronium).*

Muscle relaxants have low lipid solubility and are highly ionized at physiologic pH. When clinical doses of relaxants are given, insignificant amounts are transferred across the placenta to the fetus.

Succinylcholine, administered to the mother in doses of 2 to 3 mg/kg, is detectable in fetal blood and may cause alterations in the electromyograph, but it has no depressant effects on neonatal respiration. When a massive dose (10 mg/kg) is administered to the mother, neonatal depression occurs. Despite reduced pseudocholinesterase in the mother, the metabolism of succinylcholine is usually not prolonged. In patients with atypical cholinesterase, prolonged maternal and neonatal respiratory depression has been reported.

Pancuronium or d-tubocurarine do cross the placenta to the fetus. Fetal blood levels of d-tubocurarine are only one tenth of maternal blood levels, and neonatal muscle weakness is not found. In clinical doses pancuronium does not affect the neonate.

Gallamine appears to be more easily transferred than the other relaxants. Relatively high fetal levels are found after clinical doses are given to

Table 24-1. The Apgar scoring system

SIGN	0	1	2
Heart rate	Absent	Less than 100/min	More than 100/min
Respiratory effort	Absent	Slow, irregular	Good, crying
Muscle tone	Limp	Some flexion of extremities	Active motion
Reflex irritability (response to catheter in nose)	Absent	Grimace	Cough or sneeze
Color	Blue, pale	Body pink, extremities blue (acrocyanosis)	Completely pink

Each sign is evaluated individually and scored from 0 to 2 at both 1 and 5 minutes of life. The final score at each time is the sum of the individual scores. (From Apgar V: A proposal for a new method of evaluation of the newborn infant. Curr Res Anesth Analg (Cleve) 32:260-267, 1953)

the mother. Even though neonatal muscle weakness has not been reported, gallamine has not achieved popularity in obstetric anesthesia.

Shnider SM, Levinson G: Anesthesia for Obstetrics, pp 264-266. Baltimore, Williams & Wilkins, 1979

C.6. Would you hyperventilate the patient before the fetus is delivered? Why?

No. Maternal hyperventilation should be avoided during general anesthesia for cesarean section. Peng and associates reported that maternal hyperventilation was associated with fetal hypoxemia, fetal metabolic acidosis, lower 1-minute Apgar scores, and delayed onset of sustained respiration. The mechanisms include the following:

- Decreased uterine and umbilical blood flow from decreased cardiac output secondary to increased intrathoracic pressure
- Uterine vasoconstriction secondary to maternal hypocarbia and alkalosis
- Increased affinity of maternal hemoglobin for oxygen secondary to maternal alkalosis, resulting in less placental transfer of oxygen

Datta S, Alper MH: Anesthesia for cesarean section. Anesthesiology 53:150, 1980

Peng ATC, Blancato LS, Motoyama EK: Effect of maternal hypocapnia *vs* eucapnea on fetus during cesarean section. Br J Anaesth 44:1173-1178, 1972

Shnider SM, Levinson G: Anesthesia for Obstetrics, pp 262-263. Baltimore, Williams & Wilkins, 1979

C.7. Discuss the Apgar scoring system for evaluation of the newborn.

The Apgar scoring system is a quick method for evaluating the condition of the newborn in the delivery room at 1 and at 5 minutes after birth. A rating of 10 points describes the best possible condition, with 2 points each given for color, heart rate, reflex irritability, muscle tone, and respiratory effort. It is easier to remember the five signs of Apgar score as follows: **A**ppearance (color), **P**ulse (heart rate), **G**rimace (response to catheter in nose), **A**ctivity (muscle tone) and **R**espiration. The scores are shown in Table 24-1.

Apgar V: A proposal for a new method of evaluation of the newborn infant. Curr Res Anesth & Analg (Cleve) 32:260–267, 1953

C.8. If the Apgar score of the newborn is less than 3, how would you manage the newborn?

When the Apgar score is less than 3, the newborn has suffered from severe asphyxia and is usually apneic or in cardiac arrest. If there is no response to intermittent positive pressure ventilation (IPPV) with 100% oxygen by bag and mask, laryngoscopy and endotracheal intubation must be performed immediately and concomitantly with closed chest cardiac massage. The principles of newborn resuscitation should be followed: airway, breathing, circulation, drug therapy, evaluation, and maintenance of thermal environment. The following drugs may be useful:

- Sodium bicarbonate, 2 to 3 mEq/kg
- Epinephrine, 0.1 ml/kg of a 1:10,000 solution
- Isoproterenol, 4 mg/250 ml of 5% dextrose in water, IV drip
- Atropine, 0.03 mg/kg
- Calcium gluconate, 100 mg/kg given over a period of 5 to 10 minutes
- 10% dextrose in water, 100 ml/kg/24 hours
- Naloxone, 0.01 mg/kg

Gregory GA: Resuscitation of the newborn. Anesthesiology 43:225–237, 1975

C.9. How would you administer drug therapy to the newborn in the initial resuscitation?

Drugs used in the initial resuscitation of the newborn are usually administered through an umbilical vein catheter. In the acidotic, hypoxic, and hypercarbic newborn, it is often not possible to cannulate an umbilical artery because of intense vasoconstriction. Therefore, short term cannulation of the umbilical vein will provide an intravenous route for the initial stage of resuscitation. The cannula should not be inserted more than 2 cm into the umbilical vein, to avoid cannulation of a major hepatic vessel.

Ostheimer GW: Newborn resuscitation. ASA Refresher Courses in Anesthesiology 8:139–154, 1980

C.10. How do you perform closed chest cardiac massage in the newborn?

The correct method for performing closed chest cardiac massage is to place two thumbs over the midsternum and then encircle the chest with both hands so that the sernum will be depressed two-thirds of the distance to the vertebral column. Use a rate of 100 to 120 compressions per minute. The effectiveness of the cardiac massage is monitored through the umbilical artery catheter and by pupil size.

Todres ID et al: Methods of external cardiac massage in the newborn infant. J Pediatr 86:781–782, 1975

Gregory GA: Resuscitation of the newborn. Anesthesiology 43:225–237, 1975

C.11. What factors stimulate the respiratory center of the newborn to initiate the onset of rhythmic breathing?

Numerous factors stimulate the respiratory center of the newborn to initiate the onset of rhythmic breathing. They include acidosis, hypoxia, hypercarbia, cold, tactile stimulation, and umbilical cord clamping.

Ostheimer GW: Newborn resuscitation. ASA Refresher Courses in Anesthesiology 8:139–154, 1980

C.12. What is the inspiratory volume of the first breath in the newborn?

The inspiratory volume of the first breath is 20 ml to 75 ml, whereas 15 ml to 20 ml is the resting tidal volume after respirations have been established.

Ostheimer GW: Newborn resuscitation. ASA Refresher Courses in Anesthesiology 8:139–154, 1980

C.13. How much inspiratory pressure is required to expand the airless, collapsed lung after delivery of the newborn?

Expansion of the airless, collapsed lung after delivery requires higher pressure than that required to move air into the aerated lungs. It has been demonstrated that the normal infant exerts 40 to 80 cm H_2O negative pressure to overcome the collapsed lung.

Ostheimer GW: Newborn resuscitation. ASA Refresher Courses in Anesthesiology 8:139–154, 1980

C.14. Discuss the mechanism of thermoregulation in the newborn?

When the newborn is cold stressed, oxygen consumption and metabolic activity are increased. Large amounts of norepinephrine are released (in contrast to epinephrine in the adult), which activates an adipose tissue lipase to break down brown fat (so called because of its rich vascular supply) to form triglycerides, which are hydrolysed to form glycerol and nonesterified fatty acids (NEFA). The NEFA may pass out of the cell, oxidize to carbon dioxide and water in the cell (which is an exothermic or heat production reaction), or reesterify with glycerol to form triglycerides. Resynthesis of triglycerides is also an exothermic reaction.

This nonshivering thermogenesis occurs mainly in the brown fat of the newborn, which is found at an interscapular mass (the "hibernating gland"), muscles and blood vessels of the neck, clavicles and axillae, great vessels entering the thoracic inlet and abdominal viscera, especially around the kidneys and adrenals.

Stern L: Clinical aspects of thermoregulation in the newborn. Contemporary OB/GYN 13:109–134, 1979

D. Postoperative Management

D.1. When would you extubate the patient?

The patient should be extubated only after she is fully awake, able to protect her airway, and breathing adequately.

Shnider SM, Levinson G: Anesthesia for Obstetrics, p 261. Baltimore, Williams & Wilkins, 1979

D.2. The patient was not breathing adequately at the end of surgery. What are the possible causes?

- Central depression from narcotics, major tranquilizers, potent inhalation agents, or hypocarbia from mechanical or manual hyperventilation
- Peripheral neuromuscular blockade related to the following:
  - Dual block from large doses of succinylcholine infusion
  - Low pseudocholinesterase levels from pregnancy
  - Atypical cholinesterase

Shnider SM: Serum cholinesterase activity during pregnancy, labor and puerperium. Anesthesiology 26:355, 1965

25 Toxemia
Michael Tjeuw

This 27-year-old woman, para 1 gravida 2, at 38 weeks of gestation had a sharp weight gain of 6 kg. She developed a blood pressure of 180/100 torr, and 3+ albuminuria. She had been relatively normotensive.

A. Medical Disease and Differential Diagnosis

1. Outline the differential diagnosis of hypertension in pregnancy.
2. Outline the classification of toxemia of pregnancy.
3. What is the etiology and incidence of preeclampsia and eclampsia?
4. What pathophysiologic changes are seen in toxemia?
5. Outline the variety of clinical courses that this patient could develop.
6. What are the causes of maternal death?
7. Why is the fetus at greater risk in toxemia?
8. What hematologic findings can be present in toxemia?
9. When can eclamptic convulsions appear?

B. Preoperative Evaluation and Preparation

1. How would mild preeclampsia be managed?
2. How would severe preeclampsia be managed?
3. Discuss the effects of magnesium.
4. What are the side effects and toxic effects of magnesium?
5. What is the dosage and therapeutic plasma level of magnesium?
6. Discuss the interaction of magnesium with the muscle relaxants.
7. What is the antidote to magnesium?
8. How is magnesium excreted?
9. What is an oxytocin challenge test (OCT)? What is the fetal nonstress test (NST)?
10. How would you manage eclampsia?

C. Intraoperative Management

1. What anesthetic technique would you use for labor in mild preeclampsia or severe preeclampsia?
2. What are the primary advantages of continuous lumbar epidural anesthesia?
3. Discuss the problems that may be associated with epidural anesthesia.
4. Can continuous caudal epidural analgesia be used for the first stage of labor?
5. What local anesthetic agent would you use for epidural anesthesia, and why? Would you add epinephrine to it?
6. How do local anesthetic agents block the conduction of nerve impulses? Discuss the mechanism of action.
7. Is there a specific site to which local anesthetics bind?
8. How would you recognize the toxic effects of a local anesthetic in epidural anesthesia? Discuss the management of this problem.
9. The toxic effects of local anesthetics on the central nervous system (CNS) cause excitation followed by generalized CNS depression. How do you explain these effects?
10. Discuss the effects of vasopressors on uterine blood flow in obstetric patients.
11. If the patient refused regional anesthesia, what could you give her for labor pain and vaginal delivery?
12. Does the neonate from a toxemic mother present special problems and require special care?

D. Postoperative Management

1. How do you manage the patient who has had an inadvertent spinal puncture?
2. Would you perform a prophylactic epidural blood patch?
3. What are the absolute contraindications of epidural blood patch (EBP)?

A. Medical Disease and Differential Diagnosis

A.1. Outline the differential diagnosis of hypertension in pregnancy.

The current classification of hypertensive disorders of pregnancy as recommended by the American College of Obstetrics and Gynecologists is as follows:

- Preeclampsia—eclampsia
- Chronic hypertension
- Chronic hypertension with superimposed preeclampsia (or eclampsia)
- Gestational hypertension, also called late or transient hypertension of the third trimester

Shnider SM, Levinson G: Anesthesia for Obstetrics, p 224. Baltimore, Williams & Wilkins, 1979

A.2. Outline the classification of toxemia of pregnancy.

The term toxemia of pregnancy refers specifically to preeclampsia and eclampsia. Preeclampsia is a syndrome of hypertension, proteinuria, and generalized edema occurring after the 20th week of gestation and usually abating within 48 hours of delivery. Eclampsia is the occurrence of convulsions superimposed on preeclampsia.

Shnider SM, Levinson G: Anesthesia for Obstetrics, p 224. Baltimore, Williams & Wilkins, 1979

A.3. What is the etiology and incidence of preeclampsia and eclampsia?

The etiology of preeclampsia is unknown, but the following three factors are thought to be involved:

- Immunologic injury of the placenta
- Uterine ischemia
- Development of intravascular coagulation

However, it is not clear whether these factors cause toxemia or are the result of toxemia (Fig. 25–1). The incidence of toxemia is 5% to 7% of pregnancies in the United States, with a higher incidence in women of a lower socioeconomic group. Recurrences are in 30% to 60% of subsequent pregnancies. Toxemia is most commonly seen in young and elderly primigravidas, particularly in patients who have received inadequate prenatal care. There is a higher incidence of toxemia in conditions causing rapid uterine enlargement such as multiple gestations, diabetes mellitus, polyhydramnios, and hydatidiform mole.

Albright GA: Anesthesia in Obstetrics, pp 328–331. Menlo Park, CA, Addison–Wesley, 1978

Shnider SM, Levinson G: Anesthesia for Obstetrics, pp 224–225. Baltimore, Williams & Wilkins, 1979

A.4. What pathophysiologic changes are seen in toxemia?

The pathophysiologic changes of preeclampsia are thought to be due to vascular changes in the placenta during the first trimester of pregnancy. An antigen–antibody reaction between maternal and fetal tissue activates a placental vasculitis. Later in pregnancy, this leads to tissue anoxia and the release of a thromboplastin-like substance into the general circulation of the mother, causing the symptoms and signs of preeclampsia. Utero-

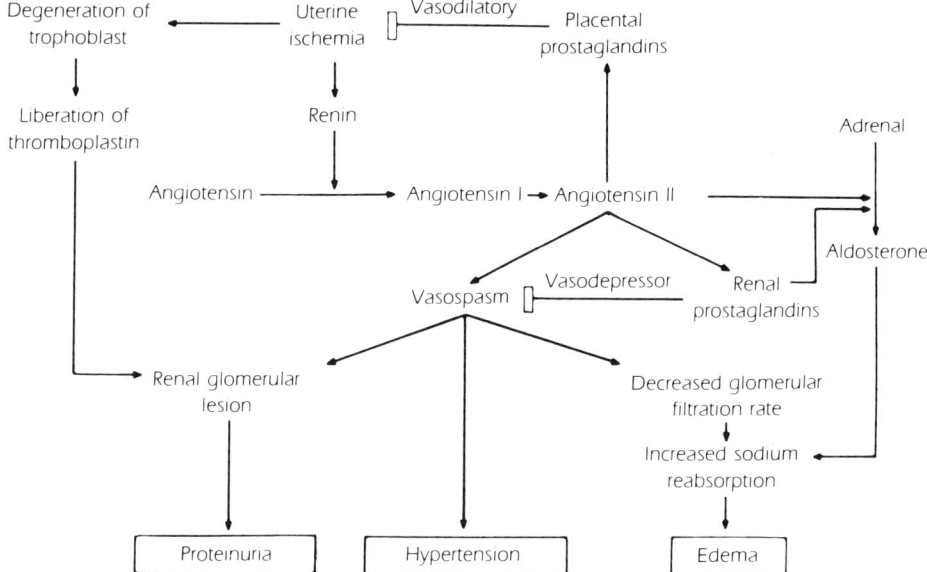

Fig. 25-1. Mechanism of toxemia. (Reprinted by permission from Speroff L: Toxemia of pregnancy, mechanism and therapeutic management. Am J Cardiology 32:587, 1973)

placental ischemia results in the excretion of a renin-like substance, which causes the increased production of angiotensin and aldosterone. It is also postulated that the synthesis of vasodilating substances, particularly the prostaglandins, may be inhibited. The resultant vasoconstriction leads to the following:
- Hypertension
- Renal glomerular lesion resulting in proteinuria
- Decreased glomerular filtration rate resulting in increased sodium reabsorption and subsequent edema

Simmon et al: The pathophysiology of hypertension in pregnancy. J Reprod Med 8:102, 1972

Speroff L: Toxemia of pregnancy: Mechanism and therapeutic management. Am J Cardiol 32:582, 1973

A.5. Outline the variety of clinical courses that this patient could develop.
- The triad of hypertension, proteinuria, and generalized edema usually characterizes preeclampsia. Occasionally, however, edema is not readily apparent.
- A blood pressure greater than 140/90 torr or a rise above normal in systolic pressure of 30 torr or diastolic pressure of 15 torr with a urine protein loss over 2 g a day are usually sufficient signs for the diagnosis of preeclampsia.

- If a blood pressure is above 160/110 torr and proteinuria exceeds 5 g a day (3+ to 4+), headache, visual disturbances, or epigastric pain may occur. These symptoms herald the development of severe preeclampsia and impending eclampsia.
- If grand mal convulsions occur in the presence of preeclampsia, a diagnosis of eclampsia is made. This condition significantly worsens the prognosis for both mother and fetus.
- There may be a hyperreflexia and increased central nervous system irritability. Toxemic coma may develop in the absence of convulsions.
- Blood uric acid levels are increased in toxemia.
- Edema of the upper airway and larynx may be exaggerated.
- Abnormalities in the coagulation system can occur and sometimes progress to disseminated intravascular coagulation.
- The uterus becomes hyperactive, and premature labor is common.
- With eclampsia and convulsions, frank pulmonary edema with congestive heart failure is common.
- Maternal asphyxiation may result from inadequate respiration or pulmonary aspiration of stomach contents, which may occur during convulsions.
- Coma with cerebral edema may follow convulsions.

Shnider SM, Levinson G: Anesthesia for Obstetrics, pp 224–226. Baltimore, Williams & Wilkins, 1979

A.6. What are the causes of maternal death?

The causes of maternal death are pulmonary edema with congestive heart failure, hypertensive cerebral encephalopathy, cerebral hemorrhage, placental abruption (abruptio placentae), renal failure, and pituitary necrosis.

Shnider SM, Levinson G: Anesthesia for Obstetrics, p 226. Baltimore, Williams & Wilkins, 1979

A.7. Why is the fetus at greater risk in toxemia?

The fetus is at greater risk in toxemia because marginal placental function, secondary to uteroplacental ischemia, may become inadequate, particularly in the presence of increased uterine activity. Newborns are often premature and small for gestational age.

Shnider SM, Levinson G: Anesthesia for Obstetrics, p 226. Baltimore, Williams & Wilkins, 1979

A.8. What hematologic findings can be present in toxemia?

The hematologic findings are variable, but may include thrombocytopenia, decreased fibrinogen levels, increased fibrin degradation products, prolonged thrombin time and prothrombin time and increased hematocrit values from hemoconcentration. These are characteristics of disseminated intravascular coagulation (DIC). There can be subclinical DIC. In severe preeclampsia or eclampsia, frank DIC may develop.

Beecham JB et al: Eclampsia, preeclampsia and disseminated intravascular coagulation. Obstet Gynecol 43:576, 1974

Pritchard JA et al: Coagulation changes in eclampsia: Their frequency and pathogenesis. Am J Obstet Gynecol 124:855, 1976

A.9. When can eclamptic convulsions appear?

Eclamptic convulsions may appear before labor, during labor, or in the early postpartum period.

Albright GA: Anesthesia in Obstetrics, p 328. Menlo Park, CA, Addison–Wesley, 1978

B. Preoperative Evaluation and Preparation

B.1. How would mild preeclampsia be managed?
- Hospitalization and bed rest
- Bed rest in the lateral decubitus position
- Fluids and adequate sodium intake
- Diuretic (controversial)

In general, therapy is aimed at the following: minimizing vasospasm; improving circulation to the uterus, placenta, and kidneys; improving intravascular volume; correcting acid–base and electrolyte imbalance; and decreasing CNS and reflex hyperactivity. Therapy, as a rule, is symptomatic. Definitive treatment consists of delivery of the fetus and the placenta. Hospitalization and bed rest in the lateral decubitus position are most effective in preventing aortocaval compression and improving uterine blood flow. Together with adequate fluids and dietary intake these measures will promote diuresis and a fall in blood pressure. The routine use of diuretics should be discouraged, except in cases of severe hypertension, congestive heart failure, severe fluid retention, or when required to potentiate the action of antihypertensive drugs. Evidence now favors adequate sodium intake with minimal, if any, sodium restriction.

Atkinson SM Jr: Salt, water and rest as a prevention for toxemia in pregnancy. J Reprod Med 9:233, 1972

Shnider SM, Levinson G: Anesthesia for Obstetrics, pp 227–230. Baltimore, Williams & Wilkins, 1979

B.2. How would severe preeclampsia be managed?

The same as the management of mild preeclampsia plus the following:
- Magnesium sulfate
- Antihypertensive drugs—hydralazine (Apresoline), reserpine, methyldopa (Aldomet), diazoxide (Hyperstat)
- Sedative anticonvulsive drugs—phenobarbital, diazepam (Valium)

Treatment is directed toward the prevention of convulsions. Parenteral magnesium sulfate is often selected for initial therapy. If the diastolic blood pressure remains over 110 torr despite magnesium therapy, antihypertensives are usually required. Hydralazine (Apresoline) is frequently used today, because of the following:

- Rapid action when given intravenously
- Short duration of action, better controllability
- Increase of renal blood flow

Reserpine can be used effectively, but it frequently causes neonatal respiratory obstruction due to nasal congestion in the newborn. Methyldopa has the disadvantage of a long latency period (6–8 hours) and may add to liver dysfunction in the mother. Diazoxide (Hyperstat), a potent antihypertensive drug, has the disadvantage of interfering with glucose metabolism and uric acid excretion. Diazoxide is also a potent inhibitor of uterine activity. Trimethaphan (Arfonad), in a continuous 0.1% infusion, can be used in a hypertensive crisis. Nitroprusside is not recommended for use in the antepartum period because it does not dilate the uterine vasculature to improve uterine blood flow. In addition, it crosses the placenta rapidly, in some animal studies, fetal cyanide toxicity and death may occur. Anticonvulsive drugs and sedatives may be required in severe preeclampsia or eclampsia. Diazepam (Valium) has been used successfully. However, diazepam may cause neonatal hypotonia, respiratory depression, and loss of body heat and regulation. In the past, heavy sedation with barbiturates and narcotics was recommended, but this frequently resulted in severe neonatal depression.

Naulty JS et al: Placental transfer and fetal toxicity of sodium nitroprusside. Abstracts of scientific papers presented at the annual meeting of the American Society of Anesthesiologists, 1976, p 543.

Shnider SM, Levinson G: Anesthesia for Obstetrics, pp 228–229. Baltimore, Williams & Wilkins, 1979

B.3. Discuss the effects of magnesium.

The effects of magnesium are as follows:

- CNS depression
- Neuromuscular blockade
- Vasodilation
- Decreased uterine hyperactivity

Magnesium is a CNS depressant. It decreases the amount of acetylcholine release at the neuromuscular junction. It diminishes the sensitivity of the end-plate to acetylcholine and it decreases the excitability of the muscle membrane. Magnesium is a mild vasodilator. It also depresses uterine hyperactivity, thus improving uterine blood flow.

Shnider SM, Levinson G: Anesthesia for Obstetrics, p 227. Baltimore, Williams & Wilkins, 1979

B.4. What are the side effects and toxic effects of magnesium?

The side effects and toxic effects of magnesium on the mother are as follows:

- Maternal muscle weakness
- Respiratory paralysis
- ECG changes—P–Q interval prolonged, QRS complex widened, sinoatrial and atrioventricular block
- Loss of deep tendon reflexes
- Cardiac arrest

The side effects on the fetus are as follows:

- Decreased muscle tone
- Respiratory depression and apnea

Magnesium therapy is associated with both maternal and neonatal side effects. Large doses can lead to maternal muscle weakness, respiratory insufficiency, and cardiac arrest. Fortunately, these complications do not usually occur until after the deep tendon reflexes are depressed (Table 25–1). Marked depression of deep tendon reflexes is an indication to decrease or omit the magnesium. Magnesium crosses the placenta. It can markedly decrease the newborn muscle tone, and may cause respiratory depression and apnea.

Shnider SM, Moya F: The Anesthesiologists, Mother and Newborn, pp 128–135. Baltimore, Williams & Wilkins, 1974

B.5. What is the dosage and therapeutic plasma level of magnesium?

Magnesium sulfate is commonly administered as a 4 g loading dose and 1 g per hour intravenously. The therapeutic range of plasma level of magnesium is 4.0 to 6.0 mEq/L. With increasing plasma levels of magnesium, side effects can occur (Table 25–1).

Shnider SM, Levinson G: Anesthesia for Obstetrics, p 227. Baltimore, Williams & Wilkins, 1979

Shnider SM, Moya F: The Anesthesiologists, Mother and Newborn, pp 128–135. Baltimore, Williams & Wilkins, 1974

Table 25–1. Effects of Increasing Plasma Magnesium Levels

OBSERVED CONDITION	mEq/L
Normal plasma level	1.5–2.0
Therapeutic range	4.0–6.0
Ecg changes (P–Q interval prolonged, QRS—complex widens)	5.0–10
Loss of deep tendon reflexes	10
Sinoatrial and atrioventricular block	15
Respiratory paralysis	15
Cardiac arrest	25

(By permission of Shnider SM, Levinson G: Anesthesia for Obstetrics © 1979, the Williams & Wilkins Co, Baltimore)

B.6. Discuss the interaction of magnesium with the muscle relaxants.

Magnesium decreases the amount of acetylcholine liberated at the nerve terminals, diminishes the sensitivity of the end-plate to acetylcholine, and decreases the excitability of the muscle membrane (membrane stabilizer). It will increase the sensitivity of the mother to both the depolarizing and the nondepolarizing muscle relaxants. The dosage of the muscle relaxants should be reduced to avoid overdosage.

Foldes FF: Factors which alter the effects of muscle relaxants. Anesthesiology 20:464, 1959

Ghoneim MM et al: Interaction between magnesium and other neuromuscular blocking agents. Anesthesiology 32:23, 1970

B.7. What is the antidote to magnesium?

Intravenous calcium may partially overcome the neuromuscular blocking properties of magnesium in both mother and newborn. Usually, 1 gm of calcium gluconate or calcium chloride is given intravenously.

Shnider SM, Levinson G: Anesthesia for Obstetrics, p 228. Baltimore, Williams & Wilkins, 1979

B.8. How is magnesium excreted?

Magnesium is excreted by the kidneys.

Shnider SM, Levinson G: Anesthesia for Obstetrics, p 228. Baltimore, Williams & Wilkins, 1979

B.9. What is an oxytocin challenge test (OCT)?

This test is widely used to confirm whether the fetus is truly in jeopardy. Oxytocin administration is started at a rate of 0.5 mu (milliunits)/min using an intravenous infusion pump. The dose of oxytocin is doubled every 15 to 20 minutes until 3 uterine contractions occur per 10 minute period. Each contraction must be of 40 to 60 seconds' duration. A *positive* OCT requires the presence of consistent late deceleration heart rate patterns, even when fewer than 3 uterine contractions occur in a 10 minute period. A *negative* OCT is diagnosed when late deceleration patterns do not occur, while uterine contractions (as described above) are adequate. A negative test is an extremely reliable predictor of fetal well-being, reassuring the obstetrician that the fetus may safely remain in the uterus for at least another week.

Ray M et al: Clinical experience with the oxytocin challenge test. Am J Gynecol 114:1–9, 1972

What is the fetal nonstress test (NST)?

Fetal movements normally increase daily from the 18th week to reach a maximum between the 29th and 38th week, and then decrease until delivery. Generally the number of daily fetal movements varies from 30 to 40. A marked reduction in fetal movements (*e.g.* 2 in a 10–12 hour period), or cessation of movement, signals serious fetal hypoxia. The nonstress test is done as follows: the mother is placed in a semi-Fowler's position. External monitors are securely fixed to the mother's abdomen with elastic belts to assess uterine pressure and fetal heart rate (FHR). Mother and fetus are monitored continuously by a two-channel recorder. Simultaneously, the observer monitors fetal movement manually by a hand placed lightly on the mother's abdomen. Each fetal movement should be accompanied by FHR acceleration. Approximately 10 movements should occur in a 30 minute period. When this does occur, the test (NST) is considered *reactive* and the fetus is in a satisfactory condition. When minimal baseline variability is found with fewer than two fetal movements in a 10 minute period, and little or no acceleration of FHR with each movement, the NST is considered *nonreactive*, and the fetus is "at risk."

Cohen H: Fetal and infant evaluation during labor and delivery. ASA Refresher Courses in Anesthesiology 7:71–86, 1979

B.10. How would you manage eclampsia?

With the development of eclampsia, the first priority is controlling grand mal convulsions and maintaining adequate ventilation and oxygenation. Initially, a small intravenous dose of a ultra-short acting barbiturate such as thiopental sodium, 50 to 100 mg, or diazepam, 5 mg, is used. It may be necessary to intubate the mother to protect the lungs from pulmonary aspiration and to control ventilation. Postictal depression may require support of ventilation to assure adequate oxygenation and to prevent respiratory acidosis. Metabolic acidosis often occurs; bicarbonate may be indicated after arterial blood gas analysis.

If cardiac failure with pulmonary edema occurs, a diuretic such as furosemide is useful and digitalization may be indicated. If cerebral edema is suspected, mannitol, and dexamethasone may be used. Further therapy is aimed at preventing additional convulsions and controlling blood pressure. If disseminated intravascular coagulation occurs, therapy includes administration of platelets, fresh frozen plasma, fresh whole blood, and occasionally heparin. The definitive therapy is the delivery of the fetus and placenta.

Shnider SM, Levinson G: Anesthesia for Obstetrics, pp 229–230. Baltimore, Williams & Wilkins, 1979

C. Intraoperative Management

C.1. What anesthetic technique would you use for labor in mild preeclampsia or severe preeclampsia?

During labor, regional anesthesia is preferred for mild preeclampsia. The use of regional analgesia in severe preeclampsia has long been debated. Pritchard and Pritchard avoided its use because of the fear of further compromising uteroplacental circulation secondary to sympathetic blockade and maternal hypotension. On the other hand, other investigators recommended continuous epidural anesthesia in severe preeclampsia to help control blood pressure, increase renal and uterine perfusion, and control pain. However, sudden falls in maternal blood pressure during epidural anesthesia can be associated with decreased uterine blood flow and fetal asphyxia. Epidural or caudal anesthesia is useful to prevent the elevation of blood pressure during a painful labor, but it should not be used as antihypertensive therapy. Epidural or caudal anesthesia per se does not increase renal or uterine blood fow. It may prevent endogenous catecholamine secretion associated with anxiety and pain, and therefore prevent further reductions in renal and uterine perfusion. The consensus of opinion today suggests that properly administered continuous lumbar epidural analgesia is, in most instances, the preferred method of analgesia for labor and vaginal delivery for preeclamptic patients under good medical control. When properly administered, epidural anesthesia is associated with minimal complications.

Alper MH et al: Anesthetic management of the high-risk pregnancy. Clin Obstet Gynecol 16:347, 1973

Hibbard BM et al: The management of severe preeclampsia and eclampsia. Br J Anaesth 49:3, 1977

Moir DD et al: Extradural analgesia during labor in patients with preeclampsia. J Obstet Gynaecol Br Commonw 79:465, 1972

Pritchard JA et al: Standardized treatment of 154 consecutive cases of eclampsia. Am J Obstet Gynecol 123:543, 1975

C.2. *What are the primary advantages of continuous lumbar epidural anesthesia?*

Its primary advantages are as follows:

- Complete maternal pain relief
- It provides excellent conditions for the obstetrician
- It can be rapidly extended to a higher level for abdominal delivery
- Minimal effects on the fetus

Shnider SM, Levinson G: Anesthesia for Obstetrics, p 321. Baltimore, Williams & Wilkins, 1979

C.3. *Discuss the problems that may be associated with epidural anesthesia.*

Problems associated with epidural anesthesia may be discussed as follows:

- Problems of the patient
  Epidural anesthesia is not suitable and is contraindicated in the following:
  - The uncooperative subject
  - The presence of skin infection of the back
  - Patients with coagulopathy
  - The presence of deformities of the spine
- Problems of technical mishaps
  - Intravascular injection. The epidural space is rich in blood vessels. These vessels may be punctured by the needle or catheter. Intravascular

injection of local anesthetic may cause convulsions and cardiopulmonary collapse. Intravascular injection is possible even when blood has not been aspirated.
- Inadvertent dural puncture. This occurs in about 1.5% to 3% of cases, even with experienced operators. Once this occurs, the incidence of postspinal headache (with a 17 gauge epidural needle) is 40%. Undetected spinal puncture with local anesthetic injection may result in "total" spinal anesthesia.
- Kinking of the catheter
- Problems of inadequate anesthesia.
Inadequate anesthesia may take a number of forms including the following:
  - The block may be successful but leave some dermatomes unanesthetized (hot spot).
  - The block may be unilateral. Sometimes this may be remedied by a further injection through the catheter with the patient lying on the unanesthetized side.
  - The block may not be high enough. This can be easily remedied by additional injection of anesthetic.
- Problems of complications
  - Hypotension
  - Toxicity of local anesthetics
  - Total subarachnoid block (total spinal anesthesia)
  - Peridural hematoma

Ostheimer GW: Prophylactic epidural blood patch. Regional Anesthesia, pp 17–19. Oct-Dec, 1979

Shnider SM, Levinson G: Anesthesia for Obstetrics, pp 93–98. Baltimore, Williams & Wilkins, 1979

C.4. Can continuous caudal epidural analgesia be used for the first stage of labor?

Yes. It was widely used and recommended for preeclampsia in the past. Its disadvantages include the following:
- Early anesthesia of the perineum
- The need for larger doses of local anesthetics
- The greater difficulty of placing the catheter
- The inability to extend the block to an adequate level to allow for cesarean section without the use of potentially toxic doses of local anesthetics

Shnider SM, Levinson G: Anesthesia for Obstetrics, p 232. Baltimore, Williams & Wilkins, 1979

C.5. What local anesthetic agent would you use for epidural anesthesia, and why? Would you add epinephrine to it?

The choice of local anesthetics for epidural anesthesia includes bupivacaine 0.25% to 0.75%, 2-chloroprocaine 2% to 3%. 2-chloroprocaine was widely used because of its broad margin of safety. The advantages are rapid onset, short duration of action, rapid hydrolysis by plasma cholinesterase in both mother and fetus, and little, if any, detectable fetal effect. It is suggested that inadvertent subarachnoid injection of 2-chloroprocaine would produce a blockade of lesser degree and duration than other local anesthetics. However, there were recent reports of adhesive arachnoiditis and cauda equina syndromes following inadvertent subarachnoid injection of 3% 2-chloroprocaine.

A recent animal study found that subarachnoid injection of 2-chloroprocaine-CE in dogs resulted in the development of neurologic dysfunction in 35% of the animals studied. Of the 15 spinal cords of the animals that received 2-chloroprocaine-CE, 13 showed subpial necrosis. Until more evidence disproves the neurotoxicity of 2-chloroprocaine-CE, we avoid using 2-chloroprocaine-CE, and use bupivacaine instead.

Bupivacaine is a long-acting local anesthetic. It has high affinity to plasma protein binding sites (95%) and little crosses the placenta. It is currently the most commonly used local anesthetic in obstetrics.

I would not add epinephrine to the local anesthetics. Chloroprocaine and bupivacaine are generally used without epinephrine in obstetric patients. Epinephrine does not significantly increase their duration of action for epidural anesthesia. The duration of action of chloroprocaine is 1 to 1½ hours, and bupivacaine acts for 2 to 3 hours. In addition, uterine activity is significantly diminished with epidural epinephrine.

Marx FG, Bassell GM: Obstetric Analgesia and Anesthesia, p 231. New York, Elsevier-Dutton, 1980

Ravindran RS et al: Prolonged neural blockade following regional analgesia with 2-chloroprocaine. Anesth Analg (Cleve) 59:447-451, 1980

Ravindran RS, Turner MS, Muller J: Neurologic effects of subarachnoid administration of 2-chloroprocaine-CE, Bupivacaine, and low pH normal saline in dogs. Anesth Analg (Cleve) 61:279, 1982

Reisner LS et al: Persistent neurologic deficit and adhesive arachnoiditis following intrathecal 2-chloroprocaine injection. Anesth Analg (Cleve) 59, No. 6:452-454, June 1980

C.6. How do local anesthetic agents block the conduction of nerve impulses? Discuss the mechanism of action.

Based on the data available at the present time, the following sequence of events is proposed for the mechanism of action of local anesthetic agents:

- Displacement of calcium ions from the nerve receptor site at the cell membrane, resulting in
- Binding of local anesthetic moiety to the receptor site, resulting in
- Blockade of the sodium channel, and reduction of the permeability of the cell membrane to sodium ions, resulting in
- Depression of the rate of depolarization of the membrane action potential, resulting in
- Failure to reach the threshold potential, resulting in

- Lack of development of propagated action potential, resulting in
- Conduction blockade.

The possible interaction of the local anesthetic agent and calcium as the initial step in the inhibition of sodium conductance is controversial.

Covino BG, Vassallo HG: Local Anesthetics—Mechanisms of Action and Clinical Use, p 34. New York, Grune & Stratton, 1976

C.7. Is there a specific site to which local anesthetics bind?

A specific site for local anesthetics at the nerve membrane has been postulated. The location of the receptors is probably at or near the sodium channel in the nerve membrane. Some postulate that receptors may be present either on the external or internal surface of the sodium channel. Substantial new evidence suggests that local anesthetics exert their sodium blocking action by plugging the internal surface (axoplasmic side) of the membrane.

Tetrodotoxin and saxitoxin have effects similar to local anesthetics, but the site of action is at the external surface of the membrane.

Covino BG, Vassallo HG: Local Anesthetics—Mechanisms of Action and Clinical Use, p 34. New York, Grune & Stratton, 1976

C.8. How would you recognize the toxic effects of a local anesthetic in epidural anesthesia? Discuss the management of this problem.

Toxic reactions to local anesthetic agents are usually due to excessive doses, rapid absorption from a vascular site, or an inadvertent intravascular injection. Hypersensitivity or idiosyncratic reactions are rare, but they may occur with local anesthetics. Although true allergic or anaphylactic reactions are also rare, they may occur, particularly with agents of the amino–ester group.

Systemic toxic reactions to local anesthetic agents primarily involve the central nervous system (CNS) and cardiovascular system (CVS).

- CNS. Local anesthetics readily cross the blood brain barrier (BBB). The initial signs usually are excitatory in nature. The premonitory symptoms include numbness of the tongue and circumoral tissue, and a generalized feeling of light-headedness, dizziness, visual and auditory disturbances, such as difficulty in focusing and tinnitus. Drowsiness, disorientation, and temporary unconsciousness may also occur. Following these premonitory signs and symptoms, overt convulsions of a tonic–clonic nature may occur. CNS depression manifested by cessation of convulsive activity, respiratory depression, and respiratory arrest may also occur.
- CVS. Local anesthetic agents exhibit a biphasic action on the CVS. Initially an increase in heart rate and blood pressure may occur. The predominant signs of cardiovascular toxicity are hypotension, due to direct vasodilatation on peripheral arterioles, and a negative inotropic

effect on the myocardium. Management of local anesthetic toxicity and convulsions is as follows:
- Establish and maintain a patent airway, sometimes endotracheal intubation is necessary.
- Assist or control ventilation using oxygen.
- Treat signs of CNS excitation with either intravenous diazepam (0.1–0.2 mg/kg) or a short acting barbiturate such as thiopental sodium (1–2 mg/kg). Succinylcholine (0.5–1 mg/kg) may be used to terminate a state of generalized convulsions. Convulsions usually last 15 to 30 seconds and are self limiting. If convulsions persist, small doses of diazepam and thiopental sodium may be administered.
- Treat hypotension with intravenous fluids and vasopressor agents such as ephedrine.

Covino BG: Pharmacology and physiology of local anesthetics. ASA Refresher Courses in Anesthesiology 5:33–45, 1977

C.9. The toxic effects of local anesthetics on the central nervous system (CNS) cause excitation followed by generalized CNS depression. How do you explain these effects?

This is explained by the fact that initially, local anesthetics selectively block inhibitory cortical neurons or synapses and allow facilitatory fibers to function unopposed, which leads to excitation and convulsions. Further increases in dosage depress both inhibitory and facilitatory pathways, thereby causing a generalized state of CNS depression.

Covino BG: Pharmacology and physiology of local anesthetics. ASA Refresher Courses in Anesthesiology 5:33–45, 1977

C.10. Discuss the effects of vasopressors on uterine blood flow in obstetric patients.

The use of vasopressors to correct maternal hypotension following regional anesthesia in the obstetric patient has been investigated both in man and animals. Studies have demonstrated that vasopressors raise maternal blood pressure, but further reduce uterine blood flow.

In studies on primates and ewes, Methoxamine (Vasoxyl) was shown to raise maternal blood pressure by increasing peripheral resistance. Both maternal cardiac output and uterine blood flow were lowered, and the deterioration of fetal acid–base status ensued.

Metaraminol (Aramine) was shown to improve maternal blood pressure and uterine blood flow in sheep. However, the fetus, which had become acidotic with the advent of hypotension, deteriorated further. Other vasopressors similarly implicated are phenylephrine (Neo-Synephrine), levarterenol (Levophed), and angiotension (Hypertensin). Mephentermine may increase uterine contractility and thus decrease uterine blood flow. In contrast, when ephedrine was used, maternal blood pressure was restored, and fetal deterioration was arrested. Fetal oxygenation improved and fetal acidosis decreased. Ephedrine is probably the vasopressor of choice in obstetric patients. The prophylactic use of ephedrine in patients undergoing cesarean section under spinal or epidural anesthesia has *not* been consistently effective in preventing hypotension.

Marx GF: Parturition and Perinatology Clinical Anesthesia Series, p 30. Philadelphia, FA Davis, 1973

C.11. If the patient refused regional anesthesia, what could you give her for labor pain and vaginal delivery?

Narcotics, if used, should be given in minimal dosage to minimize newborn depression. Tranquilizers and other adjuncts often used with narcotics should also be given in small doses. For the later part of first stage of labor and delivery, continuous administration of 30% to 40% nitrous oxide in oxygen will provide good analgesia. At delivery, pudendal block or local infiltration of the perineum will allow most forceps deliveries. Some authors suggest that paracervical block is safe to provide analgesia for the first stage of labor. However, the possibility of its causing fetal distress in the already compromised fetus leaves this open to question. In certain circumstances, general anesthesia is required for vaginal delivery.

Shnider SM, Levinson G: Anesthesia for Obstetrics, p 75. Baltimore, Williams & Wilkins, 1979

C.12. Does the neonate from a toxemic mother present special problems and require special care?

Yes. The neonate born of the toxemic mother is at high risk. He may be suffering from any of the following problems:

- Prematurity
- Small for gestational age
- Asphyxia
- Drug depression
- Meconium aspiration

Prompt and proper resuscitative measure should be available in the delivery room. He may require intensive care in the intensive care unit.

Shnider SM, Levinson G: Anesthesia for Obstetrics, p 233. Baltimore, Williams & Wilkins, 1979

D. Postoperative Management

D.1. How do you manage the patient who has had an inadvertent spinal puncture?

The incidence of postspinal puncture headache is 40% with a 17 gauge epidural needle. The patient should be informed and urged to maintain her hydration. Analgesics are given as needed. A prophylactic saline epidural injection, 30 to 50 ml, may be administered before the catheter is removed. When a spinal headache occurs, the patient is reassured, and bed rest in the supine position is ordered (except for bathroom privileges). Forced oral hydration (3000 ml daily) and oral parenteral analgesics are given as required. If severe persistent headache occurs, epidural blood patch is the treatment of choice.

Ostheimer GW: Prophylactic epidural blood patch. Regional Anesthesia, Oct-Dec, pp 17–19, 1979

D.2. Would you perform prophylactic epidural blood patch?

No. The use of prophylactic epidural blood patch is not warranted because the failure rate is quite high. Two reasons for its high failure rate (in contrast to the high success rate of therapeutic epidural blood patch) have been postulated. The autologous blood is not placed in the proper interspace to clot over the hole produced by the dural puncture, especially when the epidural catheter is used to carry the injection of blood, and the pressure or volume of leaking cerebrospinal fluids is sufficient to prevent organization of the clot over the dural defect.

Ostheimer GW: Prophylactic epidural blood patch. Regional Anesthesia, Oct-Dec, pp 17–19, 1979

D.3. What are the absolute contraindications of epidural blood patch (EBP)?

Septicemia, localized infection in the area of needle insertion, and active neurologic disease remain the absolute contraindications to epidural blood patch.

Ostheimer GW: Prophylactic epidural blood patch. Regional Anesthesia, pp 17–19, Oct-Dec, 1979

26 Breech Presentation and Fetal Distress

Michael Tjeuw

A 26-year-old woman at 36 weeks gestation, with a breech presentation, was in labor. Acute fetal distress developed, associated with prolapsed cord. An emergency cesarean section was scheduled.

A. Medical Disease and Differential Diagnosis

1. What is the incidence of breech presentation?
2. Name the different types of breech presentation.
3. What is the etiology of breech presentation?
4. How is the diagnosis of breech presentation made?
5. Are breech deliveries associated with increased maternal morbidity?
6. Why are the perinatal morbidity and mortality of the infant comparatively higher in breech deliveries than in vertex deliveries?

B. Preoperative Evaluation and Preparation

1. What is meant by baseline heart rate of the fetus?
2. What is meant by beat-to-beat variability in the fetal heart rate (FHR)?
3. Discuss the various patterns of FHR deceleration.
4. What are normal values of fetal blood gases?
5. The patient is scheduled for an emergency cesarean section. Would you premedicate this patient? What premedicants would you use, and why?

C. Intraoperative Management

1. What anesthetic technique would you use for emergency cesarean section?
2. What are the advantages and disadvantages of spinal anesthesia and epidural anesthesia for cesarean section?

3. What intravenous induction agents would you use?
4. Thiopental crosses the placenta rapidly, and it is not possible to deliver the fetus before the drug is transferred to the fetus. Why is the neonate not affected when 4 mg/kg of thiopental is given to the mother?
5. Describe the technique of general anesthesia for emergency cesarean section.
6. Does 0.5% halothane decrease uterine contractility? Discuss the effects of inhalation agents on uterine contraction.
7. If the patient vomits and aspirates during intubation, discuss the immediate management.
8. Should bronchoscopy be performed on all patients with aspiration of stomach contents?
9. Should all patients with aspiration of stomach content be treated with mechanical ventilation?
10. What criteria do you use to treat aspiration with mechanical ventilation?
11. What is Mendelson's syndrome?

D. Postoperative Management

1. The newborn Apgar score was 6. Discuss management.

A. Medical Disease and Differential Diagnosis

A.1. What is the incidence of breech presentation?

The incidence of breech presentation is approximately 3.5% of pregnancies.

Greenhill JP, Friedman EA: Biological Principles and Modern Practice of Obstetrics, p 598. Philadelphia, WB Saunders, 1974

A.2. Name the different types of breech presentation.

The three main types of breech presentations are as follows:
- Frank breech
- Complete breech
- Incomplete breech

A frank breech is one in which the lower extremities are flexed at the hips and extended at the knees so that the feet are against the face. A complete breech is one in which the fetal lower extremities are flexed at both the hips and knees so that the buttocks with the feet along side them present at the cervix. Incomplete breech presentation is one in which one or both fetal lower extremities are extended and one or both feet present in the vagina or introitus. This type is also referred to as a single or double footling breech presentation.

Frank breech is present in 60% of all breech deliveries, incomplete breech is found in 30%, and complete breech appears in 10% approximately.

Shnider SM, Levinson G: Anesthesia for Obstetrics, p 171. Baltimore, Williams & Wilkins, 1979

A.3. What is the etiology of breech presentation?

The etiology of breech presentation is not known, but several associated factors are thought to predispose to this presentation. Breech presentations are more common in premature than in full-term fetuses.
  Additional factors include the following:

- Abnormalities of the fetus (*e.g.*, hydrocephalus, anencephaly)
- Abnormalities of the uterus (*e.g.*, placenta previa, uterine anomalies)
- Others (*e.g.*, pelvic tumors, multiple fetuses, polyhydramnios)

Shnider SM, Levinson G: Anesthesia for Obstetrics, p 171, Baltimore, Williams & Wilkins, 1979

A.4. How is the diagnosis of breech presentation made?

The diagnosis of breech presentation is usually made by manual examination.

Shnider SM, Levinson G: Anesthesia for Obstetrics, p 171. Baltimore, Williams & Wilkins, 1979

A.5. Are breech deliveries associated with increased maternal morbidity?

Yes. Breech deliveries are associated with increased maternal morbidity. Compared with vertex presentations there is greater likelihood of cervical lacerations, perineal injury, shock due to intrapartum and postpartum hemorrhage, retained placenta, and infection.

Pritchard JA, MacDonald PC: Williams Obstetrics, 15th ed, pp 889–902. New York, Appleton–Century–Crofts, 1976

A.6. Why are the perinatal morbidity and mortality of the infant comparatively higher in breech deliveries than in vertex deliveries?

The perinatal mortality rate, corrected for prematurity and congenital anomalies, is almost four times higher in breech deliveries. These infants are more likely to suffer asphyxia from cord compression and intracranial hemorrhage from head trauma. Intrauterine manipulation may further increase fetal trauma and cord compression. During spontaneous breech delivery, the uncontrolled expulsion of the fragile fetal head can result in tentorial tears and brain damage. Prolapse of the umbilical cord is a significant cause of fetal mortality. The incidence of cord prolapse is 0.5%

with frank breech presentation, and 10% with incomplete or complete breech presentation.

Morgan HS et al: An analysis of 16,327 breech births. JAMA 187:262, 1964

Shnider SM, Levinson G: Anesthesia for Obstetrics, p 171. Baltimore, Williams & Wilkins, 1979

B. Preoperative Evaluation and Preparation

B.1. What is meant by baseline heart rate of the fetus?

The fetal heart rate (FHR) is normally 120 to 160 beats/min. Fetal tachycardia is defined as a sustained heart rate of more than 160 beats/min; fetal bradycardia as a sustained rate of less than 120 beats/min. Elevated rates are associated with chronic fetal distress, maternal fever, and drugs (*e.g.*, atropine administered to the mother). Fetal bradycardia is associated with congenital heart block, severe hypoxia and asphyxia, and the administration of drugs such as propranolol.

Cohen H: Fetal and infant evaluation during labor and delivery. ASA Refresher Courses in Anesthesiology 7:71–86, 1979

B.2. What is meant by beat-to-beat variability in the fetal heart rate (FHR)?

Normal beat-to-beat variability in the FHR ranges from 7 to 14 beats/min. The variability provides the single best method for evaluating the well-being of the near-term or term fetus. Absence of variability may occur in the premature fetus, in the normal mature fetus during sleep cycles, and in fetal central nervous system (CNS) depression or damage. Some variability should normally be present. Loss of variability may indicate CNS depression caused by drugs or hypoxia.

Cohen H: Fetal and infant evaluation during labor and delivery. ASA Refresher Courses in Anesthesiology 7:71–86, 1979

B.3. Discuss the various patterns of FHR deceleration.

FHR deceleration occurs in three major forms: early, late, and variable deceleration.

- Early deceleration (type I dip)—begins with the onset of a uterine contraction, has a uniform wavelike shape, attains its lowest point at the peak of the contraction, and gradually returns to the baseline as the contraction subsides. FHR usually does not fall below 100 beats/min. Deceleration in FHR is thought to be caused by vagal stimulation secondary to fetal head compression with descent of the head into the bony pelvis. Administration of large doses of atropine (1.0 mg) to the mother may ameliorate this deceleration pattern. Administration of oxygen to the mother is of no benefit. This pattern is of no serious consequences to the fetus.

- Late deceleration (type II dip)—occurs after the onset of a uterine contraction and persists beyond the contraction. It also has a uniform wavelike shape. The FHR reaches its lowest point beyond the peak of the uterine contraction. The late deceleration pattern is thought to be caused by fetal myocardial hypoxia due to uteroplacental insufficiency. Administration of oxygen to the mother (provided there is placental perfusion) will improve fetal oxygenation and will eliminate or attenuate late deceleration. When this pattern becomes repetitive and of increasing severity, the fetus becomes acidotic, and signs of severe intrauterine fetal asphyxia develop. Common causes include maternal hypotension, uterine hyperactivity or hypertonicity, and chronic uteroplacental insufficiency.
- Variable deceleration (type III dip)—is the most common pattern observed during the intrapartum period. This pattern lacks consistency in configuration and in temporal relationships to uterine contractions. It is often preceded or followed by a brief period of acceleration. Variable deceleration may begin before, during, or after the onset of a uterine contraction. Quite often the deceleration is severe, the FHR decreasing to less than 100 beats/min. Variable deceleration patterns are thought to be caused by umbilical cord compression, with severe cardiovascular reflex response in the fetus. Atropine given to the mother may diminish the severity of the deceleration. Administration of oxygen is without effect. When compression of the umbilical cord is transient, fetal acidosis rarely occurs. If compression becomes severe and prolonged, progressive fetal acidosis develops. A variable deceleration that lasts more than a minute, with an associated FHR of less than 60 beats/min, may indicate acute fetal distress and impending death *in utero*.

Cohen H: Fetal and infant evaluation during labor and delivery. ASA Refresher Courses in Anesthesiology 7:71–86, 1979

B.4. What are normal values of fetal blood gases?

- Umbilical vein
  pH, 7.32; P_{CO_2}, 40±2 torr; P_{O_2}, 29±3 torr; O_2 saturation, 70%
- Umbilical artery
  pH, 7.21; P_{CO_2}, 55±3 torr; P_{O_2} 22±2 torr; O_2 saturation, 40%

The pH of the scalp sample lies between the pH of arterial blood and that of venous blood. The fetal capillary blood pH values of 7.25 or more are classified as normal, pH 7.20 to 7.24 is defined as preacidotic, and pH 7.20 is the lowest limit of normal.

Bonica JJ: Principles and Practice of Obstetric Analgesia and Anesthesia, p 127. Philadelphia, FA Davis, 1972

Cohen H: Fetal and infant evaluation during labor and delivery. ASA Refresher Courses in Anesthesiology 7:71–86, 1979

B.5. The patient is scheduled for an emergency cesarean section. Would you premedicate this patient? What premedicants would you use, and why?

Yes. I would premedicate this patient with milk of magnesia, 30 ml by mouth. All parturients should receive oral antacid therapy every 2 hours during labor. The usual mixture is aluminum hydroxide and magnesium hydroxide. Woman scheduled to have elective cesarean section should be given a dose ½ hour before anesthesia induction. In an emergency situation, where there is not enough time for the full buffering effect to be achieved, it has been shown that a single oral dose of milk of magnesia (30 ml) or sodium citrate (15 ml) requires only 10 minutes to buffer gastric acid to a pH of greater than 2.5. Premedication with narcotics or ataractics is *not* indicated before cesarean section. The neonatal depressant effects outweigh any possible maternal benefit. Anticholinergic derivatives may be given intravenously immediately before induction if necessary.

Max FG, Bassell GM: Obstetric Analgesia and Anesthesia, p 285. New York, Elsevier–Dutton, 1980

C. Intraoperative Management

C.1. What anesthetic technique would you use for emergency cesarean section?

Conduction anesthesia is not a good choice for a real emergency cesarean section. Epidural anesthesia is time consuming. Both spinal and epidural anesthesia may precipitate hypotension and further decrease blood flow to the fetus. In the presence of fetal distress, we avoid conduction anesthesia. General anesthesia is the choice.

C.2. What are the advantages and disadvantages of spinal anesthesia and epidural anesthesia for cesarean section?

The principal advantages of spinal anesthesia for cesarean section are simplicity, speed, reliability, and minimal fetal drug exposure. The parturient remains awake, and the hazards of aspiration are minimized. Disadvantages of spinal anesthesia include the high incidence of hypotension, intrapartum nausea and vomiting, and the possibility of postlumbar puncture headache.

The advantages attributed to lumbar epidural anesthesia for cesarean delivery include the avoidance of dural puncture and the decreased incidence and severity of maternal hypotension. In either technique, blood loss is less than that associated with general anesthesia.

Datta S, Alper MH: Anesthesia for cesarean section. Anesthesiology 53:142–160, 1980

C.3. What intravenous induction agents would you use?

The commonly used agent is a thiobarbiturate, usually thiopental. A single dose of 4 mg/kg does not significantly affect the fetal outcome as measured by Apgar score.

Ketamine has been advocated for induction of anesthesia, especially in the presence of unstable maternal hemodynamics associated with blood loss. With doses as high as 1 mg/kg, Peltz and Sinclair found no deleterious effect in the newborn. Ellingson et al reported that levels of ketamine in cord blood exceeded those in maternal vein blood within 97 seconds of its injection, with maximal levels at 125 seconds. The place of ketamine in obstetrics remains unsettled.

Stovner and Vangen compared diazepam, 20 mg, with thiopental, 200 mg, and found no difference in neonatal conditions as measured by Apgar score. However, diazepam has been associated with neonatal hypotonia and increased susceptibility to cold stress.

Datta S, Alper MH: Anesthesia for cesarean section. Anesthesiology 53:142–160, 1980

Ellington A, Haram R, Sagen N et al: Transplacental passage of ketamine after intravenous administration. Acta Anaesthesiol Scand 21:41–44, 1977

Peltz B, Sinclair DM: Induction agents for caesarian section. Anaesthesia 28:37–42, 1973

Stovner J, Vangem O: Diazepam compared to thiopentone as induction agent for caesarian sections. Acta Anaesthesiol Scand 18:264–269, 1974

C.4. *Thiopental crosses the placenta rapidly, and it is not possible to deliver the fetus before the drug is transferred to the fetus. Why is the neonate not affected when 4 mg/kg of thiopental is given to the mother?*

After a single maternal intravenous dose, the drug can be detected in umbilical venous blood within 30 seconds. It reaches its peak concentration in umbilical venous blood in 1 minute and in umbilical arterial blood in 2 to 3 minutes. After 4 mg/kg of thiopental is given, the fetal brain concentration is not high. Umbilical arterial levels of thiopental are much lower than umbilical venous levels. This may be due to the fact that blood from the placenta first passes through the liver, so most of the thiopental is either cleared by the liver, or diluted by blood from the lower extremities and viscera. Other reasons are swift decline of the drug concentration in maternal blood, and nonhomogeneous distribution in the intervillous space. *Note,* after large doses of thiopental (8 mg/kg) neonates are delivered depressed.

Shnider SM, Levinson G: Anesthesia for Obstetrics, pp 263–264. Baltimore, Williams & Wilkins, 1979

C.5. *Describe the technique of general anesthesia for emergency cesarean section.*

The patient is placed on the operating table with head slightly elevated and pelvis tilted to the left by a wedge under the right hip. The abdomen is surgically prepared and draped. Blood pressure and ECG are monitored. After preoxygenation for 5 minutes and precurarization with 3 to 6 mg of d-tubocurarine, anesthesia is rapidly induced with thiopental (4 mg/kg pregnant body weight) and succinylcholine (1.0–1.5 mg/kg pregnant body weight), Cricoid pressure (Sellick's maneuver) is applied during intubation with a cuffed endotracheal tube. Anesthesia is maintained with nitrous oxide/oxygen and a succinylcholine infusion to provide adequate muscle relaxation. Halothane, 0.5%, or enflurane, 1.0%, may be added to prevent maternal awareness and recall. After delivery of the baby and clamping of the umbilical cord, narcotic or other adjuvants are administered as needed, to maintain anesthesia. Extreme care must be taken at the end of the procedure and during extubation to avoid aspiration. The patient may be extubated when she regains consciousness and there is adequate spontaneous respiration.

Ostheimer GW: Physiologic changes in the paturient. Anesthesiology Review 6, No 2:17–21, 1979

C.6. Does 0.5% halothane decrease uterine contractility? Discuss the effects of inhalation agents on the uterine contraction.

Yes. The uterine contractility is depressed by 0.5% halothane, but it is still responsive to oxytocin stimulation. Halothane, enflurane, and isoflurane are potent uterine depressants. Munson and Embro reported that halothane, enflurane, and isoflurane at equivalent minimal alveolar concentration (MAC), had the same degree of uterine depression. In our laboratory, we found that at equivalent MAC, enflurane is the most potent uterine depressant, followed by isoflurane, halothane, ether, methoxyflurane, and cyclopropane. The dose-response curves for all the above mentioned agents show a linear relationship in a semi-log plot. However, clinically there is no increased blood loss with low-dose halothane, 0.1% to 0.8%, or enflurane, 0.5% to 1.5% during cesarean section, because at these low concentrations, the uterus still responds to oxytocin stimulation.

Yao FS, Tjeuw MTB, Van Poznak A: Relative depressant effects of enflurane, isoflurane, halothane, diethylether, cyclopropane, and methoxyflurane on isolated human gravid and nongravid uterine muscle. Unpublished. Presented at the New York Academy of Medicine, May 5, 1976

Munson ES, Embro W: Enflurane, isoflurane and halothane, and isolated human uterine muscle. Anesthesiology 46:11–14, 1977

C.7. If the patient vomits and aspirates during intubation, discuss the immediate management.

If the patient vomits, the table is rapidly tilted to a 30° to 40° head-down position. When the larynx is at a higher level than the pharynx, gastric material can drain to the outside.

The mouth and pharynx should be suctioned rapidly. If solid material is found, it is scooped out. A finger wrapped in gauze is a good method. Get a clear view of the larynx, apply pressure on the cricoid, intubate, and inflate the cuff immediately to prevent further aspiration. If the condition of the patient allows, apply suction through the endotracheal tube before administering 100% oxygen by positive pressure ventilation. This is to prevent pushing aspirated material further into the bronchi. Suction should be brief (less than 15 seconds) to avoid hypoxia. Give 100% oxygen both before and after suctioning subsequently.

Bronchial irrigation is indicated only in the obstructive type of aspiration. 5 to 10 ml of normal saline are instilled into the tracheobronchial tree, followed immediately by suction. It is preceded and followed by oxygenation. The sequence is repeated until the aspirated fluid is clear. To evacuate the stomach, a nasogastric tube should be inserted. The evacuated material should be sent to the laboratory for pH determination. If the patient has bronchospasm, give aminophylline, 250 mg slowly IV, followed by 250 mg in 250 ml of 5% dextrose in water at a rate of 1 mg/kg/hr.

Abouleish E et al: Vomiting, regurgitation, and aspiration in Obstetrics. Pa Med 77:45–58, 1974

C.8. Should bronchoscopy be performed on all patients with aspiration of the stomach contents?

No. Bronchoscopy should not be performed on all patients with aspiration of stomach contents. When solid particles are causing obstruction, bronchoscopy should be performed by an experienced person. The history, physical examination, x-ray of the chest, and nature of the gastric contents help to determine the need for bronchoscopy.

Abouleish E et al: Vomiting, regurgitation, and aspiration in obstetrics. Pa Med 77:45–58, 1974

C.9. Should all patients with aspiration of stomach contents be treated with mechanical ventilation?

No. Not all patients with aspiration of stomach contents will have respiratory insufficiency or failure. Some patients have the initial cyanosis, bronchospasm, or respiratory dysfunction, and then improve spontaneously. Therefore, patients should be meticulously observed for at least 48 hours for symptoms and signs of respiratory insufficiency and treatment initiated accordingly. Chest x-ray and arterial blood gases should be followed carefully.

Abouleish E et al: Vomiting, regurgitation, and aspiration in obstetrics. Pa Med 77:45–58, 1974

C.10. What criteria do you use to treat aspiration with mechanical ventilation?

Mechanical ventilation is required if the patient shows the following signs and symptoms: dyspnea, cyanosis, tachypnea, tachycardia, tracheal tug, retraction, flaring, the use of accessory muscles of respiration, PaO_2 of less than 200 mm Hg on 100% oxygen, $PaCO_2$ higher than 50 mm Hg, arterial pH less than 7.2, increased dead space (V_D/V_T more than 60%), vital capacity less than 15 ml/kg, effective compliance less than 15 ml/cm H_2O. In such cases, intubation and institutions of intermittent positive pressure ventilation (IPPV) with positive end-expiratory pressure (PEEP) may be of great value.

The advantages of IPPV in these cases are as follows:

- It relieves the patient's exhaustion and dyspnea.
- It improves alveolar ventilation, and reduces shunting.
- It is beneficial in preventing and treating acute pulmonary edema by reducing transmural pulmonary arterial pressure.
- It allows removal of secretions by suction.

Bendixen H et al: Respiratory Care. St Louis CV Mosby, 1965

McCormick PW: The severe pulmonary aspiration syndrome in obstetrics. Proceedings of the Royal Society of Medicine 59:66, 1966

C.11. What is Mendelson's syndrome?

Mendelson's syndrome is the result of aspiration of liquid gastric juice with a pH of 2.5 or less, which produces clinical symptoms and signs of pulmonary edema, pulmonary vasoconstriction, and pulmonary hypertension. Tachypnea, cyanosis, tachycardia, wheezing, bloody frothy sputum, and arterial hypotension may also occur. The chest x-ray shows a classic picture of irregular soft mottling in the peripheral lung fields. Pulmonary compliance is decreased. There are ventilation/perfusion inequalities and significant intrapulmonary shunting.

Mendelson CL: The aspiration of stomach contents into the lungs during obstetric anesthesia. Am J Obstet Gynecol 52:191, 1946

D. Postoperative Management

D.1. The newborn Apgar score was 6. Discuss management.

The newborn with an Apgar score of 6 has generally suffered some mild asphyxia just prior to birth, and usually responds to vigorous stimulation and oxygen blown over the face. If the infant fails to do so within 60 seconds, assisted ventilation is instituted with an oxygen-enriched mixture. These infants are generally well by 5 minutes of age.

Gregory GA: Resuscitation of the newborn. Anesthesiology 43:225–237, 1975

Section Seven
The Hematologic System

27 Sickle Cell Disease
Vinod Malhotra

A 26-year-old black female was admitted for bilateral tubal ligation. She had frequent joint and bone pain, a past history of abdominal pain, and jaundice. Hematocrit 22%, blood pressure 140/60 torr, pulse 100/min.

A. Medical Disease and Differential Diagnosis

1. What was the most likely medical problem in this patient?
2. What is sickle cell disease?
3. What is sickle cell trait?
4. What does the term heterozygote imply in relation to sickle cell disease?
5. What are the clinical features of the disease?
6. What is sickle cell crisis?
7. What is the pathogenesis of sickle cell crisis?

B. Preoperative Evaluation and Preparation

1. What were the possible medically justifiable reasons for bilateral tubal ligation in this patient?
2. How would you evaluate this patient for anesthesia?
3. How would you prepare the patient for general anesthesia?
4. What is your opinion of preoperative exchange transfusion in these patients?

C. Intraoperative Management

1. What was the risk for anesthetic complications in this patient?
2. What anesthetic agents and techniques would you employ?
3. What special precautions should one take to prevent sickling in this patient?

D. Postoperative Management

1. How would you manage this patient in the immediate postoperative period?
2. What complications might occur in this patient in the immediate postoperative period?
3. What is the treatment of sickle cell crisis?

A. Medical Disease and Differential Diagnosis.

A.1. What was the most likely medical problem in this patient?

In light of the fact that this young black patient presented with a history of joint pains, abdominal pain, jaundice, and anemia, sickle cell disease was the most likely diagnosis.

Katz J, Benumof J, Kadis LB: Anesthesia and Uncommon Diseases, pp 327–328. Philadelphia, WB Saunders, 1981

A.2. What is sickle cell disease?

Sickle cell disease is a group of well-defined inherited hemoglobinopathies involving abnormal alteration of the globin moeity. Under certain conditions, especially hypoxia, the hemoglobin aggregates to give the red blood cells a crescent-shape (sickle) and hence the name.

Katz J, Benumof J, Kadis LB: Anesthesia and Uncommon Diseases, pp 325–327. Philadelphia, WB Saunders, 1981

A.3. What is sickle cell trait?

Sickle cell trait is used to describe a person who is a heterozygote for a normal hemoglobin gene (A) with an abnormal gene (S). Persons with sickle cell trait lead a normal life and do not present with symptoms, morbidity, or mortality associated with sickle cell disease.

Konotey–Ahulu FID: The sickle cell diseases. Arch Intern Med 133:612, 1974

A.4. What does the term heterozygote imply in relation to sickle cell disease?

The term heterozygote only describes the genotype of the individual and should not automatically be associated with sickle cell trait. Sickle cell trait is that heterozygous state in which there is one normal hemoglobin (A) gene and one abnormal hemoglobin (S) gene. If both the genes in the heterozygote are abnormal (*e.g.* SC, S Thal, SD), a disease state is evident. The classical sickle cell disease is homozygous for hemoglobin S and presents with the most severe form of the disease.

Konotey–Ahulu FID: The sickle cell diseases. Arch Intern Med 133:612, 1974

A.5. What are the clinical features of the disease?

Sickle cell disease is most common among the black population, although it has also been observed in Mediterraneans. It occurs in less than 1% of black Americans. The patients are young and present with the clinical picture of anemia, obstructive or hemolytic jaundice, joint and bone pains, abdominal and chest pains, lymphadenopathy, chronic leg ulcers, hematuria, epistaxis, priapism, finger clubbing, and skeletal deformities. The disease is characterized by periodic exaggeration of symptoms or sickle cell crisis.

Konotey–Ahulu FID: The sickle cell diseases. Arch Intern Med 133:612–618, 1974

A.6. What is sickle cell crisis?

Sickle cell crisis refers to the acute clinical picture due, generally, to sickling of red blood cells *in vivo*. Four main clinical types of crises have been described. They are the following:

- Vasculo-occlusive crises with organ infarction and pain
- Hemolytic crises with hematologic features of sudden hemolysis
- Sequestration syndrome with sequestration of red blood cells in liver and spleen causing their massive, sudden enlargement and an acute fall in peripheral hematocrit
- Aplastic crises with bone marrow suppression

The patient in painful crisis presents with fever, anemia, limb pain, and abdominal pain. He is tachypneic and may have enlarged liver and spleen in addition to abdominal tenderness. Peripheral blood smear shows sickle cells, and radiologic changes in the bones are evident.

Katz J, Benumof J, Kadis LB: Anesthesia and Uncommon Diseases, p 328. Philadelphia, WB Saunders, 1981

A.7. What is the pathogenesis of sickle cell crisis?

The pathogenesis of cell sickling involves the various factors that contribute to local hypoxia and acidosis. The pathogenesis is shown in Figure 27–1. Once sickling is initiated, it becomes a vicious cycle that causes more sickling unless proper remedial measures are undertaken.

Katz J, Benumof J, Kadis LB: Anesthesia and Uncommon Diseases, p 329. Philadelphia, WB Saunders, 1981

B. Preoperative Evaluation and Preparation

B.1. What were the possible medically justifiable reasons for bilateral tubal ligation in this patient?

In patients with sickle cell disease, the fetal and maternal mortality has been reported between 20% and 40%. Postpartum shock can result from

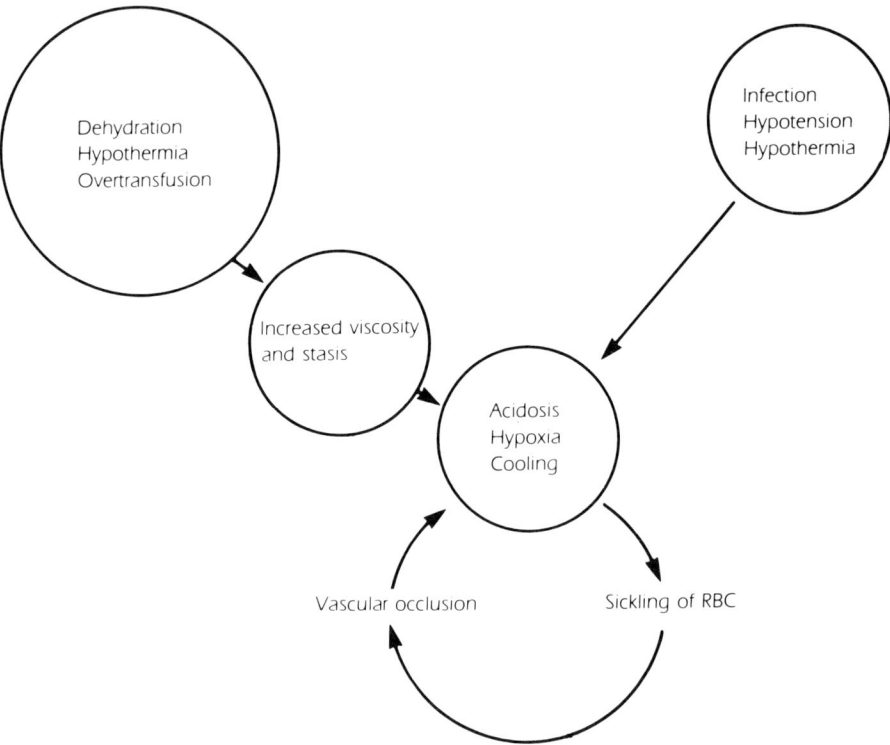

Fig. 27-1. Pathogenesis of sickle cell crisis

sudden sequestration syndrome. Because each pregnancy is fraught with danger regardless of previous pregnancies, family planning is important.

Sheehy TW, Plumb VJ: Treatment of sickle cell disease. Arch Intern Med 137:782, 1977

B.2. How would you evaluate this patient for anesthesia?

A careful history and physical examination should be done and cardiopulmonary status should be thoroughly investigated in view of cardiac and pulmonary complications in these patients. One should exclude dehydration or infection in the preoperative evaluation. The laboratory tests that should be carried out are as follows: complete blood count, prothrombin time, partial thromboplastin time, serum electrolytes, BUN, serum creatinine, urinalysis, ECG, and chest x-ray. In addition, the following specific tests should be carried out:

- Peripheral smear for evidence of sickle cells
- Sickle cell preparation
- Hemoglobin electrophoresis to determine hemoglobin S, quantitatively
- Reticulocyte count

Vandam LD: To Make the Patient Ready for Anesthesia, pp 168–169. Menlo Park, CA, Addison–Wesley, 1980

Sickle Cell Disease · 335

B.3. How would you prepare the patient for general anesthesia?

The patient's general condition should be improved and she should be well hydrated. Any infection should be treated promptly. Anemia should be treated with transfusion if hemoglobin is less than 7 g/100 ml. A hematocrit of between 25% and 30% seems to be best tolerated by these patients. Make no attempt to increase the hematocrit to normal values because increased viscosity, then, predisposes the patient to sickling.

Holzmann L, Finn H, Lichtman HC et al: Anesthesia in patients with sickle cell disease. A review of 112 cases. Anesth Analg (Cleve) 48:567, 1969

Vandam LD: To Make the Patient Ready for Anesthesia, pp 168–169. Menlo Park, CA, Addison–Wesley, 1980

B.4. What is your opinion of preoperative exchange transfusion in these patients?

Although controversy exists as to whether these patients should be exchange transfused preoperatively, we feel that for most surgical procedures, the exchange transfusion should be carried out with buffy-coat free packed red blood cells to reduce the hemoglobin S fraction to less than 40%.

Sheehy TW, Plumb VJ: Treatment of sickle cell disease. Arch Med 137:780, 1977

Vandam LD: To Make the Patient Ready for Anesthesia, pp 168–169. Menlo Park, CA, Addison–Wesley, 1980

C. Intraoperative Management

C.1. What was the risk for anesthetic complications in this patient?

This patient was anemic and might be debilitated with cardiopulmonary complications and ischemic damage to various organs. Patients with sickle cell disease often present with cardiomegaly, pulmonary hypertension and heart failure. Pulmonary infarcts and infection are common. A significant percentage of these patients also have renal and hepatic dysfunction. All these problems, in addition to the potential for sickling crisis and sequestration syndrome, pose a greater risk of complications from anesthesia. The patients at greater risk include those with homozygous state, sickle cell C disease and sickle thalassemia. In contrast, patients with sickle cell trait do not present an increased risk for anesthesia.

Holzmann L, Finn H, Lichtman HC et al: Anesthesia in patients with sickle cell disease. Anesth Analg (Cleve) 48:571, 1969

Vandam LD: To Make the Patient Ready for Anesthesia, pp 168–169. Menlo Park, CA, Addison–Wesley, 1980

C.2. What anesthetic agents and techniques would you employ?

A general inhalation anesthetic technique with the trachea intubated following adequate preoxygenation is a suitable technique. We prefer to hyperventilate these patients moderately to avoid acidosis. We use at least

40% inspired oxygen in lower abdominal and limb surgery but higher concentrations for upper abdominal and thoracic surgery or if cardiopulmonary disease is evident. As long as adequate precautions are taken to avoid complications with the understanding of the pathophysiology of this disease, almost any anesthetic technique may be employed.

Holzmann L, Finn H, Lichtman HC et al: Anesthesia in patients with sickle cell disease. Anesth Analg (Cleve) 48:571, 1969

Katz J, Benumof J, Kadis LB: Anesthesia and Uncommon Diseases, p 330. Philadelphia, WB Saunders, 1981

C.3. *What special precautions should one take to prevent sickling in this patient?*

One should avoid or correct the factors that precipitate sickling. Special precautions include the following:

- Avoid hypoxia by preoxygenating the patient and employing higher than usual concentrations of inspired oxygen.
- Prevent acidosis by maintaining adequate oxygenation and cardiac output. Prevent respiratory acidosis by hyperventilation. Administration of alkaline buffer solutions has been recommended although we have found them rarely necessary.
- Prevent stasis. This requires proper hydration and good regional blood flow. Blood viscosity should be maintained low by limiting the rise in hematocrit to 30 and by avoiding overtransfusion. Low molecular weight dextran infusion may be helpful, too. We strongly advise against the use of tourniquets even though they have been used without ill effects in the past.
- Prevent dehydration. Patients should be well hydrated and we are quite generous with fluids in these patients. However, the cardiopulmonary complications should be kept in mind and cardiac overload should be avoided. In view of possible renal dysfunction, proper electrolyte balance should be maintained.
- Prevent hypothermia. All of these patients are monitored for body temperature and should be kept warm with a body warming device not only in the operating room, but also postoperatively.
- Replace blood loss accurately to prevent anemia or overtransfusion, which may lead to increased viscosity and cardiac failure. Fresh blood is preferred to stored blood and all blood should be given through a blood warmer.

Browne RA: Anesthesia in patients with sickle cell anemia. Br J Anaesth 37:184–186, 1965

D. Postoperative Management

D.1. *How would you manage this patient in the immediate postoperative period?*

All the prophylactic steps instituted in the preoperative period and carried on intraoperatively, should be followed through in the immediate postoperative period—namely, prevention of hypoxia, acidosis, hypotension, stasis and hypothermia. Respiratory depression should be avoided and supplemental oxygen should be given during the first 24 hours after anesthesia.

Katz J, Benumof J, Kadis LB: Anesthesia and Uncommon Diseases, p 330. Philadelphia, WB Saunders, 1981

D.2. What complications might occur in this patient in the immediate postoperative period?

The incidence of postoperative respiratory infection is considerably high and is a leading cause of morbidity. Hypoxemic episodes are always a threat in that they might precipitate a sickling crisis. Sequestration syndrome with shock is a potentially lethal complication, especially in immediate postpartum phase. Patients with cardiomegaly and pulmonary hypertension are prone to heart failure. Renal and hepatic dysfunction may result in prolongation of the effects of certain drugs.

Holzmann L, Finn H, Lichtman HC et al: Anesthesia in patients with sickle cell disease. Anesth Analg (Cleve) 48:571, 1969

Katz J, Benumof J, Kadis LB: Anesthesia and Uncommon Diseases, p 330. Philadelphia, WB Saunders, 1981

D.3. What is the treatment of sickle cell crisis?

The principles of treatment of painful sickle cell crisis include the following:

- Bed rest
- Sedation
- Hydration—oral or parenteral
- Sodium bicarbonate—to treat or prevent acidosis
- Oxygen therapy if hypoxemia is suspected
- Treat any infection
- Analgesics—nonnarcotics preferably to avoid respiratory depression. Narcotics may be necessary in severe cases.
- Transfusion—partial exchange transfusions are helpful in reducing the amount of hemoglobin S and thus ameliorating the symptoms.

Sheehy TW, Plumb VJ: Treatment of sickle cell disease. Arch Intern Med 137:779–780, 1977

28 Hemophilia
Michael Tjeuw

A 2-year-old boy had a foreign body in his ear and was bleeding. He was apparently in distress. Emergency removal of the foreign body was scheduled. BP 70/50; PR 140; HCT 36; weight 16 kg.

A. Medical Disease and Differential Diagnosis

1. What was the differential diagnosis of blood coagulopathy in this two year old boy?
2. How many types of hemophilia are there?
3. What is the incidence of hemophilia A? Discuss its pathology.
4. What is von Willebrands disease?
5. What are the findings of clotting time, bleeding time, prothrombin time, and partial thromboplastin time (PTT) in patients with hemophilia, von Willebrand's disease, and thrombocytopenia?

B. Preoperative Evaluation and Preparation

1. How would you prepare the patient with classic hemophilia A for elective surgery?
2. What is meant by one unit of factor VIII?
3. How many units of factor VIII are there in one bag of cryoprecipitate?
4. Should cryoprecipitate be typed and cross-matched?
5. How does aspirin (acetyl salicylate) cause abnormal bleeding?
6. Discuss the function of platelets.
7. This child had hemorrhagic diathesis. How would you evaluate him preoperatively?
8. Would you premedicate this child? With what premedicant?

Hemophilia · 339

C. Intraoperative Management

1. What monitoring would you use on this child?
2. Discuss the pediatric anesthetic apparatus you would use.
3. Why do you need high gas flows for the Jackson–Rees system?
4. Would you plan to intubate this child?
5. What size endotracheal tube would you use?
6. How does the anatomy of a child's larynx differ from that of the adult?
7. What techniques are available for induction of anesthesia? What agents and dosage?
8. The intravenous line infiltrated. How would you induce anesthesia for this child?
9. Why wouldn't you use ketamine intramuscularly?
10. What would you see during ketamine anesthesia?
11. Draw the chemical structures of halothane, enflurane, and isoflurane.
12. Are halothane, enflurane, and isoflurane metabolized in man?
13. This child had nothing by mouth for 4 hours. Discuss fluid therapy.
14. What is the estimated blood volume in children?
15. How do body mechanisms act to conserve fluids?

D. Postoperative Management

1. After the child was extubated in the operating room, he developed laryngospasm. Discuss management.
2. The patient was suspected of having laryngeal edema. How would you confirm the diagnosis? Discuss its management.
3. What is meant by emergence delirium? What is the cause? Discuss its management.
4. How and where does scopolamine act in the central nervous system (CNS)? What is the mechanism of action of physostigmine?

A. Medical Disease and Differential Diagnosis

A.1. What was the differential diagnosis of blood coagulopathy in this two year old boy?

The differential diagnosis of blood coagulopathy includes the following:
- Hereditary coagulation factor deficiency (Table 28–1)
- Acquired coagulation factor deficiency
  - Liver disease
  - Vitamin K deficiency
- Disease state
  - Leukemia
  - Platelet deficiency or defect in function

Isselbacher KJ et al: Harrison's Principles of Internal Medicine, 9th ed, pp 278, 1560–1565. New York, McGraw–Hill, 1980

Table 28-1. Hereditary coagulation factor deficiency disorders

DEFICIENT FACTOR	PREFERRED TERM	SYNONYMS
Fibrinogen (Factor I)	Afibrinogenemia hereditary	Hypofibrinogenemia Factor I deficiency
Prothrombin (Factor II)	Hypoprothrombinemia hereditary	Factor II deficiency Prothrombin deficiency
Factor V	Factor V deficiency	Parahemophilia Owren's disease
Factor VII	Factor VII deficiency	Hypoproconvertinemia
Factor VIII	Hemophilia A	Classic hemophilia Factor VIII deficiency AHF or AHG deficiency
	von Willebrand's disease	Vascular hemophilia Pseudohemophilia Angiohemophilia
Factor IX	Hemophilia B	Christmas disease Factor IX deficiency PTC deficiency
Factor X	Factor X deficiency	Stuart deficiency
Factor XI	Factor XI deficiency	PTA deficiency Hemophilia C Rosenthal syndrome
Factor XII	Factor XII deficiency	Hageman trait
Factor XIII	Factor XIII deficiency	Fibrin stabilizing factor deficiency

A.2. How many types of hemophilia are there?

The term "hemophilia" is often confusing because it is used by some to denote specifically classic hemophilia (hemophilia A, factor VIII deficiency), by others in a slightly broader sense to include hemophilia B (Christmas disease, factor IX deficiency), and by still others in a broad sense to include all of the hereditary coagulation factor deficiencies. (see synonyms in Table 28-1). In the broad usage, the hemophilias may be defined as a group of hereditary bleeding disorders caused by deficient activity of one or another of the ten plasma clotting factors needed for normal blood coagulation.

- Hemophilia A   (Classic hemophilia)
- Hemophilia B   (Christmas disease)
- Hemophilia C   (Rosenthal syndrome)
- Parahemophilia   (Owren's disease)
- Vascular hemophilia   (von Willebrand's disease)

Hemophilia A and hemophilia B are the most common. They account for 85% to 90% of all cases of hemophilia.

Weiss AE, Brinkhouse KM: Pathogenesis and Incidence of the Hemophilia, pp 3–16. Washington, DC, National Academy of Sciences, 1973

A.3. What is the incidence of hemophilia A? Discuss its pathology.

The incidence of hemophilia A is 1:10,000 births. It is a familial disorder of blood coagulation. It is the result of functional deficiency of antihemophilic factor (factor VIII). The plasma does *not* lack antihemophilic factor. Rather, it appears to contain a nonfunctional variant of this clotting factor. The disorder is due to an x-linked recessive gene, so that the disorder occurs almost exclusively in males. The sons of a male hemophiliac are unaffected and do not transmit the disease, although all his daughters are carriers. Heterozygous females do not bleed, but half their sons have hemophilia and half their daughters are carriers. Homozygous females, very rarely encountered, have the typical disease.

Isselbacher KJ et al: Harrison's Principles of Internal Medicine, 9th ed, p 1560. New York, McGraw–Hill, 1980

A.4. What is von Willebrand's disease?

Von Willebrand's disease (vascular hemophilia) is a hemorrhagic disorder characterized by a long bleeding time, abnormal platelet aggregation, low levels of factor VIII procoagulant activity, and decreased amount of factor VIII–von Willebrand protein. The disease is transmitted by a dominant autosomal mutant gene, but has been detected more often in women than in men. The severity of symptoms varies considerably among affected members of the same family; some may be asymptomatic. Menorrhagia and postpartum bleeding are common. A unique feature of von Willebrand's disease is the *prolonged bleeding time,* an abnormality not usually seen in hemophilic-like diseases. The coagulation defect can be corrected by giving normal plasma or even giving hemophiliac plasma. One pathognomonic test for von Willebrand's disease is the response to the infusion of plasma. In contrast to the patient with hemophilia, whose factor VIII level is maximal immediately after a plasma cryoprecipitate infusion, the patient with von Willebrand's disease demonstrates the same immediate rise in factor VIII level, but then the level continues to increase for as long as 48 hours. This indicates that the patient is producing factor VIII. These patients seem to lack a factor that controls factor VIII production.

Ellison N, Jobes DR: Diagnosis of disorders of hemostasis. ASA Refresher Courses in Anesthesiology 7:93–94, 1979

Wyngaarden JB, Smith LH: Textbook of Medicine, 16th ed, p 999. Philadelphia, WB Saunders, 1982

A.5. What are the findings of clotting time, bleeding time, prothrombin time, and partial thromboplastin time (PTT) in patients with hemophilia, von Willebrand's disease, and thrombocytopenia?

The differential diagnosis of hemophilia, von Willebrand's disease and thrombocytopenia are shown in Table 28–2.

Isselbacher KJ et al: Harrison's Principles of Internal Medicine, 9th ed, pp 278–279. New York, McGraw–Hill, 1980

342 · Anesthesiology

Table 28–2. The differential diagnosis of hemophilia, von Willebrand's disease, and thrombocytopenia

	DEFICIENCY BLOOD COMPONENTS	CLOTTING TIME	PARTIAL THROMBOPLASTIN TIME	BLEEDING TIME	PROTHROMBIN TIME
Classic hemophilia	Factor VIII	Long	Long	Normal	Normal
Christmas disease	Factor IX	Long	Long	Normal	Normal
Parahemophilia	Factor V	Long	Long	Normal	Long
von Willebrand's disease	Factor VIII	Variable	Variable	Long	Normal
Thrombocytopenia	Platelets	Normal	Normal	Long	Normal

B. Preoperative Evaluation and Preparation.

B.1. How would you prepare the patient with classic hemophilia A for elective surgery?

As patients with hemophilia A have a factor VIII deficiency, they should receive factor VIII replacement therapy. Ten percent of a normal factor VIII level can prevent spontaneous bleeding; 20% is necessary to ensure hemostasis in response to trauma; more than 30% is necessary to secure hemostasis following major operations. To ensure that factor VIII levels do not drop below 30%, it is common to infuse sufficient factor VIII to raise the level to 80% to 100% of normal and then give booster doses 4 to 12 hours later. The dose required depends on many variables, such as patient weight, metabolic rate, initial plasma level of the deficient factor, and magnitude of the operation. One unit per kg of body weight normally increases the factor VIII concentration by 2%. For example, if the desired increment of factor VIII activity is 40% for a 60-kg man, the units of factor VIII needed are as follows:

$$\frac{40\%}{2\%} \times 60 \text{ kg} = 1200 \text{ units}$$

The available biological preparations are normal plasma, fresh frozen plasma, fraction I, glycine precipitate, and cryoprecipitate.

Ellison N: Diagnosis and management of bleeding disorders. Anesthesiology 47:174, 1977

Miller RD: Anesthesia, p 68. New York, Churchill–Livingstone, 1981

B.2. What is meant by one unit of factor VIII?

One unit of clotting factor VIII activity is defined as the amount present in 1 ml of fresh average normal plasma. One unit of fresh frozen plasma contains approximately 200 ml of plasma with an average of 0.7 to 0.9 unit of clotting factor activity per ml.

Conn HF et al: Current Therapy, p 274. Philadelphia, WB Saunders, 1982

B.3. How many units of factor VIII are there in one bag of cryoprecipitate?

Factor VIII content varies from different blood banks in concentrations and consistency of quality. It ranges from 60 to 126 units per bag of cryoprecipitate. Each bag contains approximately 13 ml of cryoprecipitate.

Petit CR, Klein HG: Hemophilia, Hemophiliacs and the Health Care Delivery System, p 31. Bethesda, MD, Department of Health, Education and Welfare. Publication No. (NIH) 76-871

B.4. Should cryoprecipitate be typed and cross-matched?

Cryoprecipitate is frequently administered as ABO-compatible. However, this probably is not very important, because the concentration of antibodies in cryoprecipitate is extremely low. Cryoprecipitate may contain red blood cell fragments; thus, cryoprecipitate prepared from Rh-positive individuals can possibly sensitize Rh-negative individuals to the Rh antigen.

Miller RD: Anesthesia, p 914. New York, Churchill–Livingstone, 1981

B.5. How does aspirin (acetyl salicylate) cause abnormal bleeding?

Aspirin has platelet-inhibiting activity. Aspirin blocks the adhesion of platelets to connective tissue or collagen fibers, possibly through inhibition of collagen glycosyltransferase present in membranes of platelets. Aspirin also inhibits ADP release from platelets.

Aspirin irreversibly acetylates platelet cyclooxygenase (prostaglandin synthetase). The enzyme converts arachidonic acid to prostaglandin endoperoxide intermediate PGG2. The synthesis of prostaglandins in platelets is therefore reduced. Aspirin also appears to prevent the formation of thromboxane A2 (TXA2), a potent aggregating agent, by the platelets.

Gilman AG, Goodman LS, Gilman A: The Pharmacological Basis of Therapeutics, 6th ed, pp 685–686, 691. New York, Macmillan, 1980

B.6. Discuss the function of platelets.

In response to vascular injury, platelets accumulate at the site where they come in contact with collagen-containing subendothelial basement membrane. Platelet aggregation and platelet adhesion develop simultaneously. (*Platelet aggregation* means the affinity of platelets for one another; *platelet adhesion* means the affinity of platelets for nonplatelet surfaces). Platelet aggregation culminates with the release reaction. The released substances include ADP, serotonin, platelet factor 4 (PF4), catechols, and factors that modify vascular permeability and integrity. The most potent aggregating agent is ADP. ADP makes other platelets "sticky" and causes them to aggregate and release their ADP and to form an occlusive plug that is subsequently stabilized by fibrin formation. In small injuries, the resultant platelet plug may be sufficient to seal the defect. Platelets contribute to the coagulation mechanism in the extrinsic clotting system also. The final step in the formation of a clot, clot retraction, is probably due to a contractile mechanism found in platelets.

Ellison N, Jobes DR: Diagnosis of disorders of hemostasis. ASA Refresher Courses in Anesthesiology 7:90–91, 1979

B.7. This child had hemorrhagic diathesis. How would you evaluate him preoperatively?

The best means of detecting a hemorrhagic diathesis is to take a proper history. A family history of abnormal bleeding, a history of abnormal bleeding following dental extraction or previous surgery, and a history of drug ingestion such as aspirin are important. Petechiae or prolonged bleeding following superficial trauma is usually due to vascular or platelet abnormalities, whereas subcutaneous bleeding and ecchymosis are seen in deficiencies of coagulation factors. Hemoarthrosis or deep bleeding into muscles is more likely to be seen in coagulopathy. A coagulation profile that includes a prothrombin time, activated partial thromboplastin time, platelet count, fibrinogen level, and bleeding time should be obtained. Platelet function by means of a platelet aggregometer is helpful.

Ellison N: Diagnosis and management of bleeding disorders. Anesthesiology 47:173, 1977

B.8. Would you premedicate this child? With what premedicant?

Pentobarbital 2 to 4 mg/kg may be given orally or rectally. I would avoid intramuscular injection to prevent hematoma at the injection site. I would also avoid anticholinergic agents, because the heart rate is so rapid (pulse 140/min).

Dripps RD, Eckenhoff JE, Vandam LD: Introduction to Anesthesia, the Principles of Safe Practice, 5th ed, p 45. Philadelphia, WB Saunders, 1977

C. Intraoperative Management

C.1. What monitoring would you use on this child?

I would monitor the following:

- Blood pressure, using cuff or Doppler device
- Precordial stethoscope for respiration and heart tones
- Temperature
- ECG
- Inspired oxygen concentration, using an oxygen analyzer

Miller RD: Anesthesia, p 159. New York, Churchill–Livingstone, 1981

C.2. Discuss the pediatric anesthetic apparatus you would use.

The Jackson–Rees modification of the Ayre's T-piece is commonly used for children who weigh less than 15 to 20 kg. The advantages of this system are the relatively light weight, minimal resistance, and minimal danger of malfunction due to the absence of valves. The disadvantages include the necessity for high gas flows, heat loss, and drying of the airway.

Stehling L: Anesthesia for common pediatric surgical problems. ASA Refresher Courses in Anesthesiology 8:192, 1980

C.3. Why do you need high gas flows for the Jackson–Rees system?

High fresh gas flows are needed to prevent rebreathing of carbon dioxide. The gas flows needed to prevent rebreathing are approximately 2.5 times the minute volume. The minute volumes are calculated as follows:

$$\text{Minute volume} = \text{tidal volume } (V_T) \times \text{respiratory frequency } (f)$$
$$V_T = 6\text{–}7 \text{ ml/kg}$$
$$f = \text{according to age}$$

An acceptable approximation is minute volume = weight in kg × 150

Stehling L: Anesthesia for common pediatric surgical problems. ASA Refresher Courses in Anesthesiology 8:192–193, 1980

C.4. Would you plan to intubate this child?

Yes. Because this child is scheduled as an emergency, I would assume that he has a full stomach. Also surgery of the ear would make it difficult to mask the patient.

C.5. What size endotracheal tube would you use?

This patient is 2 years old. I would use an endotracheal tube of 20 French or 4.5 mm internal diameter and 13 cm in length. For children more than 1 year of age, the following guide is useful:

$$\text{Tube size (internal diameter in mm)} = 4 + \frac{\text{Age in years}}{4}$$
$$\text{Tube size in French} = 18 + \text{age in years}$$
$$\text{Tube length (cm)} = 12 + \frac{\text{Age in years}}{2}$$

Stehling L: Anesthesia for common pediatric surgical problems. ASA Refresher Courses in Anesthesiology 8:193, 1980

C.6. How does the anatomy of a child's larynx differ from that of the adult?

The differences are the following:

- The vocal cords are higher in children (at C 2–4 level) than in adults (at C 5–6 level).
- The larynx is funnel shaped in children, and the narrowest part is at the cricoid cartilage. The narrowest part of the adult larynx is at the level of the vocal cords.
- In children, the anterior attachment of the vocal cords is inferior to the posterior attachment.

- The angle formed by the epiglottis and vocal cords is more acute in the infant than in the adult.

Dripps RD, Eckenhoff JE, Vandam LD: Introduction to Anesthesia, The Principles of Safe Practice, 5th ed, pp 379–380. Philadelphia, WB Saunders, 1977

C.7. What techniques are available for induction of anesthesia? What agents and dosage?

The available techniques are the following:
- Rectal
    Methohexital, 20 mg/kg, or thiopental sodium, 30 mg/kg
- Intravenous
    Thiopental sodium, 3–5 mg/kg, methohexital, 1–2 mg/kg, or ketamine, 1–2 mg/kg
- Intramuscular
    Ketamine, 5–10 mg/kg
- Inhalational
    Halothane, enflurane, or isoflurane

Stehling L: Anesthesia for common pediatric surgical problems. ASA Refresher Courses in Anesthesiology 8:194–195, 1980

C.8. The intravenous line infiltrated. How would you induce anesthesia for this child?

Ideally, I would intubate him awake to protect the airway because I assume he has a full stomach. However, if this is not possible, inhalational induction with a potent inhalational agent or rectal thiopental would be my choice.

C.9. Why would you not use ketamine intramuscularly?

I would avoid intramuscular injection to a hemophiliac to avoid hemotoma at the injection site.

C.10. What would you see during ketamine anesthesia?

One might see purposeless movement, eyes opening, vocalization, nystagmus, increased blood pressure, and increased heart rate.

Miller RD: Anesthesia, pp 472–473. New York, Churchill Livingstone, 1981

C.11. Draw the chemical structures of halothane, enflurane, and isoflurane.

(See Fig. 28–1.)

Gilman AG, Goodman LS, Gilman A: Goodman and Gilman's The Pharmacological Basis of Therapeutics, 6th ed, p 277. New York, Macmillan, 1980

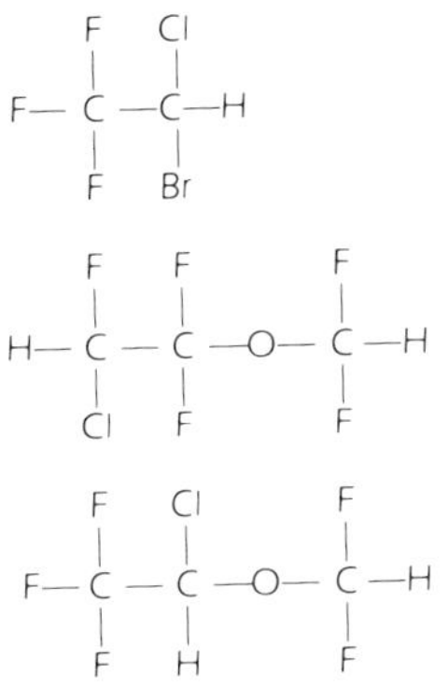

```
    F   Cl
    |   |
F — C — C — H        Halothane
    |   |
    F   Br

    F   F       F
    |   |       |
H — C — C — O — C — H    Enflurane
    |   |       |
    Cl  F       F

    F   Cl      F
    |   |       |
F — C — C — O — C — H    Isoflurane
    |   |       |
    F   H       F
```

Fig. 28-1. Chemical structures of halothane, enflurane, and isoflurane

C.12. Are halothane, enflurane, and isoflurane metabolized in man?

Yes. Approximately 12% to 20% of halothane is metabolized in man; the metabolic products are bromide, chloride, and trifluoroacetic acid. Approximately 2% of enflurane is metabolized. Approximately 0.2% of isoflurane is metabolized.

Gilman AG, Goodman LS, Gilman A: Goodman and Gilman's The Pharmacological Basis of Therapeutics, 6th ed, pp 282–285. New York, Macmillan, 1980

Holaday DA et al: Resistance of isoflurane and biotransformation in man. Anesthesiology 43, No. 3:330, 1975

C.13. This child had nothing by mouth for 4 hours. Discuss fluid therapy.

Fluid therapy may be calculated on the basis of body surface area or weight. The simplest method assumes that for maintenance fluid the average child requires approximately 4 ml/kg/hr for the first 10 kg adding 2 ml/kg/hr for the next 10 kg and 1 ml/kg/hr for weight over 20 kg. Intraoperative fluid requirement includes both maintenance fluid and replacement of the fluid deficit incurred by preoperative fasting.

This child weighs 16 kg
Maintenance fluid: 4 ml/hr × 10 + 2 ml/hr × 6 = 52 ml/hr
Deficit fluid: 52 ml/hr × 4 hr = 208 ml

This deficit fluid should be replaced over a period of 2 to 3 hours. Blood replacement regimen varies individually. Most anesthesiologists replace blood when more than 10% to 15% of the estimated blood volume is lost. Some allow the child to bleed to a calculated hematocrit of 30% without replacement. If crystalloid is used to replace the blood loss, the replacement volume is 3 to 4 times the amount of blood loss. When blood is needed, it should be replaced milliliter for milliliter, using a syringe for infusion.

Ahlergn EW: Rational fluid therapy for children. ASA Refresher Courses in Anesthesiology 7:4–5, 1979

C.14. What is the estimated blood volume in children?

The blood volume varies with age.

- Premature   100 ml/kg
- Newborn   90 ml/kg
- Small child 80–84 ml/kg
- Older child 70–80 ml/kg

Stehling L: Anesthesia for common pediatric surgical problems. ASA Refresher Courses in Anesthesiology 8:197, 1980

C.15. How do body mechanisms act to conserve fluids?

Fluids are conserved by the body to maintain adequate circulation and perfusion of the tissues. There are temporary compensatory mechanisms which conserve fluids, while the long-term mechanisms are activated to replenish and restore normal extracellular fluid volume. The temporary mechanism is transcapillary refill. If there is a decrease in circulating plasma volume, the loss is offset by an increased exchange of interstitial fluid. This refill process reduces interstitial fluid volume. There is loss of skin turgor, sunken eyeballs, and in the infant, sinking fontanelle.

The body mechanisms for conserving fluid with salt and water are primarily renal, the major one being the renin–angiotensin–aldosterone system. If salt and water are not adequately replaced, the antidiuretic hormone (ADH) is activated and the kidney absorbs the remaining water. The sympathetic nervous system is the last mechanism to be activated. If the amount of fluid loss is excessively fast or the volume is inadequate to maintain adequate circulation, the sympathetic nervous system will be activated and catecholamines are secreted to help support the circulation.

Miller RD: Anesthesia, p 877. New York, Churchill Livingstone, 1981

D. Postoperative Management

D.1. After the child was extubated in the operating room, he developed laryngospasm. Discuss management.

Laryngospasm during emergence from general anesthesia is a fairly common complication. Treatment with positive pressure applied by means of a mask and breathing bag with 100% oxygen should break the spasm in most instances. If laryngospasm persist to the point of hypoxia, a small dose of succinylcholine, 10–20 mg, IV, may be necessary to break the spasm.

Cullen DJ: Recovery room care of the surgical patient. ASA Refresher Courses in Anesthesiology 8:16, 1980

D.2. The patient was suspected of having laryngeal edema. How would you confirm the diagnosis? Discuss its management.

The first sign of laryngeal edema following extubation is a croupy cough beginning within a few minutes to a few hours. Sobbing inspiration and intercostal retraction are warning signs. Tachypnea, tachycardia, and sweating may be noted.

Management of laryngeal edema includes the following:

- Maximal humidification of inspired gases
- Administration of nebulized racemic epinephrine 2.25% (0.25–0.5 ml in 5 ml saline) during either spontaneous or positive-pressure ventilation every hour
- Administration of a steroid such as dexamethasone, 2 mg/kg, IV, was effective in reducing subglottic edema. It may be repeated every 3 hours.
- Induction of diuresis with furosemide, 10 to 20 mg, IV, has been suggested. In children, laryngeal edema can rapidly progress to complete airway obstruction. Therefore, the young patient should be observed closely in a unit staffed by experienced personnel. Equipment for performing emergency laryngoscopy, intubation, bronchoscopy, and tracheostomy must be available for immediate use.

Cullen DJ: Recovery room care of the surgical patient. ASA Refresher Courses in Anesthesiology 8:16–17, 1980

D.3. What is meant by emergence delirium? What is the cause? Discuss its management.

Emergence delirium is a phenomenon that occurs when a patient emerges from anesthesia more slowly than expected and is disoriented, uncooperative, or thrashes about. If this patient has had scopolamine as a premedicant, it is likely that scopolamine crossed the blood–brain barrier, thereby causing central nervous system (CNS) effects that can include delirium, hallucinations, and prolonged somnolence. After administration of physostigmine, 1 to 1.2 mg, IV, to patients who received scopolamine as a premedicant, 97% of the patients woke up or became orientated and cooperative within 1 to 15 minutes (average 5.8 min). It is important to note that pain or cerebral hypoxia may cause a similar picture of emergence delirium.

Cullen DJ: Recovery room care of the surgical patient. ASA Refresher Courses in Anesthesiology 8:26–27, 1980

D.4. How and where does scopolamine act in the central nervous system (CNS)? What is the mechanism of action of physostigmine?

Scopolamine competitively inhibits acetylcholine at cholinergic receptor sites in the CNS. Physostigmine is an anticholinesterase. It has tertiary ammonium ion, which crosses the blood brain barrier rapidly. Physostigmine antagonizes the effect of scopolamine by increasing the amount of acetylcholine at the cholinergic receptors. Physostigmine may also reverse the effects of major tranquilizers such as droperidol, haloperidol, and diazepam by a mechanism of action not yet known.

Cullen DJ: Recovery room care of the surgical patient. ASA Refresher Courses in Anesthesiology 8:27, 1980

Section Eight
Miscellaneous

29 Myasthenia Gravis
Alan Van Poznak

Following severe emotional stress, a 26-year-old woman had excessive fatigue upon use of voluntary muscles, particularly near the end of the day. At that time, she noticed diplopia, ptosis of the upper eyelids, and dysphagia. She was scheduled for thymectomy.

A. Medical Disease and Differential Diagnosis

1. What would the differential diagnosis include in the patient with symptoms as outlined in the case history?
2. From these myopathies, what tests would establish a diagnosis of myasthenia gravis?
3. What are the electrical events that take place during normal neuromuscular transmission? Does this sequence of events occur in the patient with myasthenia gravis?
4. What are the humoral events that take place during normal neuromuscular transmission? Does this sequence of events change in the patient with myasthenia gravis?
5. Is the basic mechanism of muscle contraction affected in myasthenia gravis? Outline the physiology of skeletal muscle contraction.

B. Preoperative Evaluation and Preparation

1. What drugs would you use to premedicate this patient? What would be your guide for this therapy?
2. Are there any laboratory data necessary for preparation of this patient for anesthesia and surgery?

C. Intraoperative Management

1. What anesthetic regimen would you choose for this patient? Why would you choose each drug?
2. What are the essential monitors to be used during thymectomy? Why?

D. Postoperative Management

1. What postanesthetic problems are likely to be encountered in this patient?
2. How would you manage ventilation, muscle power, and level of consciousness?

A. Medical Disease and Differential Diagnosis

A.1. What would the differential diagnosis include in the patient with symptoms as outlined in the case history?

The following conditions would be included in the differential diagnosis:
- Thyrotoxicosis
- Neurasthenia (neurosis)
- Progressive external ophthalmoplegia and other restricted myopathies
- Illnesses with dysarthria and dysphagia, but without ptosis or strabismus
- Myasthenic polymyopathy with hypersensitivity to neostigmine

Adams RD, Victor MV: Principles of Neurology, 2nd ed, pp 990–991. New York, McGraw–Hill, 1981

A.2. From these myopathies, what tests would establish a diagnosis of myasthenia gravis?

- What would be the response to anticholinesterase?
- What would be seen on electromyography (EMG)?
- What would be the response to the intravenous curare test?

Objective and subjective improvement are seen after edrophonium or neostigmine. The EMG would show rapid reduction in the amplitude of the compound action potential evoked during repetitive stimulation of a peripheral nerve at a rate of 3 per second (decrementing response). Marked weakness would be seen when a very small dose of curare was given intravenously.

Adams AD, Victor MV: Principles of Neurology, 2nd ed, p 990. New York, McGraw–Hill, 1981

A.3. What are the electrical events that take place during normal neuromuscular transmission? Does this sequence of events occur in the patient with myasthenia gravis?

Normal electrochemical equilibria are such that the inside of the cell is kept negative with respect to the outside by a potential difference of 70 to 90 millivolts. When an action potential occurs, the ionic fluxes are such that the interior of the cell may become positive by about 40 millivolts.

Such action potentials pass down myelinated motor axons to the motor nerve terminal, which is unmyelinated. At the motor nerve terminal, there is an abrupt slowing of propagation of the action potential together with an increased duration of the negative and positive afterpotentials. The nerve action potentials cause the end-plate potential of the muscle to change. If the threshold value is exceeded, there is then generated a muscle action potential. Excitation–contraction coupling then occurs, leading to a muscle contraction.

In myasthenia gravis, the initial motor unit potentials produced by voluntary contraction or electrical stimulation are normal. If stimuli are continued at a rate of about 3 per second, the amplitude of the potentials decreases, and then may increase somewhat. This partial block is similar to that produced by curare, and can be partially corrected with neostigmine.

Adams RD, Victor MV: Principles of Neurology, 2nd ed, p 883. New York McGraw–Hill, 1981

A.4. What are the humoral events that take place during normal neuromuscular transmission? Does this sequence of events change in the patient with myasthenia gravis?

Quanta of acetylcholine are liberated from nerve terminals by the arrival of nerve action potentials. The acetylcholine crosses the synaptic cleft and attaches to receptor sites on the sarcolemma, thereby causing the depolarization known as the end-plate potential. If the threshold is exceeded, an action potential invades the muscle cell membrane and spreads up and down its surface much like the nerve action potential. The liberated acetylcholine is hydrolyzed by cholinesterase, and then resynthesized by choline acetylase.

In myasthenia gravis, the receptors for acetylcholine are partially blocked by antibodies to the receptor substance protein. The release of transmitter substance is said to be normal, but combination with receptor substance is abnormal.

Adams RD, Victor MV: Principles of Neurology, 2nd ed, p 873. New York, McGraw–Hill, 1981

A.5. Is the basic mechanism of muscle contraction affected in myasthenia gravis? Outline the physiology of skeletal muscle contraction.

In myasthenia gravis, the basic mechanism of muscle contraction is normal. The electrical action potential spreads along the walls of the transverse tubules and to the sarcoplasmic reticulum, which releases calcium. The calcium binds to the regulatory protein troponin, thereby removing the inhibition exerted by the troponin–tropomyosin system upon the contractile protein actin. This allows an interaction to take place between the cross bridges of the myosin molecules in the thick filaments and the actin molecules of the thin filaments and enables myosin adenosine triphosphatase (ATPase) to split adenosine triphosphate (ATP) at a rapid rate, thereby providing the energy for contraction. This chemical change produces a force that causes the filaments to slide past each other. Relaxation occurs as a result of active (energy-dependent) calcium reuptake by the sarcoplasmic reticulum.

Adams RD, Victor MV: Principles of Neurology, 2nd ed, p 872. New York, McGraw–Hill, 1981

B. Preoperative Evaluation and Preparation

B.1. What drugs would you use to premedicate this patient? What would be your guide for this therapy?

I would use only those drugs necessary for management of the myasthenia gravis and the control of preoperative anxiety. A moderate dose of pentobarbital would be all that would be needed in most cases to control preoperative anxiety. Atropine could be given at that time, or it could be administered intravenously at the time of anesthetic induction.

B.2. Are there any laboratory data necessary for preparation of this patient for anesthesia and surgery?

In addition to the laboratory data necessary for all patients prior to anesthesia, this patient ought to have pulmonary function studies done and recorded.

C. Intraoperative Management

C.1. What anesthetic regime would you choose for this patient? Why would you choose each drug?

The anesthetic regime would be planned in a way to provide the least and the briefest interference with neuromuscular function. Induction would be with intravenous thiopental, followed by an inhalation mixture of oxygen–nitrous oxide, with added enflurane until tracheal intubation could be accomplished easily. No muscle relaxants would be used. Maintenance would be with light to moderate levels of agents, with early desaturation. Ventilation would be assisted or controlled.

C.2. What are the essential monitors to be used during thymectomy? Why?

In addition to the usual monitors of blood pressure and ECG, I would follow neuromuscular transmission with a peripheral nerve stimulator.

Blood gases or end-expiratory P_{CO_2} would be useful. Oxygen delivery from the anesthesia machine or the patient's exhalations should also be monitored.

D. Postoperative Management

D.1. What postanesthetic problems are likely to be encounterd in this patient?

Before extubating the patient, it is important to know that respiratory ability is adequate. This can be gauged in several ways. The neuromuscular transmission monitor will help in determining if additional neostigmine or pyridostigmine is needed. These drugs, if used, should be preceded by a dose of atropine sufficient to elevate the pulse rate by about 20%. Other measures of neuromuscular and respiratory function would also be used, such as maximal inspiratory force, grip strength, and adequate response to the head-lift test.

D.2. How would you manage ventilation, muscle power, and level of consciousness?

Until consciousness had returned, I would continue mechanical ventilation, keeping the arterial P_{CO_2} in the normal range. After the return of consciousness, I would assess muscle power and treat appropriately with atropine and neostigmine, as indicated by the neuromuscular transmission monitor and the patient's clinical responses. Analgesic narcotics would be used in the smallest doses which gave relief of postoperative pain. If any questions remained about the adequacy of ventilation, I would leave the patient intubated and on a ventilator until there was an opportunity to confer with the neurologists who would be responsible for taking care of the patient in a neurological intensive care unit.

Leventhal SR, Orkin FK, Hirsh RA: Prediction of the need for postoperative mechanical ventilation in myasthenia gravis. Anesthesiology 53:26–30, 1980

Smith CA: Postoperative management after thymectomy. Br Med J 1:309–312, 1975

30 Malignant Hyperthermia
Vinod Malhotra

A 5-year-old boy with kyphoscoliosis was scheduled for repair of strabismus under general anesthesia. Previous anesthetic history included an uneventful halothane, nitrous oxide anesthesia for bilateral myringotomy. However, the mother was very nervous because a first cousin of the boy died under anesthesia in Wisconsin the previous year.

A. Medical Disease and Differential Diagnosis

1. What was the problem of concern in this case?
2. What is malignant hyperthermia?
3. What are the clinical features of a susceptible patient?
4. Does the history of previous uneventful halothane anesthesia reasonably exlude the patient's susceptibility to malignant hyperthermia?
5. What are the clinical features of the syndrome?
6. What are the laboratory findings during an acute crisis of malignant hyperthermia?
7. What are the two clinical types of the syndrome?
8. What is the incidence of this syndrome?
9. What is the mode of inheritance of the disease?
10. What is the etiopathology of the syndrome?
11. What laboratory tests can further substantiate the susceptibility of the patient to malignant hyperthermia?

B. Preoperative Evaluation and Preparation

1. How would you prepare this patient for anesthesia and surgery?
2. What laboratory tests would you wish to obtain prior to surgery?
3. What premedication would you order?
4. In anticipation of general anesthesia, what preparations would you make?

C. Intraoperative Management

1. What anesthetic techniques and agents would you employ?
2. What anesthetic agents are contraindicated?
3. If the surgeon wishes to use local anesthesia for a procedure, what agents will you recommend?
4. Twenty minutes into the case, the patient developed increasing tachycardia with ventricular premature beats and mottled skin. What emergency measures would you take?
5. What modalities would you monitor closely during management of the crisis?

D. Postoperative Management

1. What complications may follow this syndrome?
2. What would be your follow-up on this case?
3. What would you advise the patient and the family?

A. Medical Disease and Differential Diagnosis

A.1. What was the problem of concern in this case?

The patient was a 5-year-old child with kyphoscoliosis and strabismus. There was a history of an anesthetic-related death in the family in the geographic area of Wisconsin. Therefore, in addition to the respiratory problems associated with kyphoscoliosis, he presented a likelihood of susceptibility to malignant hyperpyrexia syndrome. The supporting factors for strong suspicion were the musculoskeletal disease, the family history, and the geographic location indicated.

Henschel ED: Malignant Hyperthermia: Current Concepts, pp 10, 27. New York, Appleton–Century–Crofts, 1977.

Ryan JF: Malignant hyperthermia. ASA Refresher Courses in Anesthesiology 4:87–88, 1976

A.2. What is malignant hyperthermia?

Malignant hyperthermia, first described by Denborough in 1960, is a clinical syndrome of markedly accelerated metabolic state characterized by fever, tachycardia, tachypnea, cyanosis, and death. The clinical syndrome occurs in a susceptible patient when a triggering agent is employed.

Denborough MA, Lorell RRH: Anesthetic deaths in a family. Lancet 2:45, 1960

Ryan JF: Malignant hyperthermia. ASA Refresher Courses in Anesthesiology 4:87, 1976

A.3. What are the clinical features of a susceptible patient?

Those patients who are susceptible to developing malignant hyperthermia usually present with a family history of the disorder or musculoskeletal disorders (Table 30–1).

Britt BA: Malignant hyperthermia. International Anesthesiology Clinics 17, No. 4:63–65, 1979

A.4. Does the history of previous uneventful halothane anesthesia reasonably exclude the patient's susceptibility to malignant hyperthermia?

No, it does not. About one third of the cases occur during a second or subsequent anesthetic course.

Ryan JF: Malignant hyperthermia. ASA Refresher Courses in Anesthesiology 4:87, 1976

A.5. What are the clinical features of the syndrome?

The clinical features of this syndrome essentially represent an uncontrolled, exaggerated, hypermetabolic state triggered by the use of certain drugs. The common early manifestations include the following:

- Tachycardia—96% cases (earliest and most consistent sign)
- Tachypnea—85%
- Arrythmias
- Increased temperature—30% patients not uncommonly > 43°C (hyperthermia)
- Cyanosis—70% patients
- Skin mottling
- Profuse sweating
- Overheated CO_2 absorber
- Rigidity (not always)—80% patients
- Altered blood pressure—85% patients

Britt BA: Malignant hyperthermia. International Anesthesiology Clinics 17, No. 4:153, 1979

Henschel ED: Malignant Hyperthermia: Current Concepts, p 18. New York, Appleton–Century–Crofts, 1977

Table 30-1. Musculoskeletal disorders in patients susceptible to malignant hyperthermia

MUSKULOSKELETAL DISORDERS IN PATIENTS SUSCEPTIBLE TO MALIGNANT HYPERTHERMIA (67% of patients) (36% of relatives)
• Short stocky stature • Bulky muscles with rounded belly • Muscle hypertrophy • Atrophied muscle groups • Muscle cramps • Kyphoscoliosis • Strabismus • Joint hypermobility with spontaneous dislocations • Hernias • Club foot • Pectus carinatum • Hypoplastic mandible • Poor dental enamel

Table 30-2. The laboratory findings of acute malignant hyperthermia

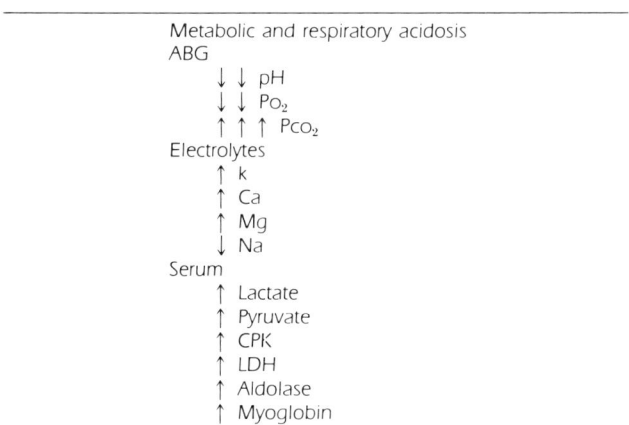

Metabolic and respiratory acidosis
ABG
↓↓ pH
↓↓ Po_2
↑↑↑ Pco_2
Electrolytes
↑ K
↑ Ca
↑ Mg
↓ Na
Serum
↑ Lactate
↑ Pyruvate
↑ CPK
↑ LDH
↑ Aldolase
↑ Myoglobin

A.6. What are the laboratory findings during an acute crisis of malignant hyperthermia?

The laboratory values, once again, reflect changes of a hypermetabolic state and muscle tissue damage (Table 30-2).

Henschel ED: Malignant Hyperthermia: Current Concepts, pp 19–25. New York, Appleton–Century–Crofts, 1977

Gronert GA: Malignant hyperthermia: Reviews. Anesthesiology 53:396–397, 1980

A.7. What are the two clinical types of the syndrome?

The syndrome has been classified as the rigid or the nonrigid type, depending on the development or absence of muscle contractures, respectively.

$$\text{MH} \begin{cases} \text{Rigid type 75\%} \\ \text{Nonrigid type 25\%} \end{cases}$$

Gronert GA: Malignant hyperthermia: Reviews. Anesthesiology 53:396, 1980

A.8. What is the incidence of this syndrome?

The estimated incidence is about 1 in 15,000 among children and 1 in 50,000 among adults. The incidence is lower in children under the age of 3 years and in the geriatric patient. The age groups most likely to be affected are from older children to the third decade. Both sexes are affected equally up to puberty, but after puberty males are affected more frequently.

Britt BA: Malignant hyperthermia. International Anesthesiology Clinics 17:134, 1979

A.9. What is the mode of inheritance of the disease?

The familial nature of the disease is well known, even though the majority of cases are nonfamilial. The genetic inheritance is autosomal dominant with reduced penetrance and variable expressivity. Recently, it has been suggested to be polygenic in origin.

Gronert GA: Malignant hyperthermia: Reviews. Anesthesiology 53:407, 1980

A.10. What is the etiopathology of the syndrome?

The best accepted theory of pathophysiology of malignant hyperthermia dictates that the defect lies in excitation–contraction coupling of calcium to the sarcolemma in the muscle. The basic defect lies in the muscle fiber involving subcellular membrane permeability of the sarcolemma and reuptake of calcium by the sarcoplasmic reticulum, which results in an inability to control calcium concentrations within the fiber. The resultant events are heat production and muscle contracture secondary to enhanced glycolysis, uncoupling of oxidative phosphorylation, and activation of actin-myosin filaments.

Britt BA: Malignant hyperthermia. International Anesthesiology Clinics 17:13–16, 1979

A.11. What laboratory tests can further substantiate the susceptibility of the patient to malignant hyperthermia?

The two tests of importance are measurement of serum creatinine-phosphokinase (CPK) and a muscle biopsy. Serum CPK levels may be greatly elevated in these patients as well as in their relatives. Therefore, a markedly elevated CPK level is of diagnostic value, but a normal CPK level is of no value because one third of the susceptible patients have normal CPK levels. Besides, CPK levels can be altered by other factors such as stress, injury, exercise, intramuscular injection, and certain drugs, as well as by collecting and measuring techniques.

With skeletal muscle biopsy, the caffeine-contracture test is the most diagnostic test for malignant hyperthermia susceptible (MHS) patients. Strips of skeletal muscle are obtained from the quadriceps. These strips are then transported in Ringer's solution to the laboratory, where isometric tensions are recorded in a bath on a polygraph. Varying concentrations of caffeine are then added to the bath, with and without halothane, and contracture tension is recorded. The rigid MHS muscle shows contracture at much lower caffeine concentrations compared with the normal muscle, in both caffeine and caffeine plus halothane baths. In contrast, the nonrigid MHS muscle requires much higher concentrations of caffeine for the same effect when compared with the normal muscle. This test is a sensitive and specific test for diagnosing MHS patients because there is little overlap between normal and MHS muscle, and this abnormality is not shared by other myopathies. The other tests that may commonly show abnormality in MHS patients, but are not diagnostic of the syndrome, include electromyography (EMG), motor unit counting, microscopic examination of muscle, electrocardiogram, echocardiogram, myocardial scan, and ATP depletion test.

Britt BA: Malignant hyperthermia. Int Anesthesiol Clin 17, No. 4:63–85, 1979

Gronert GA: Malignant hyperthermia: Reviews. Anesthesiology 53:411–412, 1980

B. Preoperative Evaluation and Preparation

B.1. How would you prepare this patient for anesthesia and surgery?

Preoperative preparation should include assessment of the patient's physical status, evaluation of laboratory findings, and specific investigations to determine the susceptibility of the patient to malignant hyperthermia. With confirmation of MHS susceptibility, the following steps should be taken:

- Admission. The patient should be admitted to the hospital at least 3 days prior to surgery. This will allow time for measurement of baseline values of vital signs and laboratory findings, as well as for prophylactic therapy.
- Dantrolene Prophylaxis. Dantrolene sodium is given orally in divided doses according to the following regimen:
    - 1st day   1 mg/kg/day
    - 2nd day   2 mg/kg/day
    - 3rd day   2 mg/kg/day
    - 4 hr preoperatively   2 mg/kg
- Sedation. The patient should be sedated the evening before and the morning of surgery with a barbiturate hypnotic.
- Intravenous Cannulation. A wide bore intravenous cannula should be inserted at least 4 to 6 hours prior to surgery to decrease the stress of induction of anesthesia.

Britt BA: Malignant hyperthermia. Int Anesthesiol Clin 17, No. 4:145, 1979

B.2. What laboratory tests would you wish to obtain prior to surgery?

The following laboratory tests should be done in addition to the muscle biopsy: complete blood count, urinalysis, serum electrolytes, serum CPK, serum GOT and GPT, LDH, ECG and, if indicated, echocardiogram, and coagulation studies.

Britt BA: Malignant hyperthermia. Int Anesthesiol Clin 17, No. 4:145, 1979

B.3. What premedication would you order?

This patient should be premedicated with a barbiturate such as pentobarbital. Belladonna alkaloids are best avoided because of the potential for causing an increase in rigidity and death during hyperthermic reaction associated with them.

Britt BA: Malignant hyperthermia. Int Anesthesiol Clin 17, No. 4:146, 1979

B.4. In anticipation of general anesthesia, what preparations would you make?

A satisfactory preparation for administering anesthesia to this patient should include measures to prevent and treat an acute crisis of malignant hyperthermia. The following should be available:

- Equipment
  - Vapor-free anesthesia machine (no vaporizers attached)
  - Fresh circuit and reservoir bag
  - Ventilator
  - ECG and blood pressure monitors
- Cooling aids
  - Hypothermia blanket
  - Crushed ice
  - Cold saline for irrigation and intravenous infusion
  - Tubes for cavity cooling
  - Bypass pump team
- Drugs
  - Anesthetic drugs, sodium bicarbonate, mannitol, furosemide, dantrolene (intravenous), procainamide, insulin—50% dextrose, heparin, propranalol

Britt BA: Malignant hyperthermia. Int Anesthesiol Clin 17, No. 4:146, 1979

C. Intraoperative Management

C.1. What anesthetic techniques and agents would you employ?

No anesthetic is completely safe in these patients; however, one should adhere to the technique that is least likely to trigger an attack. Anesthesia should be induced with a barbiturate such as thiopental sodium and the patient should be ventilated with 100% oxygen. Fentanyl should be added to ensure adequate depth of anesthesia. Topical anesthesia of the larynx and vocal cords should be achieved with an ester type of local anesthetic such as 5% cocaine spray. The trachea is then intubated without the use of a muscle relaxant. Pancuronium may be used to facilitate intubation, if absolutely necessary. Anesthetic maintenance is achieved by using oxygen and nitrous oxide, fentanyl, and pancuronium as required. Vital signs are monitored very closely, including arterial blood gases.

Britt BA: Malignant hyperthermia. Int Anesthesiol Clin 17, No. 4:146–147, 1979

C.2. What anesthetic agents are contraindicated?

In general, the anesthetic agents best avoided include potent inhalation agents, muscle relaxants, and amide type local anesthetics. Of the agents commonly employed today, the following have been implicated in triggering MH or increasing the mortality:

- Inhalation agents
  - Halothane (most commonly), enflurane, isoflurane, methoxyflurane
- Muscle relaxants
  - Succinylcholine (most frequently), d-tubocurarine, gallamine
- Local anesthetics
  - Amides, for example, lidocaine; mepivacaine
- Premedicants and other drugs
  - Belladonna alkaloids (atropine), phenothiazines, meperidine, cardiac glycosides, corticosteroids

Gronert GA: Malignant hyperthermia: Reviews. Anesthesiology 53:412, 1980

Henschel ED: Malignant Hyperthermia: Current Concepts, pp 13–15. New York, Appleton–Century–Crofts, 1977

Ryan JF: Malignant hyperthermia. ASA Refresher Courses in Anesthesiology 4:88, 1976

C.3. *If the surgeon wishes to use local anesthesia for a procedure, what agents will you recommend?*

Local anesthetics of choice are the ester type local anesthetics (*i.e.*, cocaine, procaine, chloroprocaine, and tetracaine). The amides should be avoided.

Gronert GA: Malignant hyperthermia: Reviews. Anesthesiology 53:412, 1980

C.4. *Twenty minutes into the case, the patient developed increasing tachycardia with ventricular premature beats and mottled skin. What emergency measures would you take?*

Although tachycardia may arise from other more common causes, such as light plane of anesthesia and hypovolemia, its association with mottled skin in this patient—who is susceptible to the syndrome of malignant hyperthermia—is the first key to the onset of the syndrome. This constitutes a critical emergency. The following steps should be taken immediately:

- Stop all anesthetics and surgery.
- Administer 100% oxygen.
- Hyperventilate the patient.
- Check the machine and eliminate vaporizers and soda lime from the circuit.
- If possible, get another machine with a new circuit, and no soda lime canister or vaporizer.
- Employ a nonrebreathing circuit.
- Establish lines. A wide bore cannula for CVP, arterial line (if not already in place), Foley catheter, nasogastric tube.
- Specific drug therapy. Start dantrolene sodium early while muscle per-

fusion is still present. The dose is 1 to 2 mg/kg, which may be repeated every 5 to 10 minutes to a total dose of 10 mg/kg.
- Aggressive cooling should be initiated immediately for rapidly increasing temperatures and for those above 40°C. Methods for cooling include the following: surface cooling with the patient on a cooling blanket and packed in ice; gastric, rectal, or peritoneal lavage with iced saline; iced intravenous fluids; and pump bypass with a heat exchanger. Cooling should be stopped when the patient's temperature falls below 38°C, so as to prevent inadvertent hypothermia.
- Treat acidosis with sodium bicarbonate (2 mEq/kg initial dose and titrate as necessary).
- Treat hyperkalemia, by using sodium bicarbonate, insulin, and 20% dextrose.
- Treat arrhythmias with procainamide 15 mg/kg.
- Maintain urine output with mannitol or furosemide.
- Provide energy substrate with 20% to 50% dextrose with insulin.
- Cardiorespiratory support
- Seek help in conducting the regimen.
- Monitor the pertinent signs very closely.

Britt BA: Malignant hyperthermia. Int Anesthesiol Clin 17, No. 4:153–158, 1979

Gronert GA: Malignant hyperthermia: Reviews. Anesthesiology 53:409–411, 1980

Henschel ED: Malignant Hyperthermia: Current Concepts, pp 47–54. New York, Appleton–Century–Crofts, 1977

C.5. What modalities would you monitor closely during management of the crisis?

The modalities that should be monitored closely include the following:
- Electrocardiogram
- Temperature
- Arterial blood pressure
- Urine output
- Central venous pressure
- Arterial blood gases

Britt BA: Malignant hyperthermia. Int Anesthesiol Clin 17, No. 4:156, 1979

Henschel ED: Malignant Hyperthermia: Current Concepts, p 49. New York, Appleton–Century–Crofts, 1977

D. Postoperative Management

D.1. What complications may follow this syndrome?

The late complications of malignant hyperthermia that should be looked for include consumption coagulopathy, acute renal failure, hypothermia, hyperkalemia, pulmonary edema, muscle edema and necrosis, neurological sequelae, recurrence of the syndrome.

Britt BA: Malignant hyperthermia. Int Anesthesiol Clin 17, No. 4:162, 1979

Henschel ED: Malignant Hyperthermia: Current Concepts, p 54. New York, Appleton–Century–Crofts, 1977

D.2. What would be your follow-up on this case?

The vigorous therapy started in the operating room should be continued in the immediate postoperative period. This includes maintaining the following:
- Cardiovascular stability
- Body temperature below 38°C
- Urine output
- Normal coagulation
- Acid–base and electrolyte balance

Along with the above measures, dantrolene sodium should be administered for at least 3 days after successful treatment of the syndrome.

Britt BA: Malignant hyperthermia. Int Anesthesiol Clin 17, No. 4:156, 1979

Henschel ED: Malignant Hyperthermia: Current Concepts, pp 54–55. New York, Appleton–Century–Crofts, 1977

D.3. What would you advise the patient and the family?

The patient should be warned of the dangerous nature of this syndrome and should be advised to carry an identification band at all times. The pedigree of the family should be prepared and the members should be investigated for susceptibility to this syndrome and issued medic alert bands accordingly.

Henschel ED: Malignant Hyperthermia: Current Concepts, pp 63–64. New York, Appleton–Century–Crofts, 1977

31 Prolonged Apnea
Alan Van Poznak

After eating a large meal, a young woman in the first trimester of pregnancy experienced severe lower abdominal pain, vaginal bleeding, and great weakness. In getting to the hospital, she fell down stairs and struck her head. On arrival, she was unresponsive and in frank shock. A pelvic mass was found and emergency laparotomy was proposed for presumed ruptured ectopic pregnancy.

Anesthesia was induced with a rapid sequence technique including succinylcholine. The patient remained apneic, not only throughout the procedure, but also in the recovery room. Her husband arrived and stated that several other members of the family have had similar difficulty.

A. Medical Disease and Differential Diagnosis

This case is presented to stimulate a review of several other conditions that are treated elsewhere in this book and to which the reader is referred. These include anesthesia for the patient with a full stomach, anesthesia for the patient in shock, and anesthesia for the patient with head trauma. The reader is also referred to the parts of this book which discuss the normal mechanism of neuromuscular transmission, particularly with respect to the acetylcholine theory.

1. Describe the humoral events in normal neuromuscular transmission.
2. What is acetylcholinesterase?
3. What is serum cholinesterase?
4. How does succinylcholine resemble acetylcholine?
5. How does succinylcholine differ from acetylcholine?
6. What is the incidence of atypical cholinesterase activity?
7. How many genes are known to be involved in the determination of serum cholinesterase?
8. What is the significance of cholinesterase units?
9. What is the significance of the dibucaine number?

B. Preoperative Preparation

The reader is referred to the sections on anesthesia for patients with full stomach, in shock, and with head trauma respectively. In this emergency situation there was no opportunity to be aware of the atypical cholinesterase variant.

C. Intraoperative Management

The reader is again referred to the sections mentioned above. However, the anesthesiologist should have made some attempt to have the patient regain spontaneous respiration, and should be concerned that breathing has not returned.

D. Postoperative Management

1. **What is the differential diagnosis for postoperative apnea? How would you treat it?**

A. Medical Disease and Differential Diagnosis

A.1. Describe the humoral events in normal neuromuscular transmission.

See Chapter 29, question A.4.

A.2. What is acetylcholinesterase?

Acetylcholinesterase is a relatively specific enzyme that hydrolyzes acetylcholine faster than it does other choline esters. It is found in the red cell, the central nervous system, and the neuromuscular junction. It is responsible for hydrolyzing and inactivating the acetylcholine produced during normal neuromuscular transmission. It does not hydrolyze succinylcholine, and is inhibited by the drug.

Stanbury JB, Wyngaarden JB, Fredrickson DS: The Metabolic Basis of Inherited Disease, 3rd ed, p 1730. New York, McGraw–Hill, 1972

A.3. What is serum cholinesterase?

This enzyme, also called cholinesterase, pseudocholinesterase, and nonspecific cholinesterase, hydrolyzes many choline esters including succinylcholine. It is found in many human tissues, but not in the red cell. It is synthesized in the liver. Its physiologic function is unknown, but it may hydrolyze choline esters such as propionylcholine and butyrylcholine, which may be formed by bacterial action in the gut and also by the enzyme systems responsible for the formation of acetylcholine.

Stanbury JB, Wyngaarden JB, Fredrickson DS: The Metabolic Basis of Inherited Disease, 3rd ed, p 1730. New York, McGraw–Hill, 1972

A.4. How does succinylcholine resemble acetylcholine?

Succinylcholine causes depolarization of the postsynaptic membrane.

Gilman AG, Goodman LS, Gilman A: The Pharmacological Basis of Therapeutics, 6th ed, p 225. New York, Macmillan, 1980

A.5. How does succinylcholine differ from acetylcholine?

Succinylcholine cannot be hydrolyzed by acetylcholinesterase. Instead, it must undergo much slower hydrolysis by the nonspecific plasma cholinesterase.

Stanbury JB, Wyngaarden JB, Fredrickson DS: The Metabolic Basis of Inherited Disease, 3rd ed, p 1730. New York, McGraw–Hill, 1972

A.6. What is the incidence of atypical cholinesterase activity?

It varies with the population studied, but is approximately 1:2800 in the general population of the United States, with a 1:1 male:female ratio.

Stanbury JB, Wyngaarden JB, Fredrickson DS: The Metabolic Basis of Inherited Disease, 3rd ed, p 1730. New York, McGraw–Hill, 1972

A.7. How many genes are known to be involved in the determination of serum cholinesterase?

Four alleles have been identified so far. They include the normal (N), dibucarine-resistant (D), fluoride-resistant (F), and the silent (S). These four genes can form ten genotypes, of which six produce a marked decrease in the hydrolysis of succinylcholine (D–D, F–F, S–S, D–F, D–S, F–S). (See Table 31–1.)

A.8. What is the significance of cholinesterase units?

Cholinesterase units indicate the affinity of the enzyme for the substrate. Various test substrates have been used, among them benzoylcholine and butyrylthiocholine. Unitage differs according to the laboratory method employed.

Stanbury JB, Wyngaarden JB, Fredrickson DS: The Metabolic Basis of Inherited Disease, 3rd ed, p 1734. New York, McGraw–Hill, 1972

A.9. What is the significance of the dibucaine number?

The dibucaine number is used to identify the heterozygote. Dibucaine in 10^{-5} M concentration produces the maximal difference in inhibition between the usual and atypical forms of serum cholinesterase. The term "dibucaine number" has been applied to the percentage of inhibition of serum cholinesterase. The usual homozygote has a dibucaine number of approximately 80, the atypical homozygote has a value below 30, and the heterozygote has a value between 45 and 69.

Stanbury JB, Wyngaarden JB, Fredrickson DS: The Metabolic Basis of Inherited Disease, 3rd ed, p 1731. New York, McGraw–Hill, 1972

Table 31–1. The nomenclature characteristics, frequency and suxamethonium sensitivity of the cholinesterase genotypes at the Ch_1 (E_1) locus

NOMENCLATURE		BENZOYLCHOLINE ASSAY			BUTYRYLTHIOCHOLINE ASSAY			FREQUENCY	SUXAMETHONIUM SENSITIVITY
Goedde and Baitsch (1964)	Motulsky (1964)	Dibucaine number	Fluoride number	RO2–0683 inhibition	RO2–0683 inhibition	Activity with 6% butanol			
Homozygotes									
$Ch_1^U Ch_1^U$	$E_1^u E_1^u$	80	62	95	97	100		Normal population	? 1 in 3,200 moderately sensitive
$Ch_1^D Ch_1^D$	$E_1^a E_1^a$	20	22	10	7	3		1 in 2,800	All markedly sensitive
$Ch_1^F Ch_1^F$	$E_1^f E_1^f$	65	35	80	73	3		? 1 in 300,000	? All moderately sensitive
$Ch_1^S Ch_1^S$	$E_1^s E_1^s$	—	—	—	—	—		? 1 in 140,000	All markedly sensitive
Heterozygotes									
$Ch_1^U Ch_1^D$	$E_1^u E_1^a$	60	50	65	70	74		1 in 26	? 1 in 500 moderately sensitive
$Ch_1^U Ch_1^F$	$E_1^u E_1^f$	75	52	90	87	74		? 1 in 280	? 1 in 200 moderately sensitive
$Ch_1^U Ch_1^S$	$E_1^u E_1^s$	80	62	95	97	100		? 1 in 190	Not known; probably similar to $Ch_1^U Ch_1^D$
$Ch_1^D Ch_1^F$	$E_1^a E_1^f$	50	35	55	63	11		? 1 in 29,000	? All markedly sensitive
$Ch_1^D Ch_1^S$	$E_1^a E_1^s$	20	22	10	7	3		? 1 in 20,000	All markedly sensitive
$Ch_1^F Ch_1^S$	$E_1^f E_1^s$	65	35	80	73	3		? 1 in 200,000	? All moderately sensitive

(Stanbury JB et al: The Metabolic Basis of Inherited Disease copyright © 1972, McGraw-Hill. With the permission of McGraw-Hill Book Company)

D. Postoperative Management

D.1. What is the differential diagnosis for postoperative apnea? How would you treat it?

- Residual anesthetic agent
- Residual narcotic
- Residual muscle relaxant
- Hypocarbia
- Results of head trauma
- Occurrence of some medical complication during anesthesia, such as stroke or embolism

Treatment of the patient would include discontinuance of anesthetics, reversal of narcotics with naloxone, reversal of nondepolarizing relaxants with atropine and neostigmine, determination of arterial blood gases and appropriate adjustment of ventilation, and such other treatment as might be appropriate for the head trauma, including steroids and hyperosmotic solutions to lessen brain swelling.

Ventilatory and circulatory support should be continued while arrangements are made for determination of cholinesterase unitage. Should these be found to indicate an atypical cholinesterase, the patient and her family should be so informed. She should also be given a letter to be transmitted to any anesthesiologist who might provide care for her in the future.

Dripps RD, Eckenhoff JE, Vandam LD: Introduction to Anesthesia: The Principles of Safe Practice, 5th ed, p 207. Philadelphia, WB Saunders, 1977

32 Burn
Michael Tjeuw

A 56-year-old man involved in an apartment fire sustained a 60% second and third degree burns to his face, neck, chest, upper and lower extremities. On the 10th day, he was scheduled for tangential excision of eschar. BP 70/40 torr; PR 140/min; temperature 40°C; HCT, 30%; weight, 71 kg.

A. Medical Disease and Differential Diagnosis

1. How do you classify the burn injury?
2. How do you express the extent of the burn injury?
3. Should the "rule of nines" be used in children?
4. What pathophysiologic alterations accompany major thermal injury?
5. What is the chance of survival for this 56-year-old patient with 60% second and third degree burns? What major factors affect his prognosis?
6. Does this patient have a smoke inhalation burn? How do you make that diagnosis?
7. What resuscitative measure would you institute immediately in this 60% burned patient?
8. What fluid formula would you use?
9. What is the definition of shock? How would you classify shock etiologically?
10. Is this patient in septic shock? What is the shock syndrome?
11. Discuss pathophysiology of septic shock.

B. Preoperative Evaluation and Preparation

1. What is ASA physical status of this patient? Why?
2. How does the ASA classify physical status?
3. What preoperative preparations would you order?

4. What is this patient's mean arterial blood pressure? How do you calculate it?
5. Would you institute therapy prior to surgery in this patient who you think is in septic shock?
6. What are the beta-1 and beta-2 adrenergic effects? How are the effects of a beta-adrenergic agonist mediated intracellularly?
7. What are the alpha-1 and alpha-2 adrenergic effects? How are these effects mediated?
8. Can you name a few alpha-adrenergic antagonists and beta-adrenergic antagonists?
9. Why do you need pulmonary artery catheterization? What other information could you derive from it?
10. How do you calculate oxygen content, oxygen availability, oxygen consumption, and oxygen extraction ratio?
11. What is meant by venous admixture?
12. Would you premedicate this patient?

C. Intraoperative Management

1. What monitoring techniques would you use in the operating room? What information would you obtain from each monitor?
2. This patient has a burn injury on the face. How would you induce anesthesia? Discuss inhalational versus intravenous agents.
3. Would you monitor the patient's body temperature? Why?
4. What methods would you institute to maintain normothermia?
5. Discuss some of the physiologic changes of hypothermia in human adult.
6. What effect does hypothermia have on total body metabolism?
7. What effect does hypothermia have on the oxygen dissociation curve?
8. What is meant by P 50?
9. Does $PaCO_2$ increase or decrease during hypothermia?
10. What is the temperature correction factor for pH?
11. Is succinylcholine contraindicated in burned patients? Why?
12. Does serum cholinesterase activity change in burn patients? Does it play any role in the hyperkalemic response to succinylcholine?
13. Is the requirement for d-tubocurarine increased in major burned patients?

D. Postoperative Management

1. What is diffusion hypoxia? How do you prevent it?

A. Medical Disease and Differential Diagnosis

A.1. How do you classify the burn injury?

Burns are classified as first, second, or third degree. First degree burns are characterized by simple erythema of the skin, with only microscopic destruction of superficial layers of the epidermis. Second degree burns or partial thickness burns extend through the epidermis into the dermis. Even when most of the epithelium is destroyed, regeneration may occur from epithelial cells surrounding hair follicles or sweat glands. Third degree burns are characterized by total, irreversible destruction of all the skin, dermal appendages, and epithelial elements. Spontaneous regeneration of epithelium is not possible, and the burns are described as fullthickness. Such burns require the application of skin grafts if the development of scar tissue is to be avoided.

Schwartz IE: Principles of Surgery, 3rd ed, p 287. New York, McGraw–Hill, 1979

A.2. How do you express the extent of the burn injury?

The extent of the burn injury is expressed as a percentage of the total body surface area displaying either second or third degree burns. It is most commonly estimated by the "rule of nines." The major anatomic portions of the adult may be divided into multiples of 9% of the body surface area. The proportion of each of these areas is estimated and the summation represents the percentage of the total body surface area burn. The percentages of body surface are as follows:

- Head and neck 9
- Right upper extremity 9
- Left upper extremity 9
- Right lower extremity 18
- Left lower extremity 18
- Anterior trunk 18
- Posterior trunk 18
- Perineum 1

Schwartz IE: Principles of Surgery, 3rd ed, p 287. New York, McGraw–Hill, 1979

A.3. Should the "rule of nines" be used in children?

The "rule of nines" may not be used to estimate total body surface area burns in children because the surface area of the head and neck in children is significantly larger than 9%, and that of the lower extremities is smaller. More precise methods such as the Lund and Browder chart may be used to provide greater accuracy by taking into account the changing proportions of the body from infancy to adulthood (Fig. 32–1).

Stein ED et al: Anesthesia for the burn patient. Weekly Anesthesiology Update 1:2, 1977.

A.4. What pathophysiologic alterations accompany major thermal injury?

The pathophysiologic alterations that accompany major thermal injury are complex. Skin, the largest organ of the body, when destroyed, has systemic impact. Thermal regulation, fluid and electrolyte homeostasis and protection against bacterial infection are affected. Immediately after a

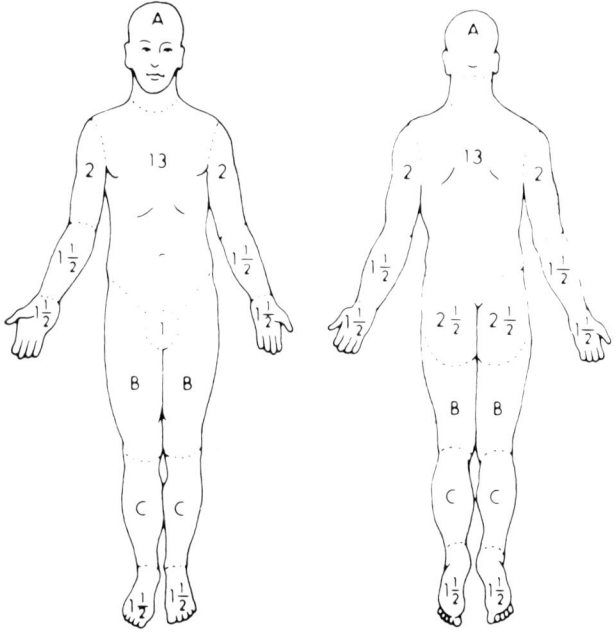

Fig. 32-1. Relative percentages of areas affected by growth. The Lund & Browder chart, which corrects body surface area estimation for different age groups. (Reprinted by permission from Stein ED, Stein JM: Anesthesia for the burn patient. Weekly Anesthesiology Update 1:2 1977)

Relative percentages of areas affected by growth (age in years)

	0	1	5	10	15	Adult
A: $\frac{1}{2}$ of head	$9\frac{1}{2}$	$8\frac{1}{2}$	$6\frac{1}{2}$	$5\frac{1}{2}$	$4\frac{1}{2}$	$3\frac{1}{2}$
B: $\frac{1}{2}$ of thigh	$2\frac{3}{4}$	$3\frac{1}{4}$	4	$4\frac{1}{4}$	$4\frac{1}{2}$	$4\frac{3}{4}$
C: $\frac{1}{2}$ of leg	$2\frac{1}{2}$	$2\frac{1}{2}$	$2\frac{3}{4}$	3	$3\frac{1}{4}$	$3\frac{1}{2}$

Total % burned _____ 2° + _____ 3° = _____

burn injury, a large amount of fluid is lost from the vascular compartment into the burn wound. Sequestration in the extravascular space results in significant hemoconcentration. Increased secretion of antidiuretic hormone (ADH) may decrease or even completely inhibit urinary output. It has been shown that during the first 4 days after a burn, an amount of albumin equal to twice the total plasma albumin content is lost through the wound. Half of this fluid remains sequestered in the extravascular space for 3 weeks or more before returning to the intravascular compartment.

The metabolic rate is markedly increased following the burn injury. Depending on the size of burn, the increase in metabolic rate can be doubled or tripled with respective increase in oxygen consumption and carbon dioxide production. This hypermetabolic state will continue for weeks or months until full skin coverage is achieved and the tissue repair

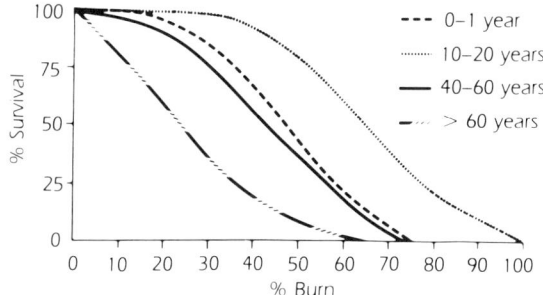

Fig. 32-2. Probability of survival from burns of various sizes for different age groups (From data compiled by the National Burn Information Exchange, Ann Arbor, Michigan) (Reprinted by permission from Stein ED, Stein JM: Anesthesia for the burn patient. Weekly Anesthesia Update 1:2, 1977)

processes are complete. Cardiac output is often decreased in major burn patients. This decrease is not entirely explained by the rapid reduction in circulating blood volume. It has been shown that a circulating myocardial depressant factor (MDF) exists in both man and laboratory animals.

Vascular integrity changes occur in other areas remote from the injury site. The entire vascular compartment in the body becomes permeable to circulating macromolecules such as dextran. This capillary leak syndrome is manifested as edema. In the lung, severe pulmonary edema can be life-threatening.

Pulmonary function decreases markedly. Functional residual capacity (FRC) is reduced. Both lung compliance and chest-wall compliance decrease markedly. The alveolar–arterial (A–a) oxygen gradient increases. Minute ventilation is increased. It can be as high as 40 L/min (normal 6 L/min).

Szyfelbein SK: Anesthetic considerations for major burn surgery. ASA Refresher Courses in Anesthesiology 8:201–216, 1980

A.5. What is the chance of survival for this 56-year-old patient with 60% second and third degree burns? What are the major factors that affect his prognosis?

The statistical probability of the survival of this patient is less than 25%, as compiled by the National Burn Information Exchange (Fig. 32–2). The major factors which affect his prognosis are as follows:

- Age
- Size and depth of burn
- Associated injuries
- Preexistent or intercurrent disease

Stein ED et al: Anesthesia for the burn patient. Weekly Anesthesiology Update 1:2, 1977.

A.6. Does this patient have a smoke inhalation burn? How do you make that diagnosis?

A patient with smoke inhalation frequently exhibits *no* physical signs or symptoms during the first 24 hours post burn. Smoke inhalation should be highly suspected in patients who were burned within an enclosed space, received burns of the face, were burned while under the influence of alcohol or drugs, or lost consciousness at the time of the accident. Such patients are most likely to have inhaled large amounts of smoke prior to being evacuated from the scene of the fire. Diagnosis is dependent on a high index of suspicion and careful physical and laboratory examination. The early symptoms and signs of respiratory tract injury include singed nasal hair, burned nasal mucosa, lips, and mouth, hoarseness, wheezing, and brassy cough with soot in the sputum. The posterior pharynx may appear red, and the larynx may appear edematous. X-ray findings are usually negative immediately after injury; this is the "clear or lucid period." Laboratory tests include blood gas analysis, carboxyhemoglobin concentration, xenon scans, and fiberoptic bronchoscopy.

Schwartz IE: Principles of Surgery, 3rd ed, p 296. New York, McGraw–Hill, 1979

A.7. What resuscitative measure would you institute immediately in this 60% burned patient?

Vigorous fluid resuscitation should be instituted immediately to combat the danger of hypovolemia from translocation of intravascular volume into the burn edema, which acts as a "third space." Fluid must be administered adequately to ensure good tissue perfusion and adequate urine output. The airway should be maintained to assure adequate ventilation. If upper airway burn is involved, endotracheal intubation is indicated.

Schwartz IE: Principles of Surgery, 3rd ed, p 286. New York, McGraw–Hill, 1979

A.8. What fluid formula would you use?

Over the past 20 years, many fluid formulas have been developed as guides to initial resuscitation in hypovolemic shock following burn injury. Most utilize various combinations of crystalloid and colloid solutions, but they differ widely in the ratio of colloid to crystalloid, as well as the rate of fluid administration. Although much controversy still surrounds the use of "the solution" for resuscitation in burn shock, scientific investigation supports the need for both crystalloid and colloid solutions. It matters little which formula is used to begin such therapy, as long as it is modified according to the patient's changing requirements. The Parkland formula, popularized by Baxter, has been adopted in most burn centers and is currently the standard against which new formulas must be compared.

Parkland Formula
First 24 hours

- Electrolyte solution (lactated Ringer's)—4 ml/kg/% of second and third degree burn
- Administration rate—½ given in the first 8 hours, ¼ in the second 8 hours, ¼ in the third 8 hours
- Urine output—maintains at 30 to 70 ml/hr

Second 24 hours
- Glucose in water (D_5W)—to replace evaporative water loss and maintain serum sodium concentration of 140 mEq/L
- Colloid solution (plasma)—to maintain plasma volume in patients with more than 40% second and third degree burns
- Urine output—maintain at 30 to 100 ml/hr

Schwartz IE: Principles of Surgery, 3rd ed, p 288. New York, McGraw–Hill, 1979

A.9. What is the definition of shock? How would you classify shock etiologically?

Shock may be defined as "a clinical condition characterized by signs and symptoms which arise when the cardiac output is insufficient to fill the arterial tree with blood under sufficient pressure to provide organs and tissues with adequate blood flow." Shock of all forms appears to be invariably related to inadequate tissue perfusion. The low-flow state in vital organs seems to be the final common denominator in all forms of shock. For purposes of a working clinical classification, the etiologic classification offered by Blalock in 1934 is still useful and functional. Blalock suggested the following four categories:

- Hematogenic shock (hemorrhagic, hypovolemic)
- Neurogenic shock
- Cardiogenic shock
- Vasogenic shock (septic)

Schwartz IE: Principles of Surgery, 3rd ed, p 134. New York, McGraw–Hill, 1979

A.10. Is this patient in septic shock? What is the shock syndrome?

Yes. This patient is probably in septic shock as he has hypotension, a rapid pulse and fever, together with the natural history of his burn injury. However, more information regarding central nervous system, hemodynamic and renal status would be helpful.

- Arterial blood pressure. It is generally accepted that systolic blood pressure of less than 80 torr, or a mean pressure of less than 50 torr, is indicative of shock state.
- Cardiac output. Cardiac index of less than 2.50 L/min/M² is generally perceived to be incompatible with adequate tissue perfusion.
- Blood volume determination is unreliable in the shock state.
- Arterial blood gases. Bicarbonate of less than 20 mEq/L is highly suggestive of inadequate tissue perfusion with resulting lactic acidosis. PvO_2 of less than 30 mm Hg is suggestive of inadequate tissue perfusion.
- Urinary output of less than 0.5 to 1 ml/kg/hr is suggestive of inadequate renal perfusion.
- Evaluation of the level of consciousness can reflect cerebral perfusion. Shock syndrome is described in the presence of hypotension, rapid and thready pulse, diaphoresis, cold, pale and clammy skin, and alteration in

consciousness. However, in septic shock, the skin can be warm, pink, and dry until circulation fails completely.

Lichtiger M, Moya F: Introduction to the Practice of Anesthesia, 2nd ed, pp 404–405. Hagerstown, MD, Harper & Row, 1978

A.11. Discuss pathophysiology of septic shock.

The most frequent causative organisms are gram-positive and gram-negative bacteria. Although any agents capable of producing infection (including viruses, fungi, parasites and rickettesiae) may initiate septic shock.

Gram-Positive Sepsis and Shock

The shock state caused by gram-positive infection such as staphylococcus is due to release of exotoxins. The hemodynamic changes that occur are different from those seen in shock due to gram-negative organisms. Hypotension with peripheral vasodilation occurs, and there is no reduction of cardiac output even with progressive hypotension. Urine flow is normal. Sensorium is clear, and perfusion of other organs is not grossly impaired.

Gram-Negative Sepsis and Shock

Gram-negative sepsis as a cause of shock is a more frequent and difficult problem. There have been significant advances in our understanding of this entity, although much of the available information is still subject to controversy. The onset of shock may be abrupt and coincident with signs and symptoms of sepsis, or may occur several hours or days after recognition of an infection. The complex hemodynamic abnormalities are incompletely understood, but are probably initiated by endotoxins from the cell walls of gram-negative bacteria.

Clinically, the shock state may be characterized by a primary adrenergic response, as seen in hypovolemic shock, with hypotension, peripheral vasoconstriction and cold, clammy extremities. Earlier in the course, however, there may be an absence of adrenergic effects with warm and dry extremities and peripheral vasodilation. These diverse responses, have led to a considerable amount of confusion over the clinical manifestations of septic shock.

MacLean and associates noted two distinct hemodynamic patterns, depending on the volume status of the patient. In patients who are *normovolemic* prior to the onset of sepsis, early septic shock exhibits a hyperdynamic circulatory pattern characterized by the following:

- Hypotension
- High cardiac output
- Normal or increased blood volume
- Normal or high CVP
- Low peripheral resistance (peripheral vasodilation)
- Warm, dry extremities
- Hyperventilation and respiratory alkalosis

A typical patient with this pattern is young and previously healthy. The high cardiac output is often associated with a decrease in oxygen utilization due to arteriovenous shunting and a primary cellular defect in the utilization of oxygen.

In patients who are *hypovolemic* prior to sepsis, septic shock exhibits a hypodynamic pattern characterized by the following:
- Hypotension
- Low cardiac output
- High peripheral resistance (peripheral vasoconstriction)
- Low CVP
- Cold, cyanotic extremities

Progressive pulmonary insufficiency is characteristically seen in many patients with septic shock. Hypoxia with compensatory hyperventilation and respiratory alkalosis are seen early in the course of shock that is progressive and eventually fatal. Endotoxin may also initiate a syndrome of disseminated intravascular coagulation.

Schwartz IE: Principles of Surgery, 3rd ed, pp 174–176. New York, McGraw–Hill, 1979

B. Preoperative Evaluation and Preparation

B.1. What is ASA physical status of this patient? Why?

The ASA physical status is IV, because this patient is in septic shock and has a life-threatening condition.

B.2. How does the American Society of Anesthesiologists classify physical status?

The classification of physical status adopted by the American Society of Anesthesiologists is as follows:
- Class 1   A normal healthy patient
- Class 2   A patient with a mild systemic disease
- Class 3   A patient with a severe systemic disease that limits activity, but is not incapacitating
- Class 4   A patient with an incapacitating systemic disease that is a constant threat to life
- Class 5   A moribund patient not expected to survive 24 hours with or without operation

In the event of emergency operation, follow the number with an E.

American Society of Anesthesiologists: New classification of physical status. Anesthesiology 24:111, 1963

B.3. What preoperative preparation would you order?

Preoperative preparation should include complete blood count, platelet count, electrolytes, BUN, creatinine, coagulation studies, urinalysis, ECG, arterial and venous blood gases, cardiac output, cardiac index, central venous pressure (CVP), urinary output, pulmonary capillary wedge pressure (PCWP), and chest x-ray film.

B.4. What is this patient's mean arterial blood pressure? How do you calculate it?

The patient's blood pressure is 70/40 torr, therefore, his mean arterial blood pressure is 50 torr. Mean arterial pressure equals diastolic pressure plus one third of pulse pressure, which is the difference between systolic and diastolic pressure.

B.5. Would you institute therapy prior to surgery in this patient who you think is in septic shock?

The only effective way to reduce mortality in septic shock is to recognize and treat the infection promptly prior to the onset of shock. Once shock occurs, definitive therapy consists of controlling infection with early surgical debridement or drainage and using appropriate antibiotics. Other measures such as fluid replacement, steroid, and vasoactive drugs represent adjunctive therapy. These measures are useful to prepare the patient prior to surgery or to support the patient until the infection process is controlled.

Therapy is directed principally at improving cardiac output and tissue perfusion. A relevant history and clinical examination must be made to determine whether hypotension is present. Low central venous pressure and low pulmonary capillary wedge pressure could aid in assessing hypovolemia. A useful "challenge" test involves infusing 250 ml of fluid rapidly and observing the change in central venous pressure or pulmonary capillary wedge pressure. If hypovolemia exists, volume expansion therapy, in the form of blood, colloid or crystalloid infusion must be initiated. In some patients, volume-expansion therapy alone will not improve low cardiac output because a maximum filling pressure is reached, beyond which cardiac output can not be improved. Inotropic support becomes necessary when left atrial pressure or PCWP is excessively high from left ventricular failure.

The following inotropes may be given:
- Dopamine, 5 to 10 μg/kg/min
- Isoproterenol, 0.5 to 4.0 μg/min
- Epinephrine, 0.5 to 4.0 μg/min

We advocate dopamine as the preferred inotropic agent. Isoproterenol or epinephrine is our next choice. Dopamine in low doses (5 μg/kg/min) has specific effects on dopaminergic receptors that produce vasodilation of renal, coronary and mesenteric arterioles. Dopamine in large doses (more than 20 μg/kg/min) has more prominant alpha-adrenergic effects than beta-adrenergic effects. Often, dopamine improves urinary output even without increasing cardiac output. Hollenberg and colleagues have shown that dopamine both increases renal perfusion and shifts renal medullary blood flow to the renal cortex. When it is given in carefully titrated doses, cardiac output usually increases and left atrial filling pressure decreases. Dopamine may cause tachycardia, but it rarely produces ventricular irritability. Other supportive therapy such as correction of acidosis and ventilatory support for pulmonary insufficiency should be instituted prior to surgery.

Goldberg LI et al: Newer catecholamines for treatment of heart failure and shock: An update on dopamine and a first look at dobutamine. Prog Cardiovasc Dis 19:327–340, 1977

Goldberg LI: Cardiovascular and renal actions of dopamine: Potential clinical applications. Pharmacol Rev 24:1–29, 1972

Hollenberg NK, Adams DF, Mendall P et al: Renal vascular responses to dopamine: Hemodynamic and angiographic observations in normal man. Clin Sci 45:733–742, 1973

B.6. What are the beta-1 and beta-2 adrenergic effects? How are the effects of a beta-adrenergic agonist mediated intracellularly?

Ahlquist in 1948 postulated that the responses to catecholamines were exerted through two different types of receptors that he named alpha-adrenergic and beta-adrenergic receptors. Beta-adrenergic receptors have been further subdivided into beta-1, which mediate the positive effects on the heart, and beta-2, which mediate smooth muscle relaxation in the bronchi, vasculature, and uterus.

The effects of beta-adrenergic agonist are mediated intracellularly by the cyclic nucleotide, cyclic adenosine monophosphate (cAMP). Cyclic AMP is often referred to as the "second messenger"; the first messenger is the water soluble catecholamine agonist (ligand) that cannot cross the lipid membrane. After binding with the receptor, the agonist-receptor complex diffuses laterally along the membrane until it couples to its effector molecule, adenylate cyclase, situated on the inner leaflet of the lipid bilayer. This enzyme is activated and converts ATP into cyclic AMP (second messenger). The level of cyclic AMP is further controlled by phosphodiesterase, which hydrolyzes the cyclic AMP to an inactive molecule. Cyclic AMP activates intracellular protein kinases that phosphorylate regulatory proteins in the cell, thereby altering their activity and causing the observed biological effect (Fig. 32–3).

Maze M: Clinical implications of membrane receptor function in anesthesia. Anesthesiology 55:160–171, 1981

B.7. What are the alpha-1 and alpha-2 adrenergic effects? How are these effects mediated?

With the advent of alpha-antagonists, it is now evident that there are two classes of alpha-receptors, alpha-1 and alpha-2. The alpha-1 adrenergic receptors are postsynaptic, and their stimulation constricts vascular

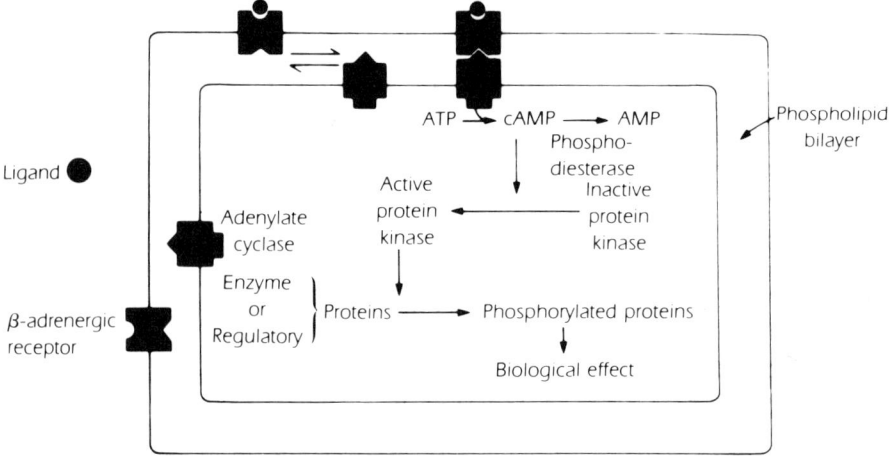

Fig. 32–3. β-adrenergic receptor (Reprinted by permission from Maze M: Clinical implications of membrane receptor function. Anesthesiology 55:163, 1981)

smooth muscle cells. Alpha-2 receptors are found on presynaptic sympathetic nerve terminals, and stimulation of these receptors causes feedback inhibition of norepinephrine release. Alpha-2 receptors are also found on platelets where they mediate platelet aggregation.

Thus far, no identifiable second messenger has been recognized for the alpha-adrenergic receptor. It is widely assumed that the combination of the alpha-agonist with the receptor generates a transmembrane message that initiates early intracellular events. Calcium flux is cited as a possible mechanism. Activation of alpha-2 adrenergic receptors on platelets results in a decreased amount of intracellular cyclic AMP through inhibition of adenylate cyclase.

Maze M: Clinical implication of membrane receptor function in anesthesia. Anesthesiology 55:160–171, 1981

B.8. Can you name a few alpha-adrenergic antagonists and beta-adrenergic antagonists?

Phenoxybenzamine and prazosin are selective alpha-1 antagonists. Phentolamine is both alpha-1 and alpha-2 antagonist. Yohimbine is a selective alpha-2 antagonist.

Propranolol and timolol are both beta-1 and beta-2 antagonists. Metoprolol and practolol are selective beta-1 antagonists, butoxamine is a selective beta-2 antagonist.

Maze M: Clinical implication of membrane receptor function in anesthesia. Anesthesiology 55:160–171, 1981

B.9. Why do you need pulmonary artery catheterization? What other information could you derive from it?

Measurements of pulmonary arterial and capillary wedge pressures are essential in critically ill patients. These measurements are critical guides to volume therapy in the treatment of low cardiac output syndromes. Disparate ventricular function occurs frequently in critically ill patients, causing right atrial pressure to correlate poorly with left atrial pressure. Pulmonary capillary wedge pressure does parallel left atrial pressure and may be used as an accurate indirect measure of the left atrial filling pressure. In isolated left ventricular failure, a low CVP may be associated with a high pulmonary capillary wedge pressure. In this case volume expansion may be contraindicated, whereas inotropic support would be crucial. In contrast, a low CVP (as in hypovolemia) or a high CVP (as in isolated right ventricular failure) may be associated with a low pulmonary capillary wedge pressure, suggesting the need for volume-expansion therapy prior to inotropic support in order to improve perfusion.

The patients who have a capillary-leak syndrome of the pulmonary vasculature should be maintained at the lowest possible wedge pressure consistent with circulatory support, in order to reduce the capillary leak. True mixed venous blood can be obtained for determination of oxygen partial pressure (PvO_2) or oxygen content (CvO_2). The four lumen catheters are capable of measuring cardiac output (CO) by thermodilution technique. This technique affords simple and repetitive determination from which many hemodynamic variables can be calculated.

$$\text{Cardiac index (CI)} = \frac{CO}{\text{Body surface area}}$$
(normal 2.8–4.2 L/min/m^2)

$$\text{Stroke index (SI)} = \frac{CI}{\text{heart rate}}$$
(normal 40–60 ml/beat/m^2)

$$\text{Left ventricular stroke work index (LVSWI)} = \frac{1.36\,(\overline{BP} - PCWP)}{100} \times SI$$
(normal 45–60 g·m/m^2)

$$\text{Right ventricular stroke work index (RVSWI)} = \frac{1.36\,(\overline{PAP} - CVP)}{100} \times SI$$
(normal 5–10 g·m/m^2)

$$\text{Systemic vascular resistance (SVR)} = \frac{\overline{BP} - CVP}{CO} \times 80$$
(normal 900–1500 dyne·sec/cm^5)

$$\text{Pulmonary vascular resistance (PVR)} = \frac{\overline{PAP} - PCWP}{CO} \times 80$$
(normal 150–250 dyne·sec/cm^5)

Cardiac function curves can be constructed for both the right side and left sides of the heart.

Forrester JS, Diamond G, McHugh TJ et al: Filling pressures in the right and left sides of the heart in acute myocardial infarction. N Engl J Med 285:190–193, 1971

Lappas D, Lell WA, Gabel JC et al: Indirect measurement of left atrial pressure in surgical patients: Pulmonary capillary wedge and pulmonary-artery diastolic pressure compared with left atrial pressure. Anesthesiology 38:394–397, 1973

Miller RD: Anesthesia, p 194. New York, Churchill Livingstone, 1981

B.10. How do you calculate oxygen content, oxygen availability, oxygen consumption, and oxygen extraction ratio?

Oxygen content = $1.34 \times Hb\ (g\%) \times O_2$ saturation + $0.003 \times PO_2$, (normal CaO_2 = 20.73 ml/100 ml, normal $C\bar{v}O_2$ = 15.76 ml/100 ml)

Oxygen availability = $CaO_2 \times CI \times 10$ (normal 600 ± 50 ml/min/M²)

Oxygen consumption = $avDO_2 \times CI \times 10$ (normal 140 ± 25 ml/min/M²)

Oxygen extraction ratio = $\dfrac{CaO_2 - C\bar{v}O_2}{CaO_2}$ (normal $26 \pm 2\%$)

B.11. What is meant by venous admixture?

Venous admixture is a measure of the fraction of the total blood flow that is not oxygenated during passage through the lungs. It is elevated in a number of conditions, including pulmonary diseases, atelectasis, pulmonary arterio–venous fistulae, diffusion abnormalities, pulmonary embolism, cardiogenic shock, and septic shock.

In order to calculate this parameter, it is necessary to know the pulmonary capillary arterial and mixed venous oxygen contents.

$$\dfrac{Qs}{Qt} = \dfrac{CcO_2 - CaO_2}{CcO_2 - C\bar{v}O_2}$$

CcO_2 = pulmonary capillary oxygen content
CaO_2 = artery oxygen content
$C\bar{v}O_2$ = mixed venous oxygen content

B.12. Would you premedicate this patient?

No. This patient is critically ill. His hemodynamic status is so unstable that any sedative-hypnotic or narcotic may further compromise his hemodynamic status. Atropine should be avoided because he is very tachycardic with a heart rate of 140.

C. Intraoperative Management

C.1. What monitoring techniques would you use in the operating room? What information would you obtain from each monitor?

- ECG to demonstrate arrhythmia and myocardial ischemia
- Indwelling arterial catheter for continuous blood pressure display and arterial blood samplings.
- Pulmonary-artery catheter for direct measurement of pulmonary artery pressure, PCWP, obtaining mixed venous blood for PvO_2 and measure-

- ment of cardiac output and systemic and pulmonary resistance
- Urinary catheter to monitor hourly urinary output and urinary electrolytes
- Esophageal or rectal temperature
- Oxygen analyzer to monitor inspired oxygen concentration

C.2. *This patient has a burn injury on the face. How would you induce anesthesia? Discuss inhalational versus intravenous agents.*

One should anticipate a difficult intubation because burns on the face may cause severe edema on the face, pharynx, or larynx. The safest way to secure the airway is to use awake intubation with topical anesthesia and sedation. Once the airway is secured, anesthetize the patient with N_2O-O_2 narcotic and a muscle relaxant such as pancuronium. Narcotics such as morphine, demerol, and fentanyl do not depress the myocardium, whereas inhalational agents depress the myocardium in a dose-related manner. If inhalational agents are chosen, the concentration should be carefully titrated to prevent loss of cardiovascular compensation.

C.3. *Would you monitor the patient's body temperature? Why?*

Massively burned patients with loss of skin have constant evaporation from open surfaces. They tend to develop severe intraoperative hypothermia. This tendency is exaggerated by the effects of general anesthesia on the temperature-regulating centers and vasodilation and by the cool, relatively dry environment of the operating room. The infusion of large amount of intravenous fluids at room temperature also contributes to the development of hypothermia.

C.4. *What methods would you institute to maintain normothermia?*

Methods to maintain normothermia involve active warming as well as prevention of heat loss. We administer all fluids and blood through the blood-warming coils. A thermal mattress is placed under a single-layer sterile sheet on the operating table and prewarmed. Room temperature is maintained between 24° and 27°C with a relative humidity above 50%. The areas of the patient's body not immediately involved in the surgery must be covered.

C.5. *Discuss some of the physiologic changes of hypothermia in human adult.*

The physiologic changes in hypothermia in human adults are complex. The following table illustrates some of the major changes observed during controlled hypothermia at various temperatures in human adults (Table 32–1).

C.6. *What effect does hypothermia have on total body metabolism?*

Metabolic rate obeys Van't Hoff's law, that is, oxygen consumption rises or falls exponentially with progressively increased or decreased temperature. The metabolic rate increases or decreases approximately twofold with each rise or fall of 10°C in body core temperature.

Collins VJ: Principles of Anesthesiology, 2nd ed, p 751. Philadelphia, Lea & Febiger, 1976

C.7. What effect does hypothermia have on the oxygen dissociation curve?

The oxygen dissociation curve shifts to the left with hypothermia. Oxygen combines easily with hemoglobin, but dissociates only at unusually low tissue partial pressure of oxygen (PO_2). This results in a reduced release of oxygen by hemoglobin. However, the shift to the left is compensated by two factors, namely an increase in solubility of oxygen in the plasma and an increase in carbon dioxide dissolved in the plasma. The increased acidity also tends to shift the curve to the right. Hypothermia per se does not lead to oxygen debt in the tissues if the perfusion is adequate.

Blair E: Clinical Hypothermia, p 57. New York, McGraw–Hill, 1964

C.8. What is meant by P 50?

P 50 is defined as oxygen tension at which 50% of hemoglobin is saturated at 37°C, PCO_2 40 torr, and pH, 7.40. Normal P 50 is approximately 27 mm Hg. In hypothermia, P 50 is lowered, which means the oxygen dissociation curve is shifted to the left. The oxygen affinity to hemoglobin is increased. The clinical application of P 50 is not clear at present; in fact, some doubt that there is any clinical usefulness for the measurement.

Shapiro BA et al: Clinical Application of Blood Gases, 2nd ed, pp 87–88. Chicago, Year Book Medical Publishers, 1977

Table 32–1. Physiologic observations during controlled hypothermia in human adults

TEMPERATURE		36–35° C (98–95° F)	35–32° C (95–90° F)	32–29° C (90–85° F)	29–27° C (85–80° F)
Level of consciousness		Complete	Calm	Stuporous	Unconscious
Response to commands		Good	Fair	Occasional	None
Reflex excitability	Shivering	++++	+	0	0
	Eyelid blink	++++	++	0	0
	Swallowing	++++	++	+	0
	Pharyngeal	++++	+++	+	0
	Skin stimulation	++++	+++	+	0
	Laryngeal	++++	+++	++	+
Cardiac rate		80	60–80	50–60	40–50
ECG changes		None	Slow rate	Bradycardia Occasional PVC	Prolonged QT Interval
Systolic pressure (Approximate percent reduction)		20%	30%	40%	50%
Diastolic pressure (Approximate percent reduction)		15%	25%	35%	40%
Muscular tone		No change	Slightly decreased	Marked decrease	Completely relaxed
Respiratory rate (Approximate percent reduction)		10%	40%	45%	50%

(Reprinted by permission from Collins VJ: Principles of Anesthesiology, 2nd ed, p 753. Philadelphia, Lea & Febiger, © 1976)

C.9. Does PaCO₂ increase or decrease during hypothermia?

If ventilation is held constant as body temperature is reduced, $PaCO_2$ decreases as a result of the interaction of decreased metabolism, increased dead space, and increased solubility of carbon dioxide during hypothermia.

The effects of solubility or hypothermia on blood gas values are easily confused. The blood solubility of carbon dioxide increases with decreasing temperature. More carbon dioxide molecules dissolve in the liquid phase and less molecules exist in the gas phase during hypothermia than during normothermia. Therefore, PCO_2 is lower when the same blood specimen is measured at hypothermia than at normothermia. For example, if the PCO_2 is 40 torr, at 37°C, the PCO_2 of the same blood measured at 25°C will be 23.6 torr. The correction factor can be found in a normogram. Note that it is not necessary to correct for temperature. The uncorrected value in management for the hypothermic patient appears to be preferable (see Chapter 7, question C.II-26).

Nunn JF: Applied Respiratory Physiology, 2nd ed, p 456. London, Butterworth & Co, 1977

Ream AK et al: Temperature correction of PCO_2 and pH in estimating acid–base status. Anesthesiology 56:41–44, 1982

C.10. What is the temperature correction factor for pH?

The temperature correction factor is $0.015\,pH$ units for each degree centigrade change in temperature. The pH value increases as the temperature is decreased. For example, if the pH is 7.40 at 37°C, it will be 7.55 when the same blood sample is measured at 27°C. ($7.40 + 0.015 \times 10 = 7.55$). Again, it is important to note that the temperature correction of pH is not necessary. The uncorrected pH value should be used if one assumes normal pH to be 7.40.

Nunn JF: Applied Respiratory Physiology, 2nd ed, p 456. London, Butterworth & Co, 1977

Ream AK et al: Temperature correction of PCO_2 and pH in estimating acid–base status. Anesthesiology 56:41–44, 1982

C.11. Is succinylcholine contraindicated in burned patients? Why?

Succinylcholine is unequivocally contraindicated in the burned patients. Intravenous injection of succinylcholine may cause a significant transient increase in serum potassium (up to 10 mEq/L) and cardiac arrest. This potassium releasing action of succinylcholine begins about 5 to 15 days after thermal injury and persists for 2 to 3 months, irrespective of degree and size of burn injury.

The mechanism responsible for this response is unclear. Gronert postulated that the abrupt release of potassium is related to increased chemosensitivity of the muscle membrane, which is due to development of receptor sites in the extra-junctional areas. Succinylcholine can produce a potentially lethal efflux of potassium in the presence of increased sensitivity.

Gronet GA, Theye RA: Pathophysiology of hyperkalemia induced by succinylcholine. Anesthesiology 43:89–99, 1975

Schaner PJ et al: Succinylcholine induced hyperkalemia in burned patients. Anesth Analg (Cleve) 48:764–770, 1969

Tolmie JD et al: Succinylcholine danger in the burned patients. Anesthesiology 28:467–470, 1967

C.12. Does serum cholinesterase activity change in burn patients? Does it play any role in the hyperkalemic response to succinylcholine?

A pronounced decrease in serum cholinesterase activity occurs after burns. Minimum levels of serum cholinesterase activity are usually reached 5 to 6 days after the burn injury. The activity may be depressed by more than 80% and can remain at a low level for months. These low levels of serum cholinesterase activity are found during the period when the burned patient is most liable to show an abnormal increase in serum potassium after succinylcholine injection (*i.e.*, 18 to 60 days after the burn injury).

Viby–Morgensen and associates found that the low serum cholinesterase activity plays no role in the hyperkalemic response to succinylcholine.

Birch et al: Changes in serum potassium response to succinylcholine following trauma. J Am Med Assoc 210, 490, 1969

Gronert GA et al: Succinylcholine-induced hyperkalemia in burned patients-II. Anesth Analg (Cleve) 48.958, 1969

Viby–Morgensen et al: Serum cholinesterase activity in burned patients-II: Anesthesia, suxamethonium, and hyperkalemia. Acta Anesthesiol Scand 19:169–179, 1975

Viby–Morgensen et al: Serum cholinesterase activity in burned patients-I: Biochemical findings. Acta Anesthesiol Scand 19:159–168, 1975

C.13. Is the requirement for d-tubocurarine increased in major burned patients?

Yes. Martyn and associates reported that burned patients needed approximately five times higher concentrations of d-tubocurarine to attain a given percentage of twitch depression than normal subjects. The cause is unknown.

Martyn JAJ et al: Increased d-tubocurarine requirement following major thermal injury. Anesthesiology 52:352–355, 1980

D. Postoperative Management

D.1. What is diffusion hypoxia? How do you prevent it?

Fink and associates in 1954 first reported diffusion hypoxia during recovery from nitrous oxide-oxygen anesthesia. A mild degree of hypoxia may develop for more than 10 minutes when nitrous oxide-oxygen anesthesia is concluded and the patient is allowed to breathe room air. The arterial oxygen saturation may fall 5% to 10% and often reaches values below 90% (PaO_2 below 60 torr). This occurs at the time when nitrous oxide is eliminated rapidly through the lungs. Nitrous oxide is 35 times more soluble in blood than nitrogen. Therefore, the amount of nitrous oxide diffused from blood to alveoli is much more than the amount of nitrogen diffused from alveoli to blood. Hence, alveolar oxygen is diluted by nitrous oxide. Diffusion hypoxia can be prevented by the inhalation of high concentrations of oxygen for several minutes before the patient is allowed to breathe room air.

Fink R et al: Diffusion anoxia during recovery from nitrous oxide-oxygen anesthesia. Fed Proc 13:354, 1954

Fink R: Diffusion anoxia. Anesthesiology 16:511–519, 1955

33 Trauma

Michael Tjeuw

A 42-year-old man involved in an automobile accident sustained fractures of the mandible and left 10th and 11th ribs. Blood appeared in the nasogastric tube. He complained of left upper quadrant abdominal pain. He was scheduled for emergency exploratory laparotomy.
BP 80/50 torr; PR 160/m; HCT 26%.
Arterial blood gases: pH 7.10, PO_2 80 torr, PCO_2 36 torr, HCO_3 18 mEq/L.

A. Medical Disease and Differential Diagnosis

1. What is the differential diagnosis of left upper quadrant abdominal pain? Why is an emergency exploratory laparotomy scheduled?
2. How do you diagnose intraperitoneal and retroperitoneal injuries?
3. What is the definition of shock? How would you classify shock etiologically?
4. What are the characteristic signs and symptoms of hemorrhagic hypovolemic shock?
5. What is the pathophysiology of hypovolemic shock?
6. How much blood loss can be tolerated before shock appears in an otherwise healthy subject?
7. What is the clinical manifestation of adult respiratory distress syndrome (ARDS)? Discuss its management.
8. In hemorrhagic shock, what fluid would you give as volume-expansion therapy? Colloid or crystalloid?
9. What are Dextran and Hetastarch (Hespan)?

B. Preoperative Evaluation and Preparation

1. Would you premedicate this patient?

C. Intraoperative Management

1. How would you monitor this patient?
2. What arteries are available for cannulation? Discuss potential complication and their incidence.
3. What anesthetic techniques would you use?
4. How would you intubate this patient?
5. After intubation, it became increasingly difficult to inflate the lungs. Discuss probable causes.
6. Tension pneumothorax is suspected. Discuss pneumothorax, its diagnosis and management.
7. The patient's condition is deteriorating despite crystalloid therapy. Properly cross-matched blood is not available yet. What would you give this patient instead?
8. If the patient has been transfused with more than 2 units of O-Rh negative uncross-matched whole blood, what precautions should you take?
9. What are the complications of a massive transfusion of acid–citrate–dextrose (ACD) blood?
10. By what means can the shift of the oxygen dissociation curve of a blood sample be quantitated?
11. What percentage of platelets is viable in ACD stored blood?
12. Would you empirically give an alkalizing agent (sodium bicarbonate) to patients receiving massive blood transfusions?
13. What percentage of labile factors V and VIII remains in the blood after 21 days of storage?
14. If the patient is awake, what are the clinical manifestations of intravascular hemolysis?
15. How would you manage a hemolytic transfusion reaction?
16. What are the signs of citrate intoxication?
17. Would you administer calcium routinely to treat possible citrate intoxication during massive infusion of ACD stored blood? Why?

D. Postoperative Management

1. What is the differential diagnosis of sinus tachycardia?
2. Discuss the causes of oliguria in the recovery room.
3. What is normal renal blood flow?
4. Are diuretics useful in the therapeutic approach to acute renal failure?

A. Medical Disease and Differential Diagnosis

A.1. What is the differential diagnosis of left upper quadrant abdominal pain? Why is an emergency exploratory laparotomy scheduled?

The differential diagnosis of left upper quadrant abdominal pain secondary to blunt trauma includes injury to spleen (26.2% in frequency), kidney (24.2% in frequency), intestines and stomach (16.2% in frequency), abdominal wall, retroperitoneal vessels, mesentery, pancreas, liver, diaphragm, lung, esophagus, and ribs.

Generally, blunt abdominal trauma leads to higher mortality rates than penetrating wounds and presents greater problems in diagnosis. Injuries to spleen, liver, kidneys, and bowel are frequently associated with other injuries such as head trauma, chest trauma, and fractures. Often the patient is unconscious because of alcoholism, shock, or associated head injury. Because this patient has left upper quadrant abdominal pain, low hematocrit, and blood in the nasogastric tube, one should highly suspect the presence of intraabdominal hemorrhage and conduct an emergency exploratory laparotomy.

Schwartz JE: Principles of Surgery, 3rd ed, p 246. New York, McGraw–Hill, 1979

A.2. How do you diagnose intraperitoneal and retroperitoneal injuries?

Intraperitoneal injuries are usually diagnosed by physical examination and can be confirmed by peritoneal lavage. Retroperitoneal injuries are more difficult to diagnose. These injuries usually require radiologic or laboratory confirmation including intravenous pyelogram, serial hematocrits, and urinalysis.

Schwartz JE: Principles of Surgery, 3rd ed, pp 248–249, 272–273. New York, McGraw–Hill, 1979

A.3. What is the definition of shock? How would you classify shock etiologically?

Shock may be defined as "a clinical condition characterized by signs and symptoms which arise when the cardiac output is insufficient to fill the arterial tree with blood under sufficient pressure to provide organs and tissues with adequate blood flow." Shock of all forms appears to be invariably related to inadequate tissue perfusion. The low-flow state in vital organs seems to be the final common denominator in all forms of shock.

For working purposes, the etiologic classification offered by Blalock in 1934 is still useful and functional. Blalock suggested the following four categories:

- Hematogenic shock (hemorrhagic, hypovolemic)
- Neurogenic shock
- Cardiogenic shock
- Vasogenic shock (septic)

Schwartz JE: Principles of Surgery, 3rd ed, p 134. New York, McGraw–Hill, 1979

A.4. What are the characteristic signs and symptoms of hemorrhagic hypovolemic shock?

The characteristic signs and symptoms of hemorrhagic hypovolemic shock are hypotension, tachycardia, pallor, cyanosis, cold, clammy skin, oliguria with high specific gravity or osmolality, decreased hematocrit, decreased central venous pressure (CVP), restlessness, anxiety, apathy, and metabolic acidosis partly compensated by respiratory alkalosis.

Schwartz JE: Principles of Surgery, 3rd ed, p 136. New York, McGraw–Hill, 1979

A.5. What is the pathophysiology of hypovolemic shock?

Cardiovascular Derangement

A decrease in circulating blood volume leads to an increase in sympathetic discharge with an outpouring of epinephrine (and nonepinephrine) from the adrenal gland. An alpha–adrenergic response causes vasoconstriction, shunting blood from the skin, viscera, and muscle, thereby preserving the coronary and cerebral circulations. There is constriction of both pre-and-post-capillary sphincters. This reduces hydrostatic pressure in the capillary bed, which allows the osmotic pressure to draw fluid back into the vascular space from the interstitial areas. This process of hemodilution serves to increase the contracted blood volume. This phase of shock is termed *ischemic anoxia* because the tissues are pale and relatively bloodless. If shock is prolonged, decreased capillary blood flow leads to increased blood viscosity and aggregation of erythrocytes. This effect is particularly evident in the splanchnic circulation of dogs, in which true thrombosis and damage to small vessels becomes prominent. Data from many sources suggest that alteration in intestinal permeability allows increased amounts of bacterial endotoxin to enter the portal circulation. The endotoxin is thus disseminated widely throughout the body, thereby enhancing vasoconstriction and contributing to terminal cardiovascular collapse. There is evidence to suggest that parenchymal damage occurs within the liver, with release of hydrolytic lysosomal enzymes.

The presence of a myocardial depressant factor (MDF) has been demonstrated. This substance is thought to arise from the pancreas during low-flow states.

Pulmonary Dysfunction

Acute respiratory failure following hemorrhagic shock has received increasing attention over the last decade. "Shock lung" and "traumatic wet insufficiency" are used to describe the pulmonary dysfunction. We now recognize that the pathophysiologic findings in the lung appear to be injury at the alveolar capillary membrane, with resulting leakage of proteinaceous fluid from the intravascular space into the interstitium and subsequently into alveolar spaces resulting in pulmonary edema. Wilson has described the presence of aggregates of platelets and leukocytes that appear to obstruct pulmonary capillary blood flow. These blood elements break down and release vasoactive substances and lysosomal enzymes that damage the pulmonary parenchyma. These pathologic changes result in an atelectatic, hemorrhagic necrotic and edematous lung. These changes are not peculiar to shock states, but are seen in a variety of conditions such as aspiration pneumonia, fat embolization, oxygen toxicity, and following cardiopulmonary bypass. Collectively they have all been categorized as "adult respiratory distress syndrome" (ARDS). The prominent derangements in pulmonary function associated with ARDS are as follows:

- Hypoxia, which is unresponsive to increased oxygen concentration
- Decreased pulmonary compliance, which clinically appears as "stiff lungs"
- A fall in resting lung volume, specifically, functional residual capacity

Acid–Base Disturbances

Metabolic acidosis is a virtually universal occurrence in shock. Decreased capillary perfusion due to peripheral vasoconstriction and impaired oxygen transport in low-flow states lead to anaerobic metabolism with an accumulation of CO_2 and lactic acid in the interstitial space. Normal blood buffering capacity cannot cope with this increased acid load. Because of low-flow to the kidneys, renal excretion of hydrogen ions is also impaired. The patient responds by a compensatory hyperventilation. The acidosis produces dilatation of the precapillary sphincters, whereas postcapillary sphincters are still constricted. As a result, blood can now enter the capillary beds. Because blood cannot exit normally, it pools and floods the capillary beds. Erythrocyte stasis and aggregation increase, causing sludging and an increase in capillary hydrostatic pressure. High capillary hydrostatic pressure leads to the escape of fluid into the interstitial space. Eventually, capillary wall integrity is lost and whole blood escapes into the tissues. This leads to a dramatic decrease in effective circulating blood volume, and the stage of "irreversible shock" is reached.

Kirby RM: Pathophysiology and treatment of shock. ASA Refresher Courses in Anesthesiology 1:69–83, 1973

A.6. How much blood loss can be tolerated before shock appears in an otherwise healthy subject?

In a previously normal 70 kg man, an acute blood loss of 500 ml (10% blood volume) is tolerated reasonably well, and compensation is generally adequate without replacement of this lost blood volume. However, losses in excess of 1000 ml (20% blood volume) are associated with moderately severe shock requiring replacement therapy. Failure to replace blood volume when losses are over 40% of blood volume is generally associated with "irreversible shock."

Schwartz JE: Principles of Surgery, 3rd ed, p 139. New York, McGraw–Hill, 1979

A.7. What is the clinical manifestation of adult respiratory distress syndrome (ARDS)? Discuss its management.

ARDS may occur under a variety of circumstances. It is manifested in a spectrum of clinical severity from mild dysfunction to progressive, eventually fatal, pulmonary failure.

For descriptive purposes the clinical picture can be divided into four arbitrary stages.

Stage 1. Injury, Resuscitation, and Alkalosis
This stage immediately follows the initial injury and is characterized by spontaneous hyperventilation with hypocapnia, diminished pulmonary compliance, mixed metabolic and respiratory alkalosis, and a normal chest x-ray.

Stage 2. Circulatory Stability and Beginning of Respiratory Difficulty
This occurs after apparent stabilization of vital signs and adequate tissue perfusion. This stage is characterized by persistent hyperventilation with progressive hypocapnia, hypoxemia, increasing pulmonary shunt fraction, progressive increase in compliance, and increased cardiac output. This may persist for several hours to days. Recognition and therapeutic intervention at this point is believed to be extremely important.

State 3. Progressive Pulmonary Insufficiency

Stage 4. Terminal Hypoxemia and Acidosis with Asystole

The hallmarks of the clinical syndrome are as follows:

- Hypoxemia, which is relatively unresponsive to increased oxygen concentration indicating ventilation/perfusion imbalance and shunting
- Decreased pulmonary compliance
- Chest x-ray changes, characteristically minimal in the early stages

Interstitial edema and diffuse infiltrates appear with progression of the syndrome that may progress to areas of consolidation or atelectasis in both lungs.

Management of ARDS should include monitoring of pulmonary function, ventilatory support, maintenance of cardiovascular stability, and drugs. Monitoring of pulmonary function can be conveniently divided into the following three general areas:

- Evaluation of oxygenation—F_1O_2, PaO_2, and A-a DO_2
- Ventilation—$PaCO_2$ and minute volume
- Mechanics—Respiratory rate (RR), vital capacity, effective compliance, maximal inspiratory force

Therapeutic maneuvers could theoretically be directed at the following:

- Manipulating pulmonary blood flow by increasing the perfusion to the well-ventilated units and decreasing the perfusion to the poorly ventilated units
- Directly reducing the capillary leak by reversing the membrane injury
- Indirectly reducing the interstitial edema

- Improving ventilation of poorly ventilated segments, and preventing further alveolar filling or collapse

The last maneuver is most practical and is used clinically to support and increase alveolar volume.

A volume ventilator with positive end-expiratory pressure (PEEP) is most often chosen for the treatment of ARDS. It can affect reexpansion of atelectatic alveoli, improve arterial oxygenation, and reduce F_iO_2 to avoid the possibility of oxygen toxicity.

The cardiovascular system should be stabilized. Diuretics such as furosemide have been used to reduce the amount of pulmonary edema. There is no conclusive proof that steroids should be part of the specific therapy, although data indicate that steroids may be effective in fat embolism, septic shock, and aspiration of gastric acid.

Schwartz JE: Principles of Surgery, 3rd ed, pp 155–157. New York, McGraw–Hill, 1979

A.8. In hemorrhagic shock, what fluid would you give as volume-expansion therapy? Colloid or crystalloid?

If hemorrhagic shock has developed, blood transfusion is naturally the preferred treatment. Much work is being done on whether whole blood or component therapy should be used, or whether fine-screen filtration might reduce the problem of acute respiratory failure and capillary damage from pulmonary edema associated with massive transfusion. Leukocytes may cause an immune response in the lung, which leads to capillary leakage and pulmonary edema. Component therapy will probably become more important as blood banking capability improves. There is a dilemma about the type of nonblood containing fluid that should be given to patients in shock.

Pulmonary Function

Administering balanced salt solution without protein may reduce serum albumin and enhance pulmonary edema. Conversely, administering a colloid solution, particularly to patients who have a capillary leak syndrome, is likely to cause albumin to equilibrate across the alveolar capillary membrane and into the interstitium of the lung. If the interstitial oncotic pressure rises, more volume is retained in the lung, exacerbating pulmonary edema. Large molecules such as albumin or dextran have been shown to cross damaged capillary endothelium and enter the interstitium of the lung in humans. No doubt crystalloid solutions will leak into the lung, but with healing of the lung or with diuresis and fluid restriction, the crystalloid fluid can be mobilized and removed from the lungs. Therefore, administration of albumin to increase serum albumin concentration is undesirable in the presence of alveolar capillary damage because any gradient that develops will drive albumin into the pulminary interstitium, thereby further aggravating pulmonary edema.

Renal Function

Following hemorrhagic shock, Siegal and associates found that saline resuscitation maintained urinary output at normal levels in baboons, whereas colloid resuscitation did not restore normal urinary output until all shed blood had been returned. Suggestive evidence of tubular dysfunction was also found in the albumin-resuscitated group. Further documentation of renal function following shock managed with fluid resuscitation is needed; however, from our experience, those patients receiving large volumes of blood and Ringer's lactate solution maintain far better renal function postoperatively than those who receive large amounts of blood and colloid solution.

Carrico CJ et al: Fluid resuscitation following injury: Rationale for the use of balanced salt solutions. Crit Care Med 4:46–54, 1976

Moss GS et al: Colloid or crystalloid in the resuscitation of hemorrhagic shock: A controlled clinical trial. Surgery 89:434–525, 1981

Virgilio RW et al: Crystalloid *vs* colloid resuscitation: Is one better? A randomized clinical study. Surgery 85:129–139, 1979

A.9. What are Dextran and Hetastarch (Hespan)?

Dextran is the synthetic plasma expander. Dextran 40, which has a mean molecular weight of 40,000, and Dextran 70, which has a mean molecular weight of 70,000, are both available either in normal saline or 5% glucose solution. These solutions are slightly hyperoncotic with respect to plasma. Therefore they expand the intravascular volume. These solutions are less expensive than blood products. The major drawback of dextran in surgical patients is its effects on the clotting mechanism. Dextran is associated with decreased platelet coagulability. It interferes with blood typing and cross-matching procedures. However, this effect is seldom clinically significant in patients receiving less than 1.5 liters of dextran per day (20 ml/kg/day).

Hydroxyethyl starch (Hespan) is another synthetic plasma expander that is now available for clinical use. It has an average molecular weight of 450,000. Recent work has demonstrated that hydroxyethyl starch is an effective plasma expander with colloidal properties similar to those of albumin. It is relatively inexpensive. Clinical experience is still lacking in terms of its potential for widespread use. It may have the same action as dextran on the blood coagulation mechanism.

Gilman AG, Goodman LS, Gilman A: The Pharmacological Basis of Therapeutics, 6th ed, pp 860–861. New York, Macmillan, 1980

Lazrove S et al: Hemodynamic, blood volume, and oxygen transport responses to albumin and hydroxyethyl starch infusions. Crit Care Med 8:302, 1980

B. Preoperative Evaluation and Preparation

B.1. Would you premedicate this patient?

No. This patient is critically ill because he is in hemorrhagic shock. He is anemic, hypotensive, and acidotic. Any sedative or narcotic may further compromise his hemodynamic status. Atropine should be avoided because he is very tachycardic, with a heart rate of 160/min.

C. Intraoperative Management

C.1. How would you monitor this patient?

Monitoring this patient in hemorrhagic shock should include blood pressure, ECG, CVP, temperature, urine output, serial hematocrit, and arterial blood gases. Arterial catheterization would be desirable to obtain blood for gas analysis and direct monitoring of blood pressure. Pulmonary artery catheterization would be indicated to monitor pulmonary capillary wedge pressure as an indirect measurement of left atrial pressure.

C.2. What arteries are available for cannulation? Discuss potential complications and their incidence.

The arteries available are as follows:
- Radial artery. This is the most commonly used artery that is easily cannulated with few major complications. Good collateral circulation usually exists, so thrombosis is not a serious complication.
- Ulnar artery. This artery may be used when the radial artery has been shown to be dominant. Three percent of healthy patients may have absent ulnar pulses bilaterally. Cannulation of the ulnar artery is technically more difficult than cannulation of the radial or the dorsalis pedis because of difficulties in palpation and immobilization.
- Dorsalis pedis. This artery lies superficially on the dorsum of the foot. It serves as a good alternative to the radial or ulnar arteries. This artery is nonpalpable in 5% of children and is absent in 12% of adults. Cannulation of this artery is easy to perform, reliable, and safe.
- Brachial artery. The incidence of brachial artery thrombosis following catheterization is quite high (17%). Continuous "on line" oxygen monitoring will necessitate cannulation of the brachial artery.
- Other arteries such as superficial temporal, axillary, femoral, and posterior tibial arteries can be cannulated.

Miller RD: Anesthesia, pp 177–178. New York, Churchill Livingstone, 1981

C.3. What anesthetic techniques would you choose to use?

Circulating blood volume should be adequately restored prior to surgery. However, if surgery must be started prior to the correction of hypovolemia, when the rate of blood loss exceeds the rate of fluid replacement, the induction of anesthesia should proceed with great care; bear in mind that the patient has unstable cardiovascular function. The suggested anesthetic technique would be an intravenous technique. The patient is preoxygenated with 100% oxygen, and anesthesia should be induced with thiopental or ketamine. For endotracheal intubation, succinylcholine or a nondepolarizing muscle relaxant such as pancuronium, 0.1 mg/kg, may be used.

Anesthesia is maintained with nitrous oxide, oxygen, and a narcotic agent such as morphine, demerol, or fentanyl. Ventilation is controlled with a respirator. Reversal of muscle relaxant at the end of the procedure can be achieved with neostigmine or pyridostigmine. The patient may be extubated when respiratory function is judged adequate and when protective laryngeal and pharyngeal reflexes have returned.

C.4. How would you intubate this patient?

Because his mandible is fractured, one should expect a difficult intubation. The safest way to secure the airway would be to use an awake intubation. One should treat him as though he has a full stomach because this is an automobile accident and an emergency case. If reduction of mandibular fractures is planned, nasotracheal intubation is preferable.

C.5. After intubation, it became increasingly difficult to inflate the lungs. Discuss possible causes.

One should suspect the following causes:

- Obstruction of the anesthesia circuit
- Obstruction of the endotracheal tube
- Obstruction of the trachea and bronchus
- Pneumothorax
- Pulmonary edema

C.6. Tension pneumothorax is suspected. Discuss pneumothorax, its diagnosis and management.

Air can enter the pleural cavity in a number of ways. If there is a free communication with the atmosphere, whether through a bronchopleural fistula or a wound in the chest wall, the pneumothorax is described as open pneumothorax. If there is no communication, it is a closed pneumothorax. A particularly dangerous type of pneumothorax is that in which air can enter but cannot escape (ball-valve), leading to a tension pneumothorax. In an anesthetized patient, a pneumothorax may be open, closed, or under tension. Tension pneumothorax should be suspected during anesthesia if it is increasingly difficult to inflate the lungs, especially for this patient who has fractured ribs. The patient may present with cyanosis, hypotension, tachycardia, or bradycardia. Pneumomediastinum and subcutaneous emphysema may or may not be present.

Once a tension pneumothorax is suspected, percussion of the chest will usually reveal the side that is affected. No time should be wasted for x-ray confirmation. A wide bore needle should be passed into the pleural space on the affected side. This should be connected to a water sealed chest bottle (Pleurovac) as soon as possible.

C.7. The patient's condition is deteriorating despite crystalloid therapy. Properly cross-matched blood is not available yet. What would you give him?

Hemorrhagic shock is best managed by administration of whole blood. In this situation, there is a major blood loss and crystalloid solutions do not maintain circulation. If there is no acute need for red cells (HCT greater than 25) colloid should be infused up to a total of approximately 1250 ml. After infusion of 1250 ml of colloid, the patient will become significantly hemodiluted and need blood transfusion. The available colloid solutions are as follows:

- Albumin
- Plasma protein fraction (PPF)
- Dextran
- Hetastarch (Hespan)

If a blood transfusion is needed, the following guidelines should be followed for use of uncross-matched blood.

- Partially cross-matched blood. When using uncross-matched blood, it is best to obtain at least a partial cross-match. This is done by adding the patient's serum to donor's red blood cells, centrifuging and reading for macroscopic agglutination. This procedure takes 5 to 10 minutes and will eliminate hemolytic reactions due to ABO incompatibility.
- Group specific uncross-matched blood. If the patient's blood group is identified during the current hospitalization, one can use uncross-matched ABO/Rh group type specific blood.
  Note, do not trust blood groupings from historical records, relatives, or ambulance drivers, etc.
- Type O-Rh negative (universal donor) uncross-matched packed red cells. This should be used prior to O-Rh negative whole blood because red cells have small volumes of plasma and are virtually free of hemolytic anti-A and anti-B antibodies.

Brzica SM: Treatment of disorders of hemostasis. ASA Refresher Courses in Anesthesiology 7:57–58, 1979

C.8. If the patient has been transfused with more than 2 units of O-Rh negative uncross-matched whole blood, what precautions should you take?

If the patient has been transfused with more than 2 units of O-Rh negative uncross-matched whole blood, *do not* switch to group specific blood even after the blood bank verifies proper blood group. Switching may lead to major intravascular hemolysis of donor's red cells by increasing titers of anti-A and anti-B antibodies, which cause potential lethal complications. Continued use of O-Rh negative whole blood leads to minor hemolysis of recipient's red cells resulting in hyperbilirubinemia as the only complication. The patient is not switched to the correct A or B blood group for approximately 2 weeks following the use of more than 2 units of O-Rh negative whole blood.

Brzica SM: Treatment of disorders of hemostasis. ASA Refresher Courses in Anesthesiology 7:58, 1979

C.9. What are the complications of a massive transfusion of acid–citrate–dextrose blood (ACD)?

Problems associated with massive transfusion therapy are many. They include the following:

- The oxygen dissociation curve is shifted to the left. This has been attributed to the rapid depletion of erythrocyte inorganic phosphates, namely, 2,3-DPG.
- Coagulopathy—excessive oozing is frequently seen after rapid infusion of large amounts of ACD stored bank blood. Causes include dilutional thrombocytopenia, low levels of factors V (proaccelerin) and VIII (AHG), and disseminated intravascular coagulation (DIC).
- Hemolytic transfusion reactions by transfusion of incompatible blood. In anesthetized patients, the usual clinical manifestations of hemolytic reaction are abolished. Hypotension, abnormal bleeding, urticaria, and blood-tinged urine should suggest that incompatible blood may have been transfused.
- Hypothermia. Administration of cold blood can decrease the body temperature. Therefore, we recommend warming blood through plastic coils immersed in a warm water bath.
- Hyperkalemia. After 7 days of storage, ACD blood has a potassium content of 12 mEq/L, which progressively increases to 32 mEq/L by 21 days of storage. Several authors have found that significant hyperkalemia rarely occurs during rapid transfusion of bank blood to adults; although it is common during exchange transfusion in the newborn. In fact, we observed that after massive transfusion, the potassium level is variable; it can be increased, decreased, or normal.
- Citrate intoxication. Citrate intoxication is not caused by the citrate alone, but rather by citrate binding of calcium. The signs of citrate intoxication are therefore, those of hypocalcemia.
- Posttransfusion hepatitis. Incidence of posttransfusion hepatitis was estimated at about 15 per 1000 patients receiving blood. The frequency varies from area to area. The incidence increases when multiple-donor plasma or fibrinogen is also given.
- Adult respiratory distress syndrome (ARDS). The etiology of ARDS is unknown. Many etiologic factors are probably involved. One factor may be pulmonary vascular obstruction from infusion of unfiltered debris in the bank blood. Another appears to be a hypersensitivity reaction. The

presence of eosinophilia helps confirm the diagnosis of pulmonary hypersensitivity reaction.

Miller RD: Complications of massive blood transfusions. Anesthesiology 39:82–93, 1973

C.10. By what means can the shift of the oxygen dissociation curve of a blood sample be quantitated?

Shift of the oxygen dissociation curve of a blood sample can be quantitated by means of the P 50 values. The P 50 refers to the partial pressure of oxygen at which hemoglobin is 50% saturated with oxygen; therefore, a low P 50 indicates a leftward shift in the curve. Normal P 50 of blood is 26.5 torr, and the normal level of 2,3-DPG is about 4.8 μM/ml of erythrocytes.

Miller RD: Complications of massive blood transfusions. Anesthesiology 39:82–93, 1973

Miller RD: Transfusion therapy and associated problems. ASA Refresher Courses in Anesthesiology 1:101–113, 1973

C.11. What percentage of platelets is viable in ACD stored blood?

- After 3 hours   60% viable platelets
- After 24 hours   12% viable platelets
- After 48 hours   2% viable platelets

Miller RD: Complications of massive blood transfusions. Anesthesiology 39:82–93, 1973

C.12. Would you empirically give an alkalizing agent (sodium bicarbonate) to patients receiving massive blood transfusions?

The pH of ACD stored blood is 6.5. Infusion of acidic ACD blood to patients who are probably already in acidosis from hypovolemic shock may augment the acidosis. Howland and Schweizer suggested that 44.6 mEq of sodium bicarbonate be given intravenously for every 5 units of transfused ACD blood. Collins and Miller concluded in their studies that the empiric administration of sodium bicarbonate is not indicated. Our study on burned patients agrees with Miller's result. We found that the metabolic acid–base response to massive blood transfusions of ACD blood is very variable. It seems illogical to give sodium bicarbonate empirically to patients receiving massive blood transfusions. Serial arterial blood gas analysis is strongly recommended for proper management of acid–base balance.

Collins JA, Simmons RL et al: The acid–base status of seriously wounded combat casualties: II. Resuscitation with stored blood. Am Surg 173:6–18, 1971

Howland WS, Schweizer O: Physiologic compensation for storage lesion of bank blood. Anesth Analg (Cleve) 44:8–16, 1965

Miller RD, Tong MJ, Robbins TO: Effects of massive transfusion of blood on acid–base balance. JAMA 216:1762–1765, 1971

C.13. What percentage of labile factors V and VIII remain in the blood after 21 days of storage?

Factors V and VIII decrease gradually to 20% to 50% of normal after 21 days of storage. Infusion of large amounts of stored blood rarely dilutes factors V and VIII to below 50% of normal. Only 5% to 20% of the normal amount of factor V and 30% of factor VIII are necessary for hemostasis. Therefore, it is unlikely that a hemorrhagic diathesis would occur from deficiencies of factors V and VIII during massive transfusions of stored whole blood.

Miller RD: Complications of massive blood transfusions. Anesthesiology 39:82–93, 1973

C.14. If the patient is awake, what are the clinical manifestations of intravascular hemolysis?

The immediate symptoms, which begin after 50 ml or less of blood have been transfused, include a throbbing headache, severe lumbar pain (almost pathognomonic), precordial pain, dyspnea, anxiety, and restlessness. Signs include flushed face, then cyanosis, distended neck veins, initial slowing of the pulse, followed by a rapid thready pulse, diaphoresis, cold and clammy skin, and profound shock usually within an hour. Bleeding may follow DIC, which results from the release of erythrocytic thromboplastic substances. Oliguria, anuria, and acute renal failure may supervene.

Isselbacher RJ et al: Harrison's Principles of Internal Medicine, 9th ed, p 1575. New York, McGraw-Hill, 1980

C.15. How would you manage a hemolytic transfusion reaction?

As soon as a hemolytic transfusion reaction is suspected, the transfusion should be stopped, and the following procedures should be carried out:

- Save the remaining donor blood for further testing.
- Draw a venous blood sample from the patient. This sample and the donor's blood are returned to the blood bank for regrouping and cross-matching. A hemolytic antibody is sought by direct and indirect Coomb's test.
- A sample of urine is inspected for free hemoglobin.
- The presence of free hemoglobin in the plasma is inspected. Pink plasma indicates at least 20 mg free hemoglobin/100 ml.
- Give Mannitol (25 grams) intravenously with IV fluid to maintain aurine output of over 100 ml/hr. If the urine output falls below 100 ml/hr, the initial dose of Mannitol may be repeated, but not more than 100 grams in any 24 hour period.

If hypotension develops, hypovolemia should be corrected. Vasopressor drugs and sodium bicarbonate are given, if necessary. If acute ranal failure occurs, fluid therapy may have to be limited or modified.

Freitag JJ, Miller LW: Manual of Medical Therapeutics, 23rd ed, pp 291–292. Boston, Little Brown & Co, 1980

C.16. What are the signs of citrate intoxication?

The signs of citrate intoxication are those of hypocalcemia, including hypotension, narrow pulse pressure, elevated left ventricular end-diastolic pressure and central venous pressure, and prolonged QT interval.

Miller RD: Complications of massive blood transfusions. Anesthesiology 39:82–93, 1973

C.17. Would you administer calcium routinely to treat possible citrate intoxication during massive infusion of ACD stored blood? Why?

Routine administration of calcium is not indicated; hypocalcemia rarely occurs, probably because humans can mobilize calcium rapidly from bone tissue and metabolize large amounts of citrate. Citrate is metabolized by entering into the Kreb's tricarboxylic acid cycle, with production of sodium bicarbonate. If there is evidence of hypocalcemia (prolonged QT interval and hypotension), calcium gluconate may be given 100 mg every 3 minutes up to 1 to 2 g.

Miller RD: Complications of massive blood transfusions. Anesthesiology 39:82–93, 1973

D. Postoperative Management

D.1. What is the differential diagnosis of sinus tachycardia?

The differential diagnosis of sinus tachycardia includes the following:
- A normal response to hypotension, hypovolemia, adrenocortical insufficiency, and anaphylaxis
- The presence of catecholamine release from anxiety and from painful stimuli
- Fever, sepsis, and malignant hyperthermia
- Endocrine abnormalities (i.e., pheochromocytoma, thyrotoxicosis)
- Hypercarbia and hypoxia
- Congestive heart failure and pulmonary embolism

D.2. Discuss the causes of oliguria in the recovery room.

Oliguria is defined arbitrarily as the production of less than 400 ml of urine in 24 hours. When oliguria occurs, it is a functional manifestation of a variety of clinical entities referred to as acute renal failure (ARF). The syndrome of acute renal failure may be classified into the following three groups:
- Prerenal ARF (hypovolemic). There is no structural damage to the kidney. The reduction in renal blood flow results in a reduced filtration rate and a decrease in urinary flow. It is reversible with volume expansion. However, if untreated, it can progress to the ischemic form of acute tubular necrosis.
- Renal ARF (acute tubular necrosis). There is structural damage to the

renal tubules. The damage may be due to ischemia or nephrotoxic substances.
- Postrenal ARF (obstruction of urinary outflow). Pus, tubular debris, clots of blood, and crystalluria can cause acute bilateral obstruction of the ureters. The flow of urine is completely suppressed in contrast to the low flows found in prerenal and renal disease.

One must determine the cause of the oliguria because the management can vary greatly. To identify the cause of oliguria, a careful assessment of the urinary sediment is important. Presence of renal tubular cells, renal tubular cell casts, and pigmented granular casts is strong evidence for the diagnosis of acute tubular necrosis. A normal urinary sediment supports a diagnosis of hypovolemic renal failure. In addition, certain laboratory data may be useful to determine the causes of acute renal failure (see Table 23-1). Other data such as central venous pressure, pulmonary artery diastolic pressure, and pulmonary capillary wedge pressure can give valuable information as to the state of hydration.

Harries JD: Evaluation of renal function. ASA Refresher Courses in Anesthesiology 4:39–50, 1976

D.3. What is normal renal blood flow?

Normal renal blood flow is 1100 to 1200 ml/min, equal to 20% to 25% of cardiac output. Renal blood flow to the cortex is 400 ml/100g/min, whereas the medulla receives less than 50 ml/100g/min.

Larson CP et al: Effects of anesthetics on cerebral, renal, and splanchnic circulations. Anesthesiology 41:172–173, 1974

D.4. Are diuretics useful in the therapeutic approach to acute renal failure?

After all means to improve urinary output have failed, diuretics provide useful diagnostic information about the ability of the kidneys to produce urine. Mannitol 12.5 to 25 g followed by furosemide 5–40 mg may be given. If these diuretics are successful in increasing urinary output, renal function is not totally lost, and sufficient renal perfusion exists to allow production of urine. However, oliguria that does not respond to diuretics suggests that further efforts to improve renal function will fail, assuming cardiac output has been maintained. Note that diuretics are not given to induce diuresis, to force urinary output, or to comfort the physician that renal perfusion is improved; rather, they are given to diagnose whether the patient is capable of forming any urine whatsoever. A few studies suggest that large doses of furosemide may normalize the distribution of renal blood flow, shifting it from the medulla back to the cortex. Other studies suggest that diuretics may revert oliguria to nonoliguric renal failure. However, survival is not improved after diuretic therapy.

Cantarovich F, Galli C, Genedetti L et al: High dose of Furosemide in established acute renal failure. Br Med J 4:449–450, 1973

Frazier HS, Yager H: The clinical use of diuretics. N Engl J Med 288:246–249, 455–458, 1973

34 Porphyria
Michael Tjeuw

This 23-year-old woman complained of abdominal pain and vomiting for 3 days. Her white blood count was 18,000 and temperature 38.6°C. Because of tenderness and splinting of the right side of the abdomen, an abdominal exploration was done, which proved negative. Anesthesia for the laparotomy was thiopental sodium and nitrous oxide oxygen. Gallamine was used for muscle relaxation. Anesthesia and immediate recovery were uneventful. On the third postoperative day, she developed intense motor weakness and complained of cold and numb lower extremities.

A. Medical Disease and Differential Diagnosis

1. What is the differential diagnosis of right sided abdominal pain?
2. What is the significance of negative exploration? Name a few conditions that mimic the acute abdomen.
3. Discuss the classification of the porphyrias and the incidence of occurrence.
4. What is the basic metabolic defect of porphyria?
5. What are the pathologic changes in the nervous system and the liver?
6. What are the clinical manifestations of acute intermittent porphyria?
7. What factors have been implicated in triggering an acute attack of intermittent porphyria?
8. What are the characteristic laboratory findings in hereditary hepatic porphyria?
9. Outline the treatment for an acute attack of intermittent porphyria.
10. What is the prognosis in acute intermittent prophyria?

B. Preoperative Evaluation and Preparation

1. This patient returned 2 years later for an elective incisional herniorrhaphy. How would you prepare her for anesthesia?

2. Would you give her premedicants?

C. Intraoperative Management

1. What anesthetic technique would you choose? Discuss general versus regional anesthesia.
2. What agents would you use for induction and maintenance of anesthesia?
3. What anesthetic drugs are reportedly safe and do not precipitate an attack in hereditary hepatic porphyria?
4. A breathing induction technique with halothane-nitrous oxide-oxygen was chosen for this patient. Why were two inhalation anesthetic agents used?
5. Draw the curves of the uptake of halothane and nitrous oxide in the alveoli in relation to time.
6. Why does the concentration of nitrous oxide rise so rapidly and that of halothane rise so slowly in the alveoli?
7. Are alveolar concentrations of nitrous oxide and halothane affected by changes in ventilation?
8. Are alveolar concentrations of nitrous oxide and halothane affected by changes in cardiac output?
9. What is meant by "the concentration effect" in uptake of inhalation anesthetics?
10. What is the definition of MAC (minimum alveolar concentration)?
11. What physiologic factors may alter MAC?
12. What factors have little or no influence on MAC?
13. If the surgeon requests more relaxation, what muscle relaxant would you use?
14. Name a few nondepolarizing muscle relaxants and discuss mechanism of action, metabolism, and excretion.
15. Do nondepolarizing muscle relaxants cross the blood brain barrier?
16. What are the side-effects of d-tubocurarine?

D. Postoperative Management

1. What antagonist would you use to reverse the neuromuscular blockade by d-tubocurarine? What are the dosage and duration of action?
2. What criteria do you use to assess the recovery from the effect of muscle relaxants?

A. Medical Disease and Differential Diagnosis

A.1. *What is the differential diagnosis of right sided abdominal pain?*

Abdominal pain may be caused by a great variety of gastrointestinal and intraperitoneal diseases. Because of overlapping nerve distribution, the pain may be secondary to extraperitoneal disorders. The differential diagnosis of right sided abdominal pain includes many conditions *e.g.,* appendicitis, cholecystitis, perforated ulcer, diverticulitis, regional enteritis, pancreatitis, intestinal obstruction, renal colic, hepatitis, ectopic pregnancy, salpingitis, ovarian cyst or torsion, and endometriosis.

Schwartz SI: Principles of Surgery, 3rd ed, p 1042. New York, McGraw–Hill, 1979

A.2. What is the significance of negative exploration? Name a few conditions that mimic the acute abdomen.

The negative abdominal exploration suggests that the cause of pain may be extraabdominal in origin. The following conditions mimic the acute abdomen:

- Intrathoracic—pneumonia, myocardial ischemia
- Neurogenic—spinal cord tumors, tabes dorsalis, herpes zoster
- Metabolic—uremia, porphyria, diabetic acidosis, Addisonian crisis
- Hematogenous—leukemia, sickle cell crisis
- Toxins—drugs, lead poisoning, bacterial toxins
- Psychogenic

Schwartz SI: Principles of Surgery, 3rd ed, p 1043. New York, McGraw–Hill, 1979

A.3. Discuss the classification of the porphyrias and the incidence of occurrence.

The porphyrias may be classified as follows:

Erythropoietic Porphyrias—due to excessive production of porphyrin in the bone marrow

- Congenital erythropoietic prophyria
- Erythropoietic protoporphyria

Hepatic Porphyrias—due to excessive production of porphyrin in the liver

- Hereditary—autosomal dominant trait
  - Acute intermittent porphyria (Swedish type)—75%
  - Variegate porphyria (South African type)—20%
  - Coproporphyria—5%
- Porphyria cutanea tarda
- Acquired and secondary porphyrinuria

Erythrohepatic Protoporphyria

The incidence of the hepatic porphyrias varies according to geographic area and ethnic factors.

- The world wide incidence is estimated at 1:100,000.
- In Sweden, the incidence is estimated at 1.5:100,000.
- In Poland, the incidence is estimated at 1.8:100,000.
- In Finland, the incidence is estimated at 2.3:100,000.
- In Western Australia, the incidence is estimated at 2.4:100,000.

The highest incidence, 1:1000, has been reported in Lapland and in South Africa's white population. In Northern Ireland it is 1:5000. It is very rare in blacks. It is more common in women in the third or fourth decades of life, but rarely occurs before puberty.

Silva G: Porphyrias. Anesth Rev 6, No 5:52. New York, McNamara, 1979

Wyngaarden JB, Smith LH: Textbook of Medicine, 16th ed, p 1122. Philadelphia, WB Saunders, 1982

A.4. What is the basic metabolic defect of porphyria?

The prophyrias are biochemically characterized by an over-production and increased secretion of porphyrins and their metabolic precursors. This hyperbiosynthesis of porphyrins is the result of a failure of the regulatory mechanisms controlling heme biosynthesis in either the bone marrow (erythropoietic porphyrias) or the liver (hepatic porphyrias). The aminolevulinic acid synthetase enzyme (ALA-s), which is the initial enzyme of the pathway for porphyrin synthesis, is increased. The increase of ALA-s results in an increase of aminolevulinic acid and porphobilinogen and consequently an increase in urinary and fecal excretion of porphyrins or their precursors. Porphyrins, as well as their precursors, are pharmacologically inactive. Whether or not porphyrin is a neurotoxin will have to be investigated further. Only the hepatic porphyrias are of clinical significance to the anesthesiologist.

Katz J, Benumof J, Kadis LB: Anesthesia and Uncommon Disease, 2nd ed, p 24. Philadelphia, WB Saunders, 1981

A.5. What are the pathologic changes in the nervous system and the liver?

The pathologic changes in the nervous system include the following:
- Scattered demyelination of all types of peripheral nerves
- Chromatolysis of motor nerve cells in the spinal cord and medulla
- Demyelination of the cerebrum and cerebellum

In the acute phase, there may be central lobular necrosis of the liver.

Dundee JW et al: The hazard of thiopental anaesthesia in porphyria. Anesth Analg (Cleve) 41:567–574, 1962

A.6. What are the clinical manifestations of acute intermittent porphyria?

- Gastrointestinal tract. Moderate to severe abdominal pain, often colicky, is frequently the initial or most prominent symptom. The pain may be localized, generalized, or radiating to the back, but the abdomen is usually soft. Severe vomiting and persistent constipation are frequent symptoms. Prolonged vomiting may cause dehydration, oliguria, and azotemia.
- Nervous system. Neurologic disturbances are frequently, although not always, associated with abdominal manifestations. Symptoms may involve the central, peripheral, or automatic nervous system.

Peripheral neuropathy is usually predominantly motor, may be asymmetrical, and may vary from mild weakness in one extremity to complete flaccid quadriplegia. Sensory disorders such as hypoesthesia or hyperesthesia may occur.

Cranial nerve involvement leads to optic atrophy, ophthalmoplegia, facial palsy, dysphagia, and vocal cord paresis. Weakness of the abdominal, intercostal, or diaphragmatic musculature may progress to respiratory paralysis. Death, if it occurs, is usually caused by bulbar involvement with resultant respiratory insufficiency.

Psychiatric disturbances may include nervousness, emotional instability, personality changes, hysteria, psychoses, and confusional states. More severe CNS involvement, delirium, coma, and epileptic seizures may occur.

Autonomic involvement may present with sinus tachycardia, hypertension, and nonspecific ECG changes. This may be due to vagal neuropathy.

Wyngaarden JB, Smith LH: Textbook of Medicine, 16th ed, p 1124. Philadelphia, WB Saunders, 1982

A.7. What factors have been implicated in triggering an acute attack of intermittent porphyria?

An acute attack may be triggered by certain drugs that can alter hepatic porphyrin synthesis. Other factors include infection, menstruation, pregnancy, or ingestion of alcohol. Drugs that have been implicated as porphyria-inducing drugs are as follows:

Drugs Used in Anesthesia

- Barbiturates
- Nonbarbiturate sedative and hypnotic drugs, meprobamate, chlordiazepoxide, ethinamate, glutethimide, methyprylon, and carbromal
- The steroid configuration drugs, such as hydroxydione, althesin, (alfaxalone and alfadolone) pancuronium
- Ethyl alcohol
- Hydantoin anticonvulsants, such as diphenylhydantoin (which is also an antiarrhythmic drug)
- Nikethamide (central nervous system-cardiorespiratory stimulant)
- Pentazocine

Drugs Not Used in Anesthesia

- Sulfonamides
- Sex hormones, estrogens
- Antipyretic, analgesic, antiinflammatory drugs, such as aminopyrine and antipyrene
- Griseofulvin
- Hypoglycemic sulfonylureas, tolbutamide, and chlorpropamide

- Metapyrone (inhibitor of adrenal steroid synthesis)
- Ergot preparations
- Methyldopa

Katz J, Benumof J, Kadis LB: Anesthesia and Uncommon Disease, 2nd ed, p 29. Philadelphia, WB Saunders, 1981

A.8. What are the characteristic laboratory findings is hereditary hepatic porphyria?

The most characteristic laboratory findings is excessive aminolevulinic acid (ALA) and porphobilinogen (PBG) in the urine. In the Watson–Schwartz or Hoesch tests, PBG reacts with Ehrlich's reagent (dimethylamino benzaldehyde in HCl) to form a red complex that is not extractable with n-butanol. By contrast, the red color produced by Ehrlich aldehyde with urobilinogen or indole is readily extractable with butanol. During acute episodes of porphyria, the Watson–Schwartz test is almost always strongly positive. Positive test results should be confirmed by quantitation of urinary PBG by ion-exchange column chromatography. Freshly passed urine may be normal in color, because it contains relatively little preformed uro-and coproporphyrin. It darkens on standing because of conversion of PBG and other precursors to porphyrins and porphobilin (a dark brown pigment of unknown structure).

Wyngaarden JB, Smith LH: Textbook of Medicine, 16th ed, p 1124. Philadelphia, WB Saunders, 1982

A.9. Outline the treatment for an acute attack of intermittent porphyria.

There is *no* specific treatment for acute intermittent porphyria; therapy remains symptomatic and prophylactic. The acute pain and psychic manifestations usually can be alleviated or controlled with phenothiazines, reserpine, or meperidine. Oral chlorpromazine is preferred for abdominal and muscle pain. Acute attacks often can be aborted by prompt administration of carbohydrate ("glucose-effect"). Administration of intravenous glucose or fructose, 10 to 15 g per hour for 24 hours, may result in striking remissions. When recurrent manifestations are related to the menstrual cycle, prolonged androgenic suppression has given promising results. Supportive treatment is of great importance. Normal homeostasis should be maintained. Dehydration, electrolyte and acid–base imbalance should be corrected. If bulbar signs are present, respiratory paralysis should be anticipated and a mechanical respirator should be available. Infection should be prevented or controlled, avoiding sulfonamides. Drugs known to have triggered an acute attack of porphyria should also be avoided. Tachycardia and hypertension can be controlled with propranolol.

If acute manifestations fail to respond to these measures within 48 hours, treatment with hematin (hydroxyheme) is indicated with the rationale that it compensates for the genetic impairment of endogenous heme synthesis. The solution consists of pyrogen-free hemin (ferriprotoporphyrin IX chloride) dissolved in aqueous sodium carbonate (10 grams per liter), adjusted to pH 8.0 with HCl and sterilized by membrane filtration. It is infused slowly into the largest available vein at a maximal dose of 3 mg per kilogram given at 12-hour intervals. Apart from phlebitis at the site of infusion (in 4 per cent of cases), complications have been rare. Renal toxicity may occur if the maximal recommended dose is exceeded. A clinical and biochemical response (decreased excretion of PBG) may be expected within 72 to 96 hours after starting hematin treatment, and maximal benefit after a total of 10 to 12 doses. With cessation of hematin treatment, a rise in urinary PBG may occur, although the patient's clinical condition usually remains stable.

Wyngaarden JB, Smith LH: Textbook of of Medicine, 16th ed, pp 1124–1125. Philadelphia, WB Saunders, 1982

A.10. What is the prognosis in acute intermittent porphyria?

In the earlier literature, the prognosis of acute intermittent porphyria was very grave, with a mortality of 80% within 5 years of the first attack. More recent reports set it around 25%. Death occurs most frequently during the second and third decades. Beyond this age, manifestations tend to be less severe. As a result of hematin therapy and modern intensive care, the prognosis is much improved.

Wyngaarden JB, Smith LH: Textbook of Medicine, 16th ed, p 1125. Philadelphia, WB Saunders, 1982

B. Preoperative Evaluation and Preparation

B.1. This patient returned 2 years later for an elective incisional herniorrhaphy. How would you prepare her for anesthesia?

Preparation for anesthesia must include an extensive neurological workup and a thorough evaluation of bulbar functions and associated respiratory reserve. Tachycardia and hypertension should be corrected. Fluid, electrolytes, and acid–base abnormalities should be normalized.

Katz J, Benumof J, Kadis LB: Anesthesia and Uncommon Disease, 2nd ed, p 30. Philadelphia, WB Saunders, 1981

B.2. Would you give her premedicants?

Premedication with morphine or meperidine appears to be safe. Barbiturates are absolutely contraindicated. Atropine is reportedly safe; small amounts can be given, if needed.

Katz J, Benumof J, Kadis LB: Anesthesia and Uncommon Disease, 2nd ed, pp 28–30. Philadelphia, WB Saunders, 1981

C. Intraoperative Management

C.1. What anesthetic technique would you choose? Discuss general versus regional anesthesia.

I would choose general anesthesia. Regional anesthesia is best avoided because of the scattered occurrence and unpredictable onset of central and peripheral neuropathy in porphyria. New lesions in the nervous system might unjustly be attributed to the injection of local anesthetic. The ideal general anesthetic has not yet been developed. The identity of most anesthetic drugs that might trigger an attack has been determined, but the information is based on limited experience. There is inadequate information concerning the volatile anesthetic agents. Precipitating activity may occur because of the enzyme induction.

Katz J, Benumof J, Kadis LB: Anesthesia and Uncommon Disease, 2nd ed, p 30. Philadelphia, WB Saunders, 1981

C.2. What agents would you use for induction and maintenance of anesthesia?

All barbiturate drugs such as thiopental sodium, thiamylal, and methohexital (Brevital) are absolutely contraindicated. Dundee reported 16 thiopental anesthetics in patients with acute intermittent porphyria. All 16 patients became paralyzed and seven died. A breathing induction with a volatile anesthetic agent may be the choice. If rapid induction is required, ketamine may be the best choice. Although its safety is not established, limited clinical experience with ketamine is promising. For maintenance, the choice lies between a narcotic nitrous oxide-oxygen technique and volatile anesthetic agents and muscle relaxants.

Dundee JW et al: The hazard of thiopental anaesthesia in porphyria. Anesth Analg (Cleve) 41:567–574, 1962

C.3. What anesthetic drugs are reportedly safe and do not precipitate an attack in hereditary hepatic porphyria?

The following lists of drugs are reported to be safe for use in hereditary hepatic porphyria:
- Tranquilizers—chlorpromazine, promazine, promethazine
- Analgesics—morphine, meperidine, mefenamic acid
- Sedative–hypnotics–narcotics—paraldehyde, chloral hydrate, propanidid
- Local anesthetics—procaine
- General anesthetics—nitrous oxide, cyclopropane, diethyl ether, halothane, enflurane
- Muscle relaxants—succinylcholine, decamethonium, d-tubocurarine, gallamine
- Anticholinergics—atropine

- Anticholinesterase—neostigmine
- Antihypertensives—tetraethylammonium, pentolinium, rauwolfia alkaloids, sodium nitroprusside, nitroglycerine
- Antitachycardics—neostigmine, propranolol
- Ketamine

On purely theoretical grounds, the safety of neostigmine has been questioned because of the anticholinesterase property possessed by some triggering insecticides; however, in practice, neostigmine has proven to be safe. Muscle relaxants are not associated with triggering activity. Pancuronium is best avoided because of its steroidal configuration and capacity for biotransformation. Whether volatile anesthetic agents such as halothane and enflurane may precipitate an acute attack is inconclusive. There is inadequate information to establish their triggering activity, though it may occur through enzyme induction.

Katz J, Benumof J, Kadis LB: Anesthesia and Uncommon Disease, 2nd ed, pp 28–30. Philadelphia, WB Saunders, 1981

C.4. A breathing induction technique with halothane-nitrous oxide-oxygen was chosen for this patient. Why were two inhalation anesthetic agents used?

Two inhalation anesthetics were used to accelerate the breathing induction. Epstein and associates suggested that uptake of a large volume of a first or primary gas (usually nitrous oxide) accelerates the alveolar rate of rise of a second gas given concomitantly. This is known as "the second gas effect" and it accelerates the breathing induction.

The second gas effect can be explained by two factors, a concentrating effect and an increase in inspired ventilation. The loss of volume associated with the uptake of the first gas (nitrous oxide) by pulmonary circulation increases the concentration of the second gas (halothane). The uptake of the first gas creates a negative pressure that draws more gas mixture into the lungs.

Eger EI II: Anesthetic Uptake and Action, p 116. Baltimore, Williams & Wilkins, 1974

Epstein RM et al: Influence of the concentration effect on that uptake of anesthetic mixtures: The secong gas effect. Anesthesiology 25:364–371, 1968

C.5. Draw the curves of the uptake of halothane and nitrous oxide in relation to time.

Figure 34–1 illustrates that the approach of the alveolar concentration (FA) to the concentration inspired (FI) varies inversely with solubility. It is slower with a more soluble agent, such as halothane, but quickly nears 100% with nitrous oxide. The curves have different heights according to blood solubility, but are similar in shape. The rapid upswing to point A in the halothane curve is due to unopposed ventilation; a slower continuing

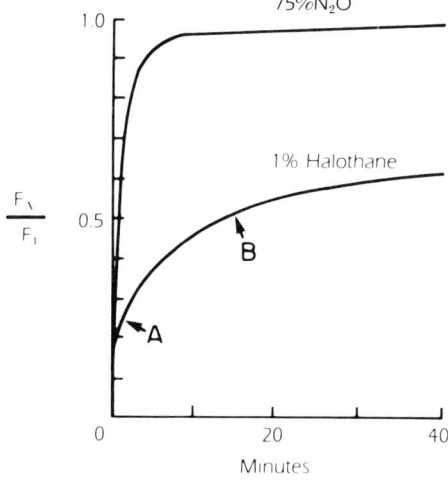

Fig. 34–1. Alveolar concentrations of halothane and nitrous oxide. (Adapted with permission from Eger EI: Anesthetic Uptake and Action, p 91. Baltimore. Williams & Wilkins, 1974)

upswing to point B is due to uptake by vessel rich groups such as brain, heart, kidney, and splanchnic vessel beds. The line continues with a slower uptake by muscle and fat.

Eger EI II: Anesthetic Uptake and Action, p 91. Baltimore, Williams & Wilkins, 1974

C.6. Why does the concentration of nitrous oxide rise so rapidly and that of halothane rise so slowly in the alveoli?

The blood gas partition coefficient or blood solubilities of the gases play an important role. The blood gas partition coefficient of nitrous oxide is 0.47 and that of halothane is 2.3. Because nitrous oxide is less soluble in the blood, the alveolar concentration of nitrous oxide rises more rapidly. Halothane has a greater blood/gas partition coefficient. The greater the uptake of anesthetic, the lower the alveolar concentration.

Eger EI II: Anesthetic Uptake and Action, pp 82–83. Baltimore, Williams & Wilkins, 1974

C.7. Are alveolar concentrations of nitrous oxide and halothane affected by changes in ventilation?

Yes. An increase in alveolar ventilation causes a more rapid rise in alveolar concentration of halothane and nitrous oxide. Although the qualitative changes are the same for both gases, there are quantitative differences. The more soluble the anesthetic, the greater the effect of a ventilatory change. Thus, alveolar nitrous oxide is less affected by alteration of ventilation, while halothane is more affected by ventilatory changes.

Eger EI II: Anesthetic Uptake and Action, p 123. Baltimore, Williams & Wilkins, 1974

C.8. Are alveolar concentrations of nitrous oxide and halothane affected by changes in cardiac output?

Yes. An increase in cardiac output causes a *decrease* in rise of alveolar concentration of halothane and nitrous oxide. As with changes in ventilation, the qualitative changes differ. The magnitude of the effect is related to the blood solubility of the anesthetics. The more soluble anesthetic such as halothane is more affected, and the less soluble nitrous oxide is less affected.

Eger EI II: Anesthetic Uptake and Action, p 131. Baltimore, Williams & Wilkins, 1974

C.9. What is meant by "the concentration effect" in uptake of inhalation anesthetics?

The concentration effect means that the higher the inspired anesthetic concentration, the more rapid the rise of alveolar concentration: inspired concentration ratio (FA/FI). For example, if the inspired concentration of an anesthetic gas is 10%, it takes 10 minutes to reach an alveolar concentration of 10%. Because of the concentration effect, when the inspired concentration is 20%, it takes *less than* 10 minutes to reach an alveolar concentration of 20%. The concentration effect, like the second gas effect, results from two factors: a concentrating effect and an augmentation of inspired ventilation.

Eger EI II: Anesthetic Uptake and Action, pp 113–116. Baltimore, Williams & Wilkins, 1974

C.10. What is the definition of MAC (minimum alveolar concentration)?

MAC is defined as the minimum alveolar concentration of anesthetic at 1 atmosphere that produces immobility in 50% of those patients or animals exposed to a noxious stimulus. It is a measure of anesthetic potency.

Eger EI II: Anesthetic Uptake and Action, p 1. Baltimore, Williams & Wilkins, 1974

C.11. What physiologic factors may alter MAC?

The factors that may alter MAC are as follows:
- Body temperature changes. Hypothermia reduces MAC for all agents. Hyperthermia increases MAC. This data supports the clinical impression that very little anesthetic is required for hypothermic patients and more anesthetic is required for febrile patients.
- Thyroid function changes. Hyperthyroidism raises the MAC, while hypothyroidism does not significantly lower the MAC.
- Age. MAC is decreased in older patients and increased in neonates.

Eger EI II: Anesthetic Uptake and Action, pp 11–13. Baltimore, Williams & Wilkins, 1974

C.12. What factors have little or no influence on MAC?

The following factors have little or no influence on MAC:

- The effect of variable stimulis. Different stimuli, such as electrical current, the tail clamp, or skin incisions, all require the same alveolar concentration to suppress movement.
- Species. There is very little variability of the average MAC from species to species or even from one class of animals to another.
- Duration of anesthesia does not affect MAC.
- Sex. There are no differences between MAC in human males and females.
- Acid–base changes fail to alter the MAC.
- Hypoxia and isovolemic anemia do not influence MAC until they attain levels that produce decompensation of the body defenses against oxygen deprivation.
- Hypertension and hypotension fail to affect MAC, until reduction of blood pressure is one-third to one-half of the control.

Eger EI II: Anesthetic Uptake and Action, pp 3–11. Baltimore, Williams & Wilkins, 1974

C.13. If the surgeon requests more relaxation, what muscle relaxant would you use?

Muscle relaxants are *not* associated with triggering activity. Therefore, both depolarizing and nondepolarizing muscle relaxants may be used. We prefer nondepolarizing relaxants such as d-tubocurarine or gallamine for muscle relaxation.

Katz J, Benumof J, Kadis LB: Anesthesia and Uncommon Disease, 2nd ed, pp 28–30. Philadelphia, WB Saunders, 1981

C.14 Name a few nondepolarizing muscle relaxants and discuss mechanism of action, metabolism, and excretion.

D-tubocurarine, pancuronium, gallamine, and alcuronium are nondepolarizing relaxants. The mechanism of action of nondepolarizing muscle relaxants is competitive action at the neuromuscular junction. In brief, a nondepolarizing muscle relaxant combines with the cholinoceptor sites at the postjunctional membranes and thereby blocks the transmitter action of acetylcholine. The metabolism of d-tubocurarine is variable. In man, about 1/3 of d-tubocurarine is excreted in the urine over a period of several hours, and a variable amount is metabolized. The metabolism of alcuronium is not yet understood. Gallamine is almost entirely excreted by the kidney, with no apparent metabolic degradation. Pancuronium is approximately 70% excreted by the kidney, 30% is metabolically degraded.

Gilman AG, Goodman LS, Gilman A: The Pharmacological Basis of Therapeutics, 6th ed, p 230. New York, Macmillian, 1980

Somogyi AA et al: Disposition kinetics of pancuronium in patients with total biliary obstruction. Br J Anaesth 49:1103–1107, 1977

C.15. Do nondepolarizing muscle relaxants cross the blood brain barrier?

No. Nondepolarizing muscle relaxants do not cross the blood brain barrier, because they are quaternary ammonium, highly ionized charged molecules and water soluble. They are lipoid-insoluble and therefore cannot penetrate the cell membranes or pass the blood brain barrier into the central nervous system.

Gissen AJ: Clinical use of muscle relaxants. ASA Refresher Courses in Anesthesiology 1:57–58, 1973

C.16. What are the side-effects of d-tubocurarine?

Rapid intravenous injection of large doses of d-tubocurarine may cause hypotension, at times precipitously. This hypotension has been implicated to be caused by sympathetic ganglionic blockade and histamine release. Histamine release may result in hypotension, skin flush, and bronchospasm. This is undoubtedly true in dogs, but it has not been clearly demonstrated in man.

Gissen AJ: Clinical use of muscle relaxants. ASA Refresher Courses in Anesthesiology 1:62, 1973

Gilman AG, Goodman LS, Gilman A: The Pharmacological Basis of Therapeutics, 6th ed, pp 227–228. New York, Macmillian, 1980

D. Postoperative Management

D.1. What antagonist would you use to reverse the neuromuscular blockade by d-tubocurarine? What are the dosage and duration of action?

The anticholinesterases such as neostigmine, edrophonium, and pyridostigmine are commonly used to antagonize the neuromuscular blockade caused by curare like drugs.

Neostigmine (2–3 mg in the adult) is usually effective in antagonizing the residual blockade. Its onset of action is rapid following intravenous administration. The peak effect is at 10 minutes and the antagonism may last from 1 to 1½ hours. It must be administered slowly and preceded by atropine, 1 mg, in order to block the muscarinic effect of neostigmine. The total dose of neostigmine should not exceed 5 mg as neuromuscular blockade may be produced by this drug at higher doses.

Edrophonium at doses of 10 to 20 mg has a faster effect and weaker muscarinic effect than neostigmine. It is not necessary to administer atropine with these doses. However, the duration of action is short (10–15 minutes), limiting its usefulness for antagonizing the long-acting nondepolarizing relaxants.

Pyridostigmine, at intravenous doses of 10 to 25 mg, is an effective antagonist like neostigmine. It must also be administered with atropine, even though it has less muscarinic activity than neostigmine. Its peak effect is within 15 to 30 minutes. Its slightly longer duration of action does not appear to offer an advantage over neostigmine.

Lichtiger M, Moya F: Introduction to the Practice of Anesthesia, 2nd ed, pp 67–69. Hagerstown, MD, Harper & Row, 1978

D.2. What criteria do you use to assess the recovery from the effect of muscle relaxants?

Estimation of the extent of recovery of neuromuscular function is most important with regard to the respiratory system. Adequate vital capacity or tidal volume is not sufficient evidence of recovery from the effect of a muscle relaxant. The patient must show enough respiratory muscle power to clear his airway of obstruction or secretion. This can be demonstrated if the following occur:

- A patient can exert an inspiratory force of more than 20 cm H_2O
- A patient can raise his head on command and sustain for a short period (e.g., 5 seconds)
- A patient can sustain contraction in response to a tetanic stimulus of 50 to 100 H_2 for 5 seconds
- A patient has a "train-of-four" ratio of greater than 65%

Gissen AJ: Clinical use of muscle relaxants. ASA Refresher Courses in Anesthesiology 1:61, 1973

35 Cleft Palate
Marjorie J. Topkins

A newborn male was noted at birth to have a cleft lip and palate. Birth weight was 2960 g. Apgar score was 7 at 1 minute, and 9 at 5 minutes. Mild icterus was noted on the second day.

A. Medical Disease and Differential Diagnosis

1. What are a cleft lip and a cleft palate?
2. What is the etiology of a cleft lip or a cleft palate?
3. What is the incidence of a cleft lip with or without a cleft palate? Is there a sex difference in the incidence of cleft lip and palate? Are there racial differences in the incidence of cleft lip and cleft palate?
4. Discuss the pathophysiology of the cleft lip and cleft palate in the neonate and the older child (*i.e.,* 5 years).
5. What other conditions are associated with a cleft lip and palate?
6. What is Pierre Robin syndrome?
7. What is Treacher Collins syndrome?
8. Why are Pierre Robin and Treacher Collins mentioned at this time?
9. What surgical procedures are anticipated for this child? Discuss indications, timing, and complications of closure of the lip and palate.

B. Preoperative Evaluation and Preparation

1. What information do you need prior to closure of a cleft lip and a cleft palate?
2. What preoperative orders are needed?

C. Intraoperative Management

1. What monitors will you need for cheiloplasty and palatoplasty?
2. Discuss anesthetic agents for cheiloplasty and palatoplasty. Discuss the use of epinephrine and halothane.
3. Discuss the induction and anesthetic management for cheiloplasty and palatoplasty.
4. What are the reported complications of this type of surgery and anesthesia?
5. Discuss hemostasis during this procedure.
6. What is velopharyngeal incompetence?
7. How can velopharyngeal incompetence be diagnosed?
8. What is the relationship of tonsillectomy and adenoidectomy to velopharyngeal incompetence?
9. Briefly describe the operation known as push back and pharyngeal flap.
10. How does a pharyngeal flap affect your anesthetic management or any subsequent anesthetic administered to this patient?
11. In one sentence, what is the crucial problem of anesthesia for cleft palate? Enumerate the consequences of failure.

D. Postoperative Management

1. What complications of cleft lip and cleft palate surgery may be seen in the recovery room?
2. How do you protect the airway postoperatively?

A. Medical Disease and Differential Diagnosis

A.1. What are a cleft lip and a cleft palate?

Simply, a cleft lip or cleft palate is a defect in the lip or palate. These two entities can occur alone or together. The cleft lip can be classified anatomically by inspection. The cleft can be unilateral or bilateral. It can be complete or incomplete. The cleft may be associated with nasal deformity, most commonly columellar shortening or deformity, absence of the nasal floor, and deformity of the ala nasi.

The cleft palate is divided into prepalatal clefts and postpalatal clefts. The incisive foramen marks the boundary between these two. The development of prepalatal and postpalatal clefts are embryologically different. Prepalatal clefts involve the anterior palate, the alveolus, the lip, the nostril floor, and the ala nasi. They can be complete or incomplete. Postpalatal clefts are posterior to the incisive foramen. They can be complete or incomplete depending on whether or not they extend all the way through the soft and hard palates to the incisive foramen. The third type of palatal cleft is the submucosal cleft in which a bone defect exists without a mucosal defect. The most common cleft of the palate is a left complete cleft of the prepalatal and palatal structures. The second most common is a midline cleft of all the soft palate and part of the hard palate without a cleft in the prepalatal area.

Grabb WC, Smith JW: Plastic Surgery, pp 159, 160, 183. Boston, Little, Brown & Co, 1973

A.2. What is the etiology of a cleft lip or a cleft palate?

Prepalatal clefts are caused by a lack of mesodermal development. Three mesodermal islands, one central and two lateral, are described. When these mesodermal elements fail to develop and fuse prepalatal clefts result. Palatal clefts are caused when the palatal ridges fail to migrate medially, contact, and fuse. The palatal ridges are vertical in the 7 week embryo and lie lateral to the tongue. The tongue drops down and the shelves rotate upward to the horizontal position and fuse from anterior to posterior to form an intact palate in the 12 week embryo.

Grabb WC, Rosenstein SW, Bzock KR: Cleft Lip and Palate, pp 54–65. Boston, Little, Brown & Co, 1971

Grabb WC, Smith JW: Plastic Surgery, pp 159, 181–183. Boston, Little, Brown & Co, 1973

A.3. What is the incidence of a cleft lip with or without a cleft palate? Is there a sex difference in the incidence of cleft lip and palate? Are there racial differences in the incidence of cleft lip and cleft palate?

There is considerable variation in the reported incidence of a cleft lip with or without a cleft palate and less variation in a cleft palate alone. In general, the incidence of a cleft lip has racial as well as sex differences. The highest incidence occurs in Orientals (1.61/1000), while the lowest occurs in the American black population (0.3/1000). The incidence in Caucasians is intermediate (0.9/1000). The incidence among American Indians probably exceeds that in the Oriental. There is considerably less variation in the incidence of isolated cleft palate. The incidence ranges from 0.2 for American blacks to 0.5 in Orientals and is approximately 0.4 per 1000 live births in Caucasians. The incidence among American Indians is again somewhat higher than that of Orientals. More males are born with a cleft lip with or without cleft palate, and the severity of the defect is greater in males. More females are born with isolated cleft palate. The male to female ratio of incidence of a cleft lip with or without a cleft palate is 62 to 38 and 43 to 57 for isolated cleft palate overall. Approximately 25% of patients with cleft lips and palates have an isolated cleft lip, 50% have a cleft lip and palate and 25% have only a cleft palate.

Cooper HK et al: Cleft Lip and Palate: A Team Approach, pp 116–119. Philadelphia, WB Saunders, 1979

Millard DR: Cleft Craft Vol. I. The Unilateral Deformity, pp 63–64. Boston, Little, Brown & Co, 1976

A.4. Discuss the pathophysiology of cleft lip and palate in the neonate and the older child (i.e., 5 years).

The presence of an uncorrected cleft lip or palate in the nenoate results in feeding problems. The neonate cannot suck because the presence of the cleft makes the creation of a negative pressure difficult. If the neonate regurgitates formula up into the nose, infection of the nasopharynx and secondary ear infection may result. Respiratory problems are not usually a problem unless other congenital anomalies are present. However, upper airway obstruction can occur.

In the older child an uncorrected lip or palate results in the typical speech of the cleft palate child. Speech development may be delayed because of frustration. Psychological problems may be a considerable problem as this youngster approaches school age and peer association. The speech of this child is typically nasal with an inability to sound the so-called plosives p, k, d, t, and sibilants s, and sh.

A.5. What other conditions are associated with a cleft lip and palate?

A child with one congenital anomaly may have other anomalies which should be ruled out in the neonatal period. Associated abnormalities occur 30 times more frequently in the patient with an isolated cleft palate than in the noncleft population. Between 10% and 25% of cleft lip and palate patients have abnormalities of other organs. The Pierre Robin syndrome is frequently associated with a cleft palate as is Treacher Collins syndrome and first and second branchial arch syndrome (hemifacial microsomia).

Cooper HK: Cleft Palate and Cleft Lip: A Team Approach, pp 110–117. Philadelphia, WB Saunders, 1979

Curtis EJ: Genetic and environmental factors in the etiology of cleft lip and cleft palate. Can Dent Assoc J 23:576, 1957

Gorlin RJ et al: Facial clefting and its syndromes. Birth Defects 7:3, 1971

A.6. What is Pierre Robin syndrome?

Pierre Robin syndrome is one of the few life threatening congenital conditions of the neonatal period. The elements of this syndrome are limited to the jaw, tongue, and palate. There is retrognathia or micrognathia. The chin is displaced posteriorly due either to hypoplasia of the mandible (micrognathia) or to posterior positioning of a normal mandible (retrognathia). There is a glossoptosis due to retroposition of the mandible. The tongue falls back obstructing the airway in a ball valve fashion. The tongue may be large or there may be a relative macroglossia when compared with the micrognathia. A cleft palate is frequently present, most commonly incomplete. The lip is not usually involved. Occasionally, a high arched palate is present without a cleft. The etiology of the syndrome is divided between external pressure in utero on the anterior mandible with subsequent retardation of growth, and lack of growth potential in the mandible itself.

Grabb WC, Smith JW: Plastic Surgery, pp 115–117. Boston, Little, Brown & Co, 1979

A.7. What is Treacher Collins syndrome?

Treacher Collins syndrome or mandibulofacial dysostosis is a congenital genetic anomaly that is autosomal dominant with variable penetrance and expressivity. It occurs in approximately 1 per 10,000 live births. The common features of this syndrome are notching of the lower eyelids and underdevelopment of the malar bones. The complete form of the syndrome is manifested by antimongoloid slant of the eyelids, hypoplasia of the facial, malar, and mandibular bones, notching of the outer portion of the lower eyelid (coloboma), malformation of the external ear, occasionally involving the middle and inner ear, macrostomia with a high palate, abnormal hair at the sideburn area, blind dimples or fistulae at the corner of the mouth, and skeletal defects especially clefts of the face and palate. An incomplete form was described consisting of notching of the eyelid and hypoplasia of the molar bones. The third form, described as abortive, shows only the eyelid defect.

Pozwilla D: Pathogenesis of Treacher Collins syndrome-mandibular facial dysostosis. Br J Oral Surg 13:1, 1975

A.8. Why are Pierre Robin and Treacher Collins mentioned at this time?

Because of the small size and retrognathic position of the mandible with or without a large tongue, Pierre Robin syndrome may cause considerable difficulty in intubation. Treacher Collins syndrome produces even greater difficulty. However, anticipation of problems can prevent catastrophe.

Smith RM: Anesthesia for Infants and Children, p 411. St. Louis, CV Mosby, 1980

A.9. What surgical procedures are anticipated for this child? Discuss indications, timing, and complications of closure of the lip and palate.

The care of this child will require multiple operations and a multidisciplinary approach to the problem. He will need a pediatrician to maintain his overall health, a surgeon and anesthesiologist to accomplish the various surgeries, a speech therapist to prevent or overcome the speech deficiencies associated with clefts of the palate and an orthodontist to develop and maintain a relatively normal bite and dentition. The help of a psychologist or psychiatrist may be needed by the patient or his family.

The lip may be closed in the first week of life if there are no complicating associated conditions. This permits the parents to take home a relatively normal looking infant. Complications include breakdown of the closure with scarring of the tissues, bleeding, and infection. The rule of ten has been accepted by many plastic surgeons for timing the closure of the lip: hemoglobin 10 g or greater, 10 weeks of age, and 10 kg in weight. The hard palate can be closed anytime up to 4 or 5 years, but the soft palate should be closed prior to speech development. Therefore, the usual age has been 12 to 15 months. Others report closure of the soft palate as early as 3 to 6 months. Complications of palatal closure include bleeding, obstruction to respiration, breakdown of the sutured tissues, scarring, and persistent palatal openings. Secondary procedures may be required in later years for cosmetic purposes. These may involve the columella, the nasal tip and alae, and revision of the vermillion border. Additional procedures on the palate include the push back and pharyngeal flap operation.

Cooper HK: Cleft Palate and Cleft Lip: A Team Approach, pp 145–150. Philadelphia, WB Saunders, 1979

Grabb WC, Smith JW: Plastic Surgery, pp 192, 205–222. Boston, Little, Brown & Co, 1979

Kaplan I, Dresner J: The simultaneous repair of cleft lip and palate in early infancy. Brit J Plast Surg 27:134, 1974

B. Preoperative Evaluation and Preparation

B.1. *What information do you need prior to closure of a cleft lip and a cleft palate?*

General care of the patient with cleft lip and palate includes feeding; maintaining the airway, especially in the patient with a small or retropositioned mandible (Pierre Robin); preventing or treating middle ear disease because eustachian tube function is impaired; and searching for and investigating associated anomalies, which are 30 times higher than in the noncleft population.

Preoperative anesthetic evaluation includes the history and physical examination plus suitable laboratory data. The hemoglobin and white blood count and hematocrit plus urinalysis are minimal requirements. If Treacher Collins or Pierre Robin is suspected, an x-ray of the mandible may be helpful. Examination of the mouth may give an indication of potential intubation problems. The infant should be free of acute infection, gaining weight, have a hemoglobin 10 g% or better, and have a white blood count less than 10,000. With an open cleft palate, however, it is common to have crusting and low grade infection of the nasopharynx due to food and fluid regurgitation through the cleft. It is nearly impossible to eliminate this completely. Unless an acute inflammatory process is present, this has not led to complications.

Grabb WC, Smith JW: Plastic Surgery, pp 205–222. Boston, Little, Brown & Co, 1979

Mladic R et al: Blood volume determination in cleft lip–palate infant surgery. Plast Reconstr Surg 39:71, 1967

B.2. What preoperative orders are needed?

The preoperative orders should include restriction of oral intake. Up to 6 months of age, clear fluids may be given up until 4 hours prior to surgery. Older children less than 3 years of age may have clear fluids up till 2 a.m. No solids or milk are allowed after midnight. Children over 3 years of age are given nothing by mouth after midnight. For children 6 months of age or older, a sedative and atropine should be ordered. Pentobarbitol, 5 mg/kg, and atropine, 0.01 to 0.02 mg/kg, are given. For infants less than 6 months of age, atropine alone is sufficient. The use of atropine for its vagolytic action is important to prevent the bradycardia produced by halothane, mechanical stimulation, and succinylcholine if used for intubation. Because multiple operations may be required, the emotional trauma of each hospital experience must be minimized. Special orders include antibiotics if the infant or child has associated congenital heart disease and the typing and cross-matching of a unit of blood for palatal surgery. Cheiloplasty rarely requires blood transfusion, but blood loss has been reported as high as 200 to 300 ml in palate surgery. A unit of blood should be available, even though it is rarely administered.

Mladic R et al: Blood volume determinations in cleft lip-palate infant surgery. Plast Reconstr Surg 39:71, 1967

Smith RM: Anesthesia for Infants and Children, pp 96–101, 409, 411. St Louis, CV Mosby, 1980

C. Intraoperative Management

C.1. What monitors will you need for cheiloplasty and palatoplasty?

A suitable technique for measuring blood pressure is mandatory. In infants, the Doppler or Infrasonde transducer gives satisfactory results. In older children these techniques may be used, and in addition the Riva Rocci technique may be adequate. Temperature should be monitored per rectum or axilla and a heating-cooling blanket placed under the patient for use if necessary. A precordial stethoscope monitors both heart and respiratory sounds. It is particularly important in this patient because once surgery is begun, the anesthesiologist no longer has easy direct access to the airway. An electrocardiograph gives visual and audible evidence of the electrical activity of the heart. Blood loss should be measured accurately.

C.2. Discuss anesthetic agents for cheiloplasty and palatoplasty. Discuss the use of epineprhine and halothane.

Halothane, nitrous oxide, and oxygen can be used for both cheiloplasty and palatoplasty. To avoid the possibility of retrolental fibroplasia, the inspired oxygen concentration (F_IO_2) should not exceed 40% to 50% in normal full term infants less than 2 weeks of age and in premature infants until 3 months of age. Enflurane and isoflurane offer little over halothane except in the decreased sensitivity of the myocardium to exogenous epinephrine exhibited by the two former agents. Concentrations of epinephrine from 1:100,000 to 1:200,000 and an adult dose, not in excess of 10 ml of a 1:100,000 concentration per 10 minutes, nor more than 30 ml in an hour are recommended. *Note,* these dosages are for adults. No recommendations are available for infants and children, but the dose should be reduced, based on the patient's body weight. In practice, because the structures are very small, the total dose of epinephrine is far lower than these recommendations.

Ketamine, used without an endotracheal tube for cheiloplasty repair, is contraindicated because of the high incidence of severe laryngospasm, cardiac arrest, and vomiting followed by aspiration. Small infants react upredictably to ketamine. Local anesthesia with sedation has been used for cheiloplasty in the past, but distortion of the structures by the injected local anesthetics is unsatisfactory to some surgeons. Endotracheal anesthesia offers safe airway management.

Katz RL, Epstein RA: The interactions of anesthetic agents and adrenergic drugs to produce arrhythmia. Anesthesiology 29:763, 1968

Smith RM: Anesthesia for Infants and Children, pp 246, 409, 411. St Louis, CV Mosby, 1980

C.3. Discuss the induction and anesthetic management for cheiloplasty and palatoplasty.

For cheiloplasty, after suitable monitors are attached, the infant is induced with nitrous oxide, oxygen, and halothane. An intravenous route is established as soon as the patient is asleep. Dextrose 5% in 1/4 strength normal saline is a suitable infusate. Intubation can be facilitated with succinylcholine 1 mg/kg. If there is any possibility of difficulty with intubation, succinylcholine should not be given. Prepalatal clefts are most frequently on the left and the laryngoscope tends to fall into the cleft. Bilateral clefts often have a freely mobile premaxilla associated with them. Care must be taken to avoid traumatizing these structures. The endotracheal tube must not distort the anatomy. The tube curves over the lower lip where it is fastened in the midline. The RAE tube for oral intubation fulfills the requirement. Because it has a fixed length, care must be taken to ensure that it does not enter the right or left bronchus. A thermistor probe is placed either in the rectum or axilla. Rectal stimulation is postponed until after intubation to decrease the possibility of laryngeal reflexes. Care is taken to prevent heat loss. Cheiloplasty requires only the minimal depth of anesthesia and no muscle relaxation. The anesthesiologist sits or stands at the side of the table. The breath and heart sounds are monitored with the precordial stethoscope. It is necessary to have great cooperation between the surgeon and the anesthesiologist because the surgeon's tools and hands, and the anesthesiologist's endotracheal tube and apparatus all occupy the same very small space. The Ayre T piece and its modifications or the Mapleson system can be used. The fresh gas flow with the Ayre T piece and its modifications is two to three times the minute volume. The minute volume is equal to the tidal volume times respiratory rate. The tidal volume equals the weight in pounds times three or 7 ml/kg. The Mapleson A requires a fresh gas flow equal to the minute volume and Mapleson D requires a fresh gas flow of 1.5 times minute volume.

For palatoplasty, halothane, nitrous oxide, and oxygen is quite satisfactory. Succinylcholine can also be used. If there is suspected difficulty of intubation, as might be expected with Pierre Robin or Treacher Collins syndrome, it is best omitted. Dextrose 5% in 1/4 strength normal saline at a rate of 4 ml/kg/hr can be administered once an intravenous route is available. This is a conservative fluid allowance. Blood is rarely required. If blood losses exceed 15% to 20% of the estimated blood volume, a transfusion should be started. During the palate repair a mouth gag (Dingman or Dott) is used, and the endotracheal tube is held under the tongue blade of the gag. Again the RAE oral tube can be used. Others prefer the anode or armored tube. Great care must be taken as the gag is inserted and opened. The endotracheal tube is pushed caudad where it may impinge on the carina or enter either main bronchus. Breath sounds are monitored as the gag is opened; if any change occurs, the gag is closed and the endotracheal tube repositioned. This is repeated as often as necessary until the breath sounds are normal with the gag fully open. Relaxants are not necessary and the patient should be almost awake when extubated.

Furman EB: Specific therapy in water electrolyte and blood volume replacements in pediatric surgery. Anesthesiology 42:187, 1975

Morgan GA, Steward DJ: Airway dimensions in children with and without a cleft palate. Can Anaesth Soc J 28:500, 1981

Sklar GS, King BD: Endothracheal intubation and Treacher Collins syndrome. Anesthesiology 44:247, 1976

C.4. What are the reported complications of this type of surgery and anesthesia?

Anesthetic complications include obstruction of the endotracheal tube, inadvertent extubation during the procedure and cardiac arrest. Postanesthetic complications include airway obstruction, bleeding with or without aspiration, and pneumonia. Complications not related to anesthetic management are wound healing, diarrhea, and otitis media. The mortality has been reported at less than 0.5%. Boston Children's Hospital reported no mortalities in 4500 operations over a 35 year period.

Grabb WC et al: Cleft Lip and Palate, pp 385–386. Boston, Little, Brown & Co, 1971

Smith RM: Anesthesia for Infants and Children, p 412. St Louis, CV Mosby, 1980

C.5. Discuss hemostasis during this procedure.

Epinephrine injected into the operative site decreases bleeding. As mentioned earlier, the total dose should be far less than 10 ml of 1:100,000 in 10 minutes. During palatoplasty, large areas of denuded palate are left after mobilization of the flaps for closure. Frequently these tissues ooze postoperatively. Bleeding can jeopardize the airway unless care is taken to prevent aspiration. Induced hypotensive techniques have been tried in the past in an attempt to reduce operative bleeding. Though a good operative field resulted, more postoperative bleeding was noted. In a comparative study of anesthetic agents and blood loss, methoxyflurane appeared to produce less bleeding than other agents.

Black GW et al: Anesthesia for cleft palate repair; A comparative study of anesthetic methods. Br J Plast Surg 22:343, 1969

Katz RL, Epstein RA: Interaction of anesthetic agents and adrenergic drugs to produce cardiac arrhythmias. Anesthesiology 29:763, 1968

Tempest MN: Some observations on blood loss and harelip and cleft palate surgery. Br J Plast Surg 11:34, 1958

C.6. What is velopharyngeal incompetence?

In order to produce the plosive sounds p, k, t, d, or the sibilants s or sh, the soft palate must touch the posterior pharyngeal wall to close the nose. Failure of closure results in the typical hypernasal speech. The most common cause of this is the cleft palate, but patients with congenitally short palates and no cleft may also have this typical speech. Treatment consists of surgical lengthening of the palate by the push back operation with or without a pharyngeal flap.

Grabb WC, Smith JW: Plastic Surgery, pp 218–219. Boston, Little, Brown & Co, 1979

C.7. How can velopharyngeal incompetence be diagnosed?

The diagnosis of velopharyngeal incompetence can be suspected from the speech of the child. More objective evidence can be obtained by direct vision of the soft palate while pronouncing certain key words (kah, kah), fogging of a hand mirror placed under the nose during speech, and cinefluorographic x-rays.

Grabb WC, Smith JW, Plastic Surgery, pp 218–223. Boston, Little, Brown & Co, 1979

C.8. What is the relationship of tonsillectomy and adenoidectomy to velopharyngeal incompetence?

Because the adenoids and tonsils tend to close the nasopharynx, they prevent or decrease velopharyngeal incompetence. A youngster who had normal speech may suddenly develop hypernasality after tonsillectomy and adenoidectomy. The tonsils and adenoids, therefore, are preserved if at all possible. A cleft palate constitutes a contraindication to removal of tonsils and adenoids.

Shirkey HC: Pediatric Surgery, p 1046. St Louis, CV Mosby, 1975

C.9. Briefly describe the operation known as push back and pharyngeal flap.

The palate is incised in an inverted U or W fashion laterally and anteriorly. It is mobilized and displaced posteriorly and a flap from the posterior pharyngeal wall is elevated and attached to the palate. This results in a partial closure of the nasopharynx. Breathing can take place through lateral openings left on either side of the pharyngeal flap.

Grabb WC, Smith JW: Plastic Surgery, p 200. Boston, Little, Brown & Co, 1973

C.10. How does a pharyngeal flap affect your anesthetic management or any subsequent anesthetic administered to this patient?

The presence of this flap prohibits nasoendotracheal intubation and makes many nasal techniques difficult (*i.e.*, insertion of nasogastric tube). The amount of obstruction is related to the width of the flap. Traumatic rupture of this flap secondary to attempted nasotracheal intubation could produce bleeding, aspiration, and laryngospasm. Knowledge of prior surgery is essential to good anesthetic management.

Brown TCK, Gisk GC: Anaesthesia for Children, pp 220–221. Oxford, Blackwell Scientific Publications, 1979

Topkins MJ: Personal observations

C.11. In one sentence, what is the crucial problem of anesthesia for cleft palate? Enumerate the consequences of failure.

The establishment, maintenance, and protection of the airway is the crucial problem of anesthesia for palate surgery. Failure to establish, maintain, and protect the airway results in tachypnea, CO_2 retention, hypoxemia, increased bleeding, hypovolemia, arrhythmia, cardiac arrest, and death.

Collins V: Principles of Anesthesia, pp 1347, 1351. Philadelphia, Lea & Febiger, 1976

Miller RD: Anesthesia, pp 721, 723–725, 1310. New York, Churchill Livingstone, 1981

Wylie WD, Churchill–Davidson HC: A Practice of Anaesthesia, pp 237–238. Chicago, Year Book Medical Publishers, 1972

D. Postoperative Management

D.1. What complications of cleft lip and cleft palate surgery may be seen in the recovery room?

Complications include airway obstruction, bleeding, and hypothermia. Airway obstruction is the result of closure of the structures plus some edema secondary to trauma. In the case of the push back procedure with or without a pharyngeal flap, the obstruction is due to the new posterior position of the palate and the pharyngeal flap. Blood loss is not an anesthetic complication but replacement is the anesthesiologist's responsibility, as is prevention of aspiration. Hypothermia delays emergence and produces metabolic acidosis, respiratory and myocardial depression. The most important problem for the anesthesiologist is maintenance of the airway.

Smith RM: Anesthesia for Infants and Children, p 590. St Louis, CV Mosby, 1980

Stehling LC, Zauder HL: Anesthetic Implications of Congenital Anomalies in Children, p 136. New York, Appleton–Century–Croft, 1980

D.2. How do you protect the airway postoperatively?

Following palotoplasty, the pharynx and nasopharynx are suctioned prior to extubation. Some anesthesiologists advocate that this be done with the aid of the laryngoscope to ensure removal of any mucous, blood, or clots. If suctioning is done prior to removing the Dingman gag, the laryngoscope may not be necessary. The infant should be as awake as possible. A long traction suture is placed through the tongue and tied loosely. Traction on the suture stimulates respiration and clears the airway. Neither an oral nor nasal airway should be inserted; these could disrupt the sutures and undo all the surgical work. The traction suture is removed when the infant leaves the recovery room.

Following palate surgery, the infant is placed in the prone or lateral position with the head dependent, turned to the side, and hyperextended. This position can be achieved with a jack placed under the foot of the crib or by placing a bulky bath blanket under the hips of the infant. Any blood or mucus will accumulate in the dependent cheek or roll out the mouth.

Following cleft lip surgery, a Logan bow is frequently used to take tension off the newly sutured lip. The infant can still be placed in the lateral position. Elbow restraints are essential and are placed on the infant or child before leaving the operating room. A high humidity atmosphere is recommended postoperatively to reduce the incidence of postoperative tracheitis, but others have failed to show any correlation between the use of humidity and the incidence of tracheitis.

Grabb WC, Smith JW: Plastic Surgery, p 217. Boston, Little, Brown & Co, 1979

Koka B et al: Postintubation croup in children. Anesth Analg (Cleve) 56:501, 1977

Smith RM: Pediatric Anesthesia, pp 217, 599–601. St Louis, CV Mosby, 1980

36 The Bleeding Tonsil
Joseph F. Artusio, Jr.

A 6-year-old 20 kg boy has been in the recovery room for 2 hours following tonsillectomy under halothane anesthesia. Tonsillar bleeding has continued since arrival. The child is awake, restless, anxious, and pale. His skin is moist. Blood pressure is now 60/40 torr; pulse 160/m; respiration 36/m. He is returned to the operating room.

A. Medical Disease and Differential Diagnosis

1. Why is this child restless and anxious?
2. What level of cerebral blood flow will produce these central nervous system symptoms? What is normal cerebral blood flow for this child?
3. What is autoregulation in cerebral blood flow?
4. What is the difference between hypovolemic hypotension and shock?
5. What is the normal blood volume of this child?
6. Why is the child's blood pressure low? What factors maintain normal blood pressure?
7. Why is the child having tachycardia and tachypnea?

B. Preoperative Evaluation and Preparation

1. How would you restore the vascular volume? What fluids would you use, and how much?
2. Would you premedicate this child?

C. Intraoperative Management

1. How would you establish anesthesia in this child?
2. How would you induce the patient? Would you use a breathing induction or a rapid sequence induction?
3. How would you monitor this child?

4. What anesthetic agent would you use for maintenance?
5. When would you extubate this child?

D. Postoperative Management

1. What postanesthesia complications are most likely to occur?
2. How would you treat postoperative stridor and a hoarse cry?

A. Medical Disease and Differential Diagnosis

A.1. Why is this child restless and anxious?

This child may be restless and anxious because he has pain at the surgical site, or frightened at seeing his own blood on the bed linen. However, this restlessness may herald cerebral hypoxia associated with extensive blood loss and a low blood pressure. To determine the causes of restlessness and anxiety, the inspired oxygen fraction (F_IO_2) should be increased to 40% by face mask. This rise in F_IO_2 will cause an increase in the partial pressure of oxygen in the alveolus and will increase the oxygen diffusion gradient to blood. If hypoxia is the cause for this abnormal behavior, improved oxygenation will result in a calmer child. The anxiety will decrease significantly.

Miller RD: Anesthesia, p 1304. New York, Churchill Livingstone, 1981

A.2. What level of cerebral blood flow will produce these central nervous system symptoms? What is normal cerebral blood flow for this child?

The normal mean cerebral blood flow is 45 to 50 ml per 100 g of brain tissue. Although cerebral blood flow through the fast compartment (probably gray matter) is 75 ml per 100 g of brain tissue per minute, and 20 ml per 100 g of brain tissue per minute in the slow compartment (probably white matter), the mean cerebral blood flow is 45 to 50 ml per 100 g of brain tissue per minute. Under normal conditions, this flow will result in a cerebral venous oxygen tension fo 35 to 45 torr. If cerebral blood flow falls to the point where autoregulation cannot meet the metabolic requirements of the brain, restlessness and anxiety will occur. Cerebral blood flow in the child is similar to the adult. When shock ensues, cerebral blood flow will be maintained up to the limits of autoregulation.

Alexander SC: Anesthesia and the cerebral circulation. ASA Refresher Courses in Anesthesiology 1:4, 1973

A.3. What is autoregulation in cerebral blood flow?

Autoregulation refers to the capacity of the cerebral vasculature to alter its resistance and to maintain cerebral blood flow constant over a range of cerebral perfusion pressure changes. In humans, this range occurs between a mean arterial pressure of 50 and 150 torr. Autoregulation is modified by cerebral disease states, volatile anesthetics, and other cerebral vasodilators. High sympathetic tone states, such as those encountered during hypovolemic shock, result in a lower cerebral blood flow at a given arterial pressure than that obtained when hypotension is pharmacologically obtained with sympatholytic drugs. Thus, sympathetic neurogenic influences shift the lower end of the lower autoregulatory threshold to the right and render the brain more susceptible to hypotensive ischemia. Cerebral sympathetic stimulation also shifts the upper limit of autoregulation to the right and offers some protection against hypertensive breakthrough.

Miller RD: Anesthesia, p 802. New York, Churchill Livingstone, 1981

A.4. What is the difference between hypovolemic hypotension and shock?

The fall in blood pressure associated with a decrease in blood volume is related to a decrease in cardiac output, subsequent to a decrease in venous return to the right heart. The patient is warm and dry to the touch. Hypotension is present and the heart rate will increase in an attempt to maintain cardiac output. The state of shock develops when the body attempts to shrink the vascular bed to meet the available volume. The decrease in size of the vascular bed is the result of an elaboration of sympathomimetic amines that produce peripheral vasoconstriction. In early stages this compensatory mechanism will shift the available blood volume into critical areas of the body (brain, heart, liver, and kidney). The increase in peripheral resistance will shut off peripheral blood flow to the extremities and the surface of the body. These sympathomimetic amines are secreted by the adrenal medulla and by the peripheral sympathetic nerve endings. This protective mechanism, which maintains circulating blood volume to vital areas of the body, is salutary and life saving. However, if vascular volume is not restored, peripheral tissue hypoxia will result. Lactoacidosis ensues as an end product of anaerobic metabolism. The development of acidosis may be the cause of the irreversibility of shock when tissue hypoxia results in a failing peripheral compensation. Every attempt should be made to restore the intravascular volume to meet the needs of the vascular bed. Peripheral vasoconstriction will decrease and irreversibility will be prevented as volume is restored and anaerobic metabolism gives away to aerobic metabolism.

Isselbacher KJ et al: Harrison's Principles of Internal Medicine, 9th ed, pp 176–177. New York, McGraw–Hill, 1980

A.5. What is the normal blood volume of this child?

The blood volume of this child is approximately 100 ml/kg. This child has 2 liters of blood. If we calculate blood volume on 80 to 90 ml/kg, he has a blood volume of 1600–1800 ml.

Smith RM: Anesthesia for Infants and Children, 4th ed, p 574. St Louis, CV Mosby, 1980

A.6. Why is the child's blood pressure low? What factors maintain normal blood pressure?

There are several factors that determine the level of the blood pressure. The first is cardiac output, which is determined by stroke volume and heart rate. Second is peripheral vascular resistance, now termed afterload. Third is blood volume, and the fourth is related to venous return to the right heart or pre-load. In this patient, the main factor resulting in hypotension is related to a low blood volume due to bleeding. The body will sustain the vital circulation in the brain, heart, liver, and kidneys by increasing heart rate and will decrease the peripheral vascular bed in an attempt to accommodate the vascular bed to the decrease in blood volume until compensation fails. Then shock ensues.

Isselbacher KJ et al: Harrison's Principles of Internal Medicine, 9th ed, pp 175–177, 1029–1030. New York, McGraw–Hill, 1980

A.7. Why is the child having tachycardia and tachypnea?

Tachycardia is a response to decreased venous return and a decrease in heart filling. It is the reflex response of the cardiac accelerators to increase heart rate and maintain the cardiac output even though there is a decrease in ejection fraction. Tachypnea, again is an attempt by the body to increase respiratory rate to maintain oxygenation of the blood. If more air enters the lung per unit of time, the blood will be exposed to a higher oxygen diffusion gradient, and oxygenation of the blood will be maintained in spite of a lower blood pressure.

Isselbacher KJ et al: Harrison's Principles of Internal Medicine, 9th ed, pp 168–169, 177. New York, McGraw–Hill, 1980

B. Preoperative Evaluation and Preparation

B.1. How would you restore the vascular volume? What fluids would you use, and how much?

Because the patient is losing whole blood it is best to use whole blood replacement. However, if the patient has not been typed and cross-matched, balance salt solution may be used until whole blood is available. Fluid volume replacement with balanced salt solution will provide enough circulatory volume to maintain the cardiac output, but only for a relatively short period of time. It will leave the circulation and will enter the extravascular space. When typed and cross-matched whole blood becomes available, the patient should be transfused until the blood pressure begins to return to normal or the heart rate begins to slow. Under these circumstances, it is safe to anesthetize the patient so that the bleeder may be ligated and the source of the fluid loss stopped.

Berry FA: Pediatric fluid and electrolyte therapy. ASA Refresher Courses in Anesthesiology, 3:1:6, 1975

Brown TCK, Fisk GC: Anesthesia for Children, Including Aspects of Intensive Care, p 199. Oxford, Blackwell Scientific Publications, 1979

Miller RD: Anesthesia, p 1304. New York, Churchill Livingstone, 1981

B.2. Would you premedicate this child?

Premedication is not necessary. One does not wish to decrease the respiratory rate and depth, and the heart is already accelerated. We recommend that no premedication be given.

Dripps RD, Eckenhoff JE, Vandam LD: Introduction to Anesthesia. The principles of Safe Practice, 5th ed, p 45. Philadelphia, WB Saunders, 1977

Miller RD: Anesthesia, p 1304. New York, Churchill Livingstone, 1981

C. Intraoperative Management

C.1. How would you establish anesthesia in this child?

When it is obvious that the bleeding will not stop with the usual methods of postnasal pack and ordinary clotting, the patient should be typed and cross-matched, and, if possible, all coagulation factors should be obtained. The child will have to be reanesthetized in order to control the hemorrhage. All hanging clots should be aspirated from the pharynx. An intragastric tube should be placed to relieve the intragastric pressure, and then it may be removed, so as not to hold the cardioesophageal junction open and invite regurgitation of blood up into the pharynx. Although it is not critical at this time, it is important for the surgeon and the anesthesiologist to know from the parent if a history of recent aspirin ingestion had been missed in the original history of the patient. Under these circumstances, bleeding may be quite difficult to control.

Brown TCK, Fisk GC: Anaesthesia for Children, Including Aspects of Intensive Care, p 199. Oxford, Blackwell Scientific Publications, 1979

Davies DD: Reanaesthetizing cases of tonsillectomy and adenoidectomy because of persistent postoperative haemorrhage. Brit J Anaesth 36:248, 1964

C.2. How would you induce the patient? Would you use a breathing induction or a rapid sequence induction?

Whichever method of induction and intubation is chosen, the anesthesiologist must remember that this is essentially an induction and intubation in a patient with a full stomach. Much of the blood loss has been swallowed. Therefore, there is a significant amount of blood in the stomach. It is extremely difficult to do an awake intubation in a child who is anxious and frightened. This makes an awake intubation practically impossible. We either breathe the child to sleep or use rapid sequence for the induction. Both methods are acceptable, but both methods have risks. The rapid sequence induction is probably safer from the viewpoint of aspiration, particularly with an assistant aiding the intubation with Sellick's maneuver. But in a child with a borderline blood volume, a rapid sequence induction, particularly with a barbiturate, may produce severe hypotension and bradycardia, and cardiac arrest may ensue. A breathing induction with halothane or isoflurane is much safer. However, with this technique, there is the danger of regurgitation or vomiting of blood into the tracheobronchial tree.

Brown TCK, Fish GC: Anaesthesia for Children, Including Aspects of Intensive Care, p 199, Oxford, Blackwell Scientific Publications, 1979

Donlon JV: Anesthetic considerations during otolaryngologic surgery. ASA Refresher Courses in Anesthesiology 9:47, 1981

Smith RM: Anesthesia for Infants and Children, 4th ed, p 495. St Louis, CV Mosby, 1980

C.3. How would you monitor this child?

Blood pressure, heart rate, ECG, and body temperature measurements are all important monitors. In spite of the emergency nature of the procedure, the monitors should be applied to guide the anesthesiologist during the induction and maintenance of anesthesia. Shortcuts in monitoring invite disaster. Careful monitoring of the depth of anesthesia by the usual criteria may be difficult, and in this relatively hypovolemic child, anesthetic overdose is a real possibility. These hypovolemic children are quite sensitive to central nervous system depression and care must be taken to prevent cardiac arrest from deep anesthesia.

Donlon JV: Anesthetic considerations during otolaryngologic surgery. ASA Refresher Courses in Anesthesiology 9:46–47, 1981

C.4. What anesthetic agent would you use for maintenance?

It makes little difference which of the potent inhalation anesthetic agents you use for this patient. We certainly would prefer inhalation anesthesia to the narcotic–tranquilizer technique. The anesthesiologist can regulate the depth of anesthesia much more readily with an inhalation agent. At the end of the procedure the child should be responding, with upper airway reflex intact to protect him from aspiration of any residual blood in the upper airway.

Dripps RD, Eckenhoff JE, Vandam LD: Introduction to Anesthesia. The Principles of Safe Practice, 5th ed, p 137. Philadelphia, WB Saunders, 1977

C.5. When would you extubate this child?

If the child is not reacting on the endotracheal tube, we leave it in place until the child is safely in the recovery room. Extubation can then be done when the airway reflexes are active. If the upper airway reflexes are active, the child may be extubated in the operating room. The child must then be turned on his right side and the head made lower than the hips to prevent aspiration of blood either vomited or regurgitated from the stomach.

Donlon JV: Anesthetic considerations during otolaryngologic surgery. ASA Refresher Courses in Anesthesiology 9:47, 1981

D. Postoperative Management

D.1. What postanesthesia complications are most likely to occur?

The most likely postanesthesia complications are related to the upper airway. Because the child had to be reintubated, the danger of laryngeal edema is a distinct possibility, considering that there has been much suctioning in the upper airway. He should be watched carefully for a hoarse cry or any difficulty in respiration that causes increased work to get air in and out. Subglottic edema may occur. There is also the danger of a deficit in clotting factors following significant blood replacement. A coagulation profile should be obtained during the immediate postoperative period, particularly if pharyngeal ooze continues.

Jordan WS, Graves CL, Elwyn RA: New therapy for postintubation laryngeal edema and tracheitis in children. JAMA 212, No. 4:585, 1970

Miller RD: Anesthesia, pp 895–898. New York, Churchill Livingstone, 1981

D.2. How would you treat postoperative stridor and a hoarse cry?

There is some value in using cortisone in the immediate postoperative period to reduce the edema of the upper airway. However, high humidity, Vaponefrin, or Bronkosol nebulization with some additional oxygen in the inspired mixture is of greatest value. The croup tent, which keeps the child in a moist atmosphere, is probably the most effective means of reducing airway swelling. If edema continues, and the work of breathing increases as the airway becomes obviously obstructed, endotracheal intubation should be reinstituted. Once the child's airway is secured, a decision to perform a tracheostomy can be made.

Dripps RD, Eckenhoff JE, Vandam LD: Introduction to Anesthesia. The Principles of Safe Practice, 5th ed, pp 381, 386. Philadelphia, WB Saunders, 1977

Jordan WS, Graves CL, Elwyn RA: New therapy for postintubation laryngeal edema and tracheitis in children. JAMA 212, No 4:585–588, 1970

37 Morbid Obesity
Fun-Sun F. Yao

A 30-year-old Caucasian woman with cholelithiasis was scheduled for cholecystectomy and possible common bile duct exploration. She weighed 150 kilograms and was 150 cm tall. She was found somnolent during the preoperative visit. Her blood pressure was 150/90 torr; pulse 80/min; respiration 6 to 8/min.

A. Medical Disease and Differential Diagnosis

1. What problems exist with this patient? Define the terms overweight, obesity, moribid obesity, and normal weight.
2. What is the pickwickian syndrome?
3. What kind of metabolic problems would you expect to find in morbidly obese patients?
4. Describe the changes that occur in the following respiratory functions in morbidly obese patients:
   - Lung volumes—tidal volume, FRC, residual volume, vital capacity, inspiratory and expiratory reserve volumes, and total lung capacity
   - Compliances—lung, chest wall, total
   - Work of breathing
5. What changes occur in PaO_2 and $PaCO_2$?
6. What changes occur in Qs/QT and VD/VT? Describe the equation.
7. What changes occur in the cardiovascular system of the obese patient? Discuss cardiac output, blood volume, blood pressure, and pulmonary arterial pressure.
8. Are there any other disease entities usually associated with obesity?

B. Preoperative Evaluation and Preparation

1. How would you evaluate the patient preoperatively?
2. Interpret the following arterial blood gases: pH, 7.25; PCO_2, 50 torr; PO_2, 58 torr; HCO_3^-, 25 mEq/L on room air.

3. What is the equation for blood pH?
4. What are the normal values of blood PKa, dCO_2, HCO_3^-, and H_2CO_3?
5. Interpret the following spirometry screening test: vital capacity 2360 ml (expected 3375 ml); FEV_1/FVC, 82%; VC 70% of expected value.
6. How would you premedicate the patient? Why?

C. Intraoperative Management

1. How would you monitor the patient?
2. How would you induce anesthesia? Describe the intubation technique.
3. How would you maintain the anesthesia? What is your choice of agents?
4. What kind of muscle relaxants would you use?
5. Can regional anesthesia be used? What are the advantages and disadvantages of regional anesthesia?
6. What is the effect of narcotics on Oddi's sphincter?
7. During surgery, arterial blood gases showed pH, 7.35; PaO_2, 57 torr; $PaCO_2$, 52 torr; F_IO_2, 0.6; respirator tidal volume, 1000 ml, and rate 15/m. Ten cm H_2O PEEP was added to the circuit and the tidal volume was increased to 1200 ml. Twenty minutes later, the arterial blood gases showed pH, 7.32; PaO_2, 55 torr; $PaCO_2$ 55 torr. What is the explanation for these changes?

D. Postoperative Management

1. When are you going to extubate the patient? What are the criteria for extubation?
2. What are the major early postoperative complications in the morbidly obese patient?
3. How does position affect respiratory function in obese patients?
4. How would you prevent postoperative atelectasis?

A. Medical Disease and Differential Diagnosis

A.1. What problems exist with this patient? Define the terms overweight, obesity, morbid obesity, and normal weight.

Obesity and cholelithiasis are the main problems. *Overweight* is defined as body weight as much as 20% greater than predicted ideal weight. *Obesity* is defined as body weight more than 20 percent greater than predicted ideal weight. *Morbid obesity* is defined as body weight more than twice predicted ideal weight. Ideal normal body weight is difficult to define. It is generally based on American life insurance statistics, according to height, build, sex, and ages. The so-called body mass index (BMI), body weight in kilograms over height in meters squared, appears to be very useful. The normal BMI is 25 or less. Obesity is defined as BMI of 30 or more. In practice we use Broca Index, height in centimeters less 100 for males and less 105 for females as ideal body weight in kilograms. The ideal body weight for a man 170 cm tall is 70 kg.

Bendixen HH: Morbid obesity. ASA Refresher Courses in Anesthesiology 6:1–14, 1978

Fisher A, Waterhouse TD, Adams AP: Obesity: Its relation to anesthesia. Anesthesia 30:633–647, 1975

Vaughan RW: Obesity: Implications in anesthetic management and toxicity. ASA Refresher Courses in Anesthesiology, 9:184, 1981

A.2. What is the pickwickian syndrome?

The syndrome was named by Burwell in 1956. He felt that the first adequate description of this syndrome had been made in 1837 by Charles Dickens in the *Posthumous Papers of the Pickwick Club* in which he described an obese, somnolent boy named Joe. The complete pickwickian syndrome consists of massive obesity, somnolence, alveolar hypoventilation, periodic respiration, hypoxemia, secondary polycythemia, right heart failure, and right ventricular hypertrophy.

Burwell CB et al: Extreme obesity associated with alveolar hypoventilation—A pickwickian syndrome. Am J Med 21:811–818, 1956

Hedley–Whyte J et al: Applied Physiology of Respiratory Care, pp 301–310. Boston, Little, Brown & Co, 1976

A.3. What kind of metabolic problems would you expect to find in morbidly obese patients?

The basic problem in morbid obesity is the increase in total absolute oxygen consumption and carbon dioxide production associated with the increase in total tissue mass. The increases in metabolism show a linear relationship to body weight and body surface area. However, the basal metabolic rate in obesity is within normal limits.

White RL Jr, Alexander JK: Body oxygen consumption and pulmonary ventilation in obese subjects. J Appl Physiol 20:197–201, 1965

A.4. Describe the changes that occur in the following respiratory functions in morbidly obese patients:

- Lung volumes—tidal volume, FRC, residual volume, vital capacity, inspiratory and expiratory reserve volumes, and total lung capacity
- Compliances—lung, chest wall, total
- Work of breathing.

Tidal volume (V_T) is normal or increased in nonpickwickian obesity, decreased in pickwickian obesity. Inspiratory reserve volume (IRV) is decreased. Expiratory reserve volume (ERV) is most markedly decreased because the heavy weight of the torso decreases the normal expansive tendency of the rib cage. Residual volume (RV) is normal. Functional residual capacity (FRC) is markedly decreased because of a decrease in the expiratory reserve volume (FRC = RV + ERV). Vital capacity is decreased because of markedly decreased ERV (VC = IRV + V_T + ERV). Total lung capacity is decreased. Lung compliance is often normal, but decreased when pulmonary and circulatory complications are present. Chest wall compliance is always decreased because of the weight of the torso and the abdominal contents against the diaphragm. Total compliance is always decreased. The work of breathing is always increased because of low compliance.

Alexander JK et al: Lung volume changes with extreme obesity. Clinical Research 7:171, 1959

Bendixen HH: Morbid obesity. ASA Refresher Courses in Anesthesiology 6:1–14, 1978

A.5. What changes occur in PaO_2 and $PaCO_2$?

The most common abnormal blood gas finding in the obese patient is hypoxemia. Although hypoxemia can occur as a result of hypoventilation, most often it is due to a low ventilation–perfusion ratio. The pulmonary perfusion is increased in obese patients because of increased cardiac output, increased circulating blood volume, and pulmonary hypertension. The alveolar ventilation is decreased, secondary to airway closure, as a result of a markedly decreased expiratory reserve volume, which is often lower than the closing volume. The changes in $PaCO_2$ are variable depending on the alveolar ventilation. The following three types of alveolar ventilation are found among the morbidly obese:

- Alveolar hyperventilation in response to hypoxic drives. This is usually seen in young, active, obese patients with a $PaCO_2$ of about 35 torr.
- Alveolar hypoventilation is found in older or more obese patients with pickwickian syndrome. The $PaCO_2$ is always more than 40 torr.
- Periodic hypoventilation. The patients maintain normal or below normal $PaCO_2$ values during the daytime, but retain CO_2 at night or at rest.

Bendixen HH: Morbid obesity. ASA Refresher Courses in Anesthesiology 6:1–14, 1978

Hedley–Whyte J et al: Applied Physiology of Respiratory Care, pp 301–310. Boston, Little, Brown & Co, 1976

A.6. What changes occur in Q_S/Q_T and V_D/V_T? Describe the equation.

The intrapulmonary shunt Q_S/Q_T is always increased because of a low ventilation–perfusion ratio and as a result of airway closure, decreased FRC, hypoventilation, and increased pulmonary circulation. (Normal Q_S/Q_T is less than 5%.)

$$\text{Shunt equation: } Q_S/Q_T = \frac{CcO_2 - CaO_2}{CcO_2 - CvO_2}$$

In the absence of complications, V_D/V_T is often less than normal because of increased tidal volume and unchanged dead space.

$$\text{Bohr equation: } V_D/V_T = \frac{PaCO_2 - P\bar{e}CO_2}{PaCO_2}$$

$P\bar{e}CO_2$: mixed expired CO_2 tension

Bendixen HH: Morbid obesity. ASA Refresher Courses in Anesthesiology 6:1–14, 1978

Nunn JF: Applied Respiratory Physiology, 2nd ed, pp 228, 278. London, Boston, Butterworth & Co, 1977

A.7. What changes occur in the cardiovascular system of the obese patient? Discuss cardiac output, blood volume, blood pressure, and pulmonary arterial pressure.

Cardiac output and stroke volume increase in proportion to oxygen consumption and the degree of obesity. Blood volume is expanded when it is expressed in absolute values. However, it is contracted when calculated in terms of body weight of adipose tissue compared with lean body mass. Hypertension is more prevalent in obese people because of increased cardiac output and blood volume. The relationship between body weight and arterial pressure is greater for systolic than for diastolic pressure. Pulmonary hypertension is usually present in pickwickian obesity as a result of hypoxic pulmonary vasoconstriction and increased cardiac output. However, pulmonary arterial pressure is normal in nonpickwickian obese patients without heart or lung disease. Because of hypertension and increased cardiac output, congestive heart failure occurs in as many as 10% of obese patients.

Hedley–Whyte J et al: Applied Physiology of Respiratory Care, pp 301–310. Boston, Little, Brown & Co, 1976

Reisin E, Frohlich ED: Obesity: Cariovascular and respiratory pathophysiological alterations. Arch Intern Med 141:431–434, 1981

A.8. Are there any other disease entities usually associated with obesity?

Secondary obesity may be associated with hypothyroidism, Cushing's disease, insulinoma, and hypothalamic disorders. Although only a minority of obese patients are diabetic, 80% to 90% of nonketotic diabetics are obese. Increased insulin secretion and insulin resistance due to tissue insensitivity are well characterized features of obesity. Obesity exacerbates the diabetic state. Osteoarthritis, sciatica, varicose veins, thromboembolism, ventral and hiatal hernias, and cholelithiasis are more common in obese patients.

Isselbacher KJ et al: Harrison's Principles of Internal Medicine, 9th ed, pp 411–413. New York, McGraw–Hill, 1980

B. Preoperative Evaluation and Preparation

B.1. How would you evaluate the patient preoperatively?

Preoperative evaluation should include a detailed history, physical examination, and laboratory tests. Special attention should be paid to circulatory, pulmonary, and hepatic functions. Circulatory evaluation includes symptoms and signs of right or left ventricular failure, history of hypertension, and electrocardiogram. Respiratory evaluation should include smoking history, exercise tolerance, history of hypoventilation and somnolence, pulmonary function test with spirometry and base line arterial blood gases, and chest x-ray. Hepatic function tests should include

Table 37-1. Predicted pH at different $PaCO_2$ levels in the absence of metabolic acid–base abnormality

PCO_2	pH (approximate)
80	7.20
60	7.30
40	7.40
30	7.50
20	7.60

Note, each 10 torr decrease in $PaCO_2$ from normal increases the ph 0.1 unit. Each 20 torr increase in $PaCO_2$ from normal decreases the pH 0.1 unit.

serum albumin and globulin, SGOT, SGPT, bilirubin, alkaline phosphatase, prothrombin time, and cholesterol levels.

Katz J, Benumof J, Kadis LB: Anesthesia and Uncommon Diseases: Pathophysiologic and Clinical Correlations, 2nd ed, p 453. Philadelphia, WB Saunders, 1981

B.2. Interpret the following arterial blood gases: pH, 7.25; PCO_2, 50 torr; PO_2, 58 torr; HCO_3^-, 25 mEq/L on room air.

These blood gases indicate respiratory acidosis and metabolic acidosis with hypoxemia. HCO_3^-, 25 mEq/L is a laboratory error. A pH of 7.25 suggests acidosis, which may be respiratory or metabolic, or a combination of both. If there is no metabolic abnormality, a PCO_2 of 50 torr should produce a pH of 7.35 (Table 37–1). The difference in pH (7.35 − 7.25 = 0.10 units) is due to metabolic acidosis. For each 7 mEq/L of acid or base excess, pH changes 0.10 unit in the appropriate direction. A metabolic acidosis of 0.1 unit pH means a 7 mEq/L base deficit. The HCO_3^- is expected to be 17 mEq/L (24 − 7 = 17), but a change in PCO_2 itself will change the HCO_3^- from chemical equilibrium. Each 10 torr increase in $PaCO_2$ from normal increases the HCO_3^- 1 mEq in acute CO_2 retention and 4 mEq in a chronic situation. Therefore, we expect the HCO_3^- to be 17 + 1 = 18 mEq in acute CO_2 retention or 17 + 4 = 21 mEq in chronic CO_2 retention. The blood gas machine provides direct measurement of the pH, PCO_2, and PO_2. The HCO_3^- is usually derived from an equation or from a nomogram. If there is a discrepancy between the pH, PCO_2, and HCO_3^-, the technical error is usually in the HCO_3^-. It is important to recheck the blood gases according to clinical conditions. A $PaCO_2$ of 50 torr means alveolar hypoventilation due to decreased minute volume or increased dead space. In order to interpret PaO_2, the F_IO_2 should always be available. A PaO_2 of 100 torr may mean severe pulmonary failure if the F_IO_2 is 1.0. Hypoxemia in obese patients usually is due to increased venous admixture from decreased ventilation–perfusion ratio as a result of low FRC and hypoventilation. Metabolic acidosis with hypoxemia indicates lactic acidosis from anaerobic metabolism.

Dripps RD, Eckenhoff JE, Vandam LD: Introduction of Anesthesia: The Principals of Safe Practice, 5th ed, pp 326–327. Philadelphia, WB Saunders, 1977

B.3. What is the equation for blood pH?

The Henderson–Hasselbalch equation is: $pH = pK + \log \frac{(HCO_3^-)}{(H_2CO_3)}$

The H_2CO_3 concentration is very low and cannot be measured directly. Normal blood H_2CO_3 concentration is 0.0017 mMol/L. H_2CO_3 is proportional and not equal to dissolved CO_2. Clinically dissolved CO_2 is used to replace H_2CO_3. Therefore, pK is changed to pKa. Dissolved CO_2 is calculated as α P_{CO_2}; α, being the solubility coefficient for carbon dioxide in body fluids, is 0.031 mMol per liter per torr P_{CO_2}. For a normal P_{CO_2} of 40 torr, dissolved CO_2 is calculated to be $40 \times 0.031 = 1.2$ mMol per liter. Pka is 6.1, but this is variable with temperature and pH. The modified Henderson–Hasselbalch equation is as follows:

$$pH = pKa + \log \frac{(HCO_3^-)}{dCO_2} \quad \text{or} \quad pH = pKa + \log \frac{(HCO_3^-)}{0.031 \times P_{CO_2}}$$

Nunn JF: Applied Respiratory Physiology, 2nd ed, pp 336–337. London, Boston, Butterworth & Co, 1977

B.4. What are the normal values of blood pKa, dCO_2, HCO_3^-, and H_2CO_3?

The normal values are: pKa, 6.1; dCO_2, 1.2 mMol/1; HCO_3^-, 24 mEq/L; H_2CO_3, 0.0017 mMol/L.

Nunn JF: Applied Respiratory Physiology, 2nd ed, p 339. London, Boston, Butterworth & Co, 1977

B.5. Interpret the following spirometry screening test: vital capacity (VC) 2360 ml (expected 3375 ml); $FEV_{1.0}/FVC$, 82%; VC, 70% of expected value.

The spirometry shows mild restrictive lung disease and no evidence of obstructive lung disease. Normal vital capacity depends on sex, age, and height. The normal $FEV_{1.0}/FVC$ is greater than 80%. In restrictive lung disease, vital capacity is less than 75% of expected value. In obstructive lung disease, the $FEV_{1.0}/FVC$ is less than 75%. The expected vital capacity in liters in young adult males is equal to approximately $(height)^3$ in meters. The residual volume equals approximately 30% of vital capacity. Vital capacity can also be estimated at 65 ml/in. or 25 ml/cm height for males and 52 ml/in. or 20 ml/cm height for females.

Hand Book of Physiology, Section 3, Respiration, p 388. Washington, DC, American Physiological Society, 1964

Ayers LN, Whipp BJ, Ziment I: A Guide to the Interpretation of Pulmonary Function Tests, 2nd ed. New York, Roerig, 1978

Macklem PT: Tests of lung mechanics. N Engl J Med 293:339, 1975

B.6. How would you premedicate the patient? Why?

Only atropine sulfate, 0.6 mg, is given for premedication to prevent vagal reflex from intubation and to decrease salivary and bronchial secretions.

No sedation should be given for premedication to a pickwickian obese patient. Light sedation such as 100 mg of pentobarbital may be given to an obese nonpickwickian patient. We believe that a well-conducted preoperative visit is more important than sedation. It is important to explain to the patient the possibility of postoperative intubation and ventilator support.

Bendixen HH: Morbid obesity. ASA Refresher Courses in Anesthesiology 6:1–14, 1978

C. Intraoperative Management

C.1. How would you monitor the patient?

In addition to the routine monitors of ECG, blood pressure, esophageal stethoscope, and temperature, an arterial line is inserted for frequent assessment of blood gases and for continuous blood pressure tracing. Central venous pressure and hourly urine output are monitored to evaluate fluid balance and cardiac function. A Swan–Ganz catheter is not routinely placed for this kind of patient for surgery unless there is documented left ventricular failure. The advantages of invasive monitoring have to be weighed against the possible complications.

C.2. How would you induce anesthesia? Describe the intubation technique.

Difficult intubation is not uncommon in obese patients because of suprasternal pads of fat, short neck, and poor extension of the head. Awake intubation can be done after adequate sedation with fentanyl, droperidol, or diazepam, and topical use of local anesthetics such as 4% of lidocaine (Xylocaine) or benzocaine (Cetacaine) spray around the mouth and pharynx. After awake intubation, anesthesia may be induced with thiopental sodium. If the patient is not cooperative, a breathing induction with potent inhalation agents such as isoflurane or enflurane may be used with oxygen to keep the patient breathing spontaneously. Oral intubation under direct laryngoscopy may be tried first. If it is difficult to expose the larynx, blind nasal intubation or a fiberoptic bronchoscope may be used for intubation. Nitrous oxide is not added to the circuit before intubation to ensure that there is adequate oxygenation during a difficult intubation. The patient should not be paralyzed when there is difficulty in airway management. Succinylcholine may be used to facilitate intubation if a patent airway can be maintained by mask.

Hamm CW, Koehler LS: The implications of morbid obesity for anesthesia: Report of a series. Anesthesiology Review 6:29–35, 1979

C.3. How would you maintain the anesthesia? What is your choice of agents?

We use isoflurane and N_2O–O_2 (3:2) for maintenance. Almost all anesthetic techniques and agents have been used successfully. We prefer inhalation agents because of easy controllability of the depth of anesthesia, potentiation of muscle relaxants, and the use of high oxygen concentration when needed. Neuroleptic anesthesia may require a large amount of relaxant for adequate surgical exposure and large doses of narcotics to achieve adequate analgesia. Both of these may create postoperative respiratory difficulty. The morbidly obese patient may need a very high F_IO_2 to achieve adequate oxygenation, and a balanced technique usually depends on 50% to 70% N_2O to keep the patient unconscious.

Among the current inhalation agents, isoflurane may be the best choice because of its low biotransformation. Obesity itself increases the biotransformation of methoxyflurane, enflurane, and halothane, resulting in increased serum fluoride ion levels. Methoxyflurane should be avoided in this kind of patient and surgery.

Bently JB, Vaughn RW, Millern MS et al: Serum inorganic fluoride levels in obese patients during and after enflurane anesthesia, p 69. Presented at the 53rd Congress of International Anesthesia Research Society, Hollywood, CA, 1979

Samuelson PN, Merin RG, Tabes DR et al: Toxicity following methoxyflurane anesthesia IV, The role of obesity and effect of low dose anesthesia on fluoride metabolism and renal function. Can Anaesth Soc J 23:465–479, 1976

Young SR, Stoelting RK, Peterson C et al: Anesthesia biotransformation and renal function in obese patients during and after methoxyflurane and halothane anesthesia. Anesthesiology 42:451–457, 1975

C.4. What kind of muscle relaxants would you use?

Nondepolarizing relaxants, such as pancuronium or d-tubocurarine. Pancuronium is preferred when hypotension or bradycardia is present. Curare is preferred when there is hypertension or tachycardia. Succinylcholine, IV drip, should be avoided because of the possibility of dual block from prolonged use of a high dose of succinylcholine. A peripheral nerve stimulator should be used to monitor the extent of relaxation and to avoid overdose of relaxants to correct inadequate surgical exposure.

C.5. Can regional anesthesia be used? What are the advantages and disadvantages of regional anesthesia?

Continuous spinal anesthesia has been reported as an anesthetic approach, and this approach demands that the patient remain on his side during surgery in order to maintain adequate spontaneous ventilation. One disadvantage of regional anesthesia is that it is technically difficult to use with the obese patient, as well as time consuming because of poor landmarks and enormous distances from skin to spinal canal. Another disadvantage is inadequate spontaneous ventilation when an obese patient is in the supine position and has paralyzed abdominal muscles. Psychological stress may be another disadvantage.

In an effort to control respiration during surgery, Hamm and Koehler used continuous thoracic epidural anesthesia combined with light endotracheal general anesthesia. There were several advantages in combining epidural analgesia and light general anesthesia. This technique minimized stress to the cardiovascular system during surgery. It provided stable hemodynamic conditions, with decreased blood pressure and heart rate, decreased left ventricular stroke work, and decreased peripheral vascular resistance and oxygen consumption. It avoided using narcotics and potent inhalation agents. Postoperative emergence was rapid, which permitted early extubation. Epidural analgesia provided postoperative pain relief without respiratory depression. Even though these minor advantages were reported, routine use of the technique was not recommended by the authors of that article. We feel that general anesthesia can be easily and successfully administered, as long as the anesthetics are titrated to the needs of surgery and the patients are carefully monitored.

Gelman S, Laws HL, Potzick J et al: Thoracic epidural *vs* balanced anesthesia in morbid obesity: An intraoperative and postoperative hemodynamic study. Anesth Analg (Cleve) 59:902–908, 1980

Hamm CW, Koehler LS: The implications of morbid obesity for anesthesia: Report of a series. Anesthesiology Review 6:29–35, 1979

C.6. What is the effect of narcotics on Oddi's sphincter?

Morphine may cause spasm of Oddi's sphincter, which may interfere with intraoperative cholangiography. Demerol and fentanyl have minimal effects on the sphincter. Morphine is not a good choice for bilary tract surgery.

Gilman AG, Goodman LS, Gilman A: The Pharmacological Basis of Therapeutics, 6th ed. New York, Macmillan, 1980

C.7. During surgery, arterial blood gases showed pH, 7.35; PaO_2, 57 torr; $PaCO_2$, 52 torr; F_IO_2 0.6; respirator tidal volume, 1000 ml, and rate 15/m. Ten cm H_2O PEEP was added to the circuit and the tidal volume was increased to 1200 ml. Twenty minutes later, the arterial blood gases showed pH, 7.32; PaO_2, 55 torr; $PaCO_2$, 55 torr. What is the explanation for these changes?

Usually, PEEP increases PaO_2, and increasing the tidal volume decreases $PaCO_2$. Occasionally, PEEP and hyperventilation will paradoxically decrease PaO_2 and increase $PaCO_2$, especially in morbidly obese patients, mainly due to excessively high airway pressure, whether from the use of PEEP or because of a high tidal volume. High airway pressure may interrupt pulmonary small vessel blood flow in the uppermost parts of the lungs at peak inspiration. Interrupting the pulmonary blood flow in these ventilated alveoli results in an increase in V_D/V_T and increased $PaCO_2$. Meanwhile, the impeded blood flow will be redistributed to the areas of shunting that are not affected by the high airway pressure, resulting in an increase in Q_S/Q_T. High airway pressure also decreases venous return and cardiac output. This will further decrease PaO_2 and increase $PaCO_2$.

Bendixen HH: Morbid obesity. ASA Refresher Courses in Anesthesiology 6:1–14, 1978

D. Postoperative Management

D.1. When are you going to extubate the patient? What are the criteria for extubation?

Prophylactic ventilatory support throughout the first postoperative night may be indicated for the obese pickwickian patient. However, the obese nonpickwickian patient may be extubated as soon as the following extubation criteria are met:

- The patient is alert and awake.
- Muscle relaxants are adequately reversed.
- There are acceptable blood gases on 40% inspired oxygen: pH, 7.35–7.45; PaO_2, greater than 80 torr; $PaCO_2$, less than 50 torr.
- There are acceptable respiratory mechanics—a maximal inspiratory force of at least 25 to 30 cm H_2O; a vital capacity of more than 10 ml/kg; tidal volume more than 5 ml/kg.
- A stable circulatory status has been reached.

Hedley–Whyte J et al: Applied Physiology of Respiratory Care, pp 136–309. Boston, Little, Brown & Co, 1976

D.2. What are the major early postoperative complications in the morbidly obese patient?

The major morbidity is related to thromboembolism, wound infection, and pulmonary failure. Early ambulation is encouraged.

Isselbacher KJ et al: Harrison's Principles of Internal Medicine, 9th ed, p 416. New York, McGraw–Hill, 1980

D.3. How does position affect respiratory function in obese patients?

In the supine position, intraabdominal contents elevate the diaphragm and functional residual capacity (FRC) is decreased. Reduced FRC is associated with increases in airway closure and volume of trapped gas, resulting in an increase in venous admixture (Q_S/Q_T) and a decrease in PaO_2. Therefore, the patient should be nursed in a sitting or semi-sitting position as soon as the circulatory condition is stable. FRC increases 30% by changing from the supine position to the sitting position, both in normal man and in postlaparotomy patients. FRC decreases about 25% in both the sitting and supine position on the first postoperative day after laparotomy.

Vaughan RW, Bauer S, Wise L: Effect of position of postoperative oxygenation in markedly obese subjects. Anesth Analg (Cleve) 55:37–41, 1976

Paul DR, Hoyt JL, Boutros AR: Cardiovascular and respiratory changes in response to change of posture in the very obese. Anesthesiology 45:73–78, 1976

Tucker DH, Sieker HO: The effect of change in body position on lung volume and intrapulmonary gas mixing in patients with obesity, heart failure and emphysema. Am Rev Respir Dis 82:787–791, 1960

Hsu HO, Hickey RF: Effect of posture on functional residual capacity postoperatively. Anesthesiology 44:520–521, 1976

D.4. How would you prevent postoperative atelectasis?

Early ambulation, chest physical therapy with incentive spirometry, and effective coughing and deep breathing are encouraged to improve respiration. Prolonged recumbency is avoided because of its adverse effects on the ventilation–perfusion ratio. Careful titration of postoperative pain medication should be emphasized to prevent splinting due to pain and hypoventilation from excessive narcotics.

Hedley–Whyte J et al: Applied Physiology of Respiratory Care, pp 301–309. Boston, Little, Brown & Co, 1976

Index

Abdominal aortic aneurysm, 148-158
  arterial disease in, 153t
  intraoperative management of, 156-157
  myocardial infarction and, 149-151, 150t
  postoperative management of, 157-158
  preoperative evaluation and preparation in, 153-156
  surgery in, 155-156
Abdominal decompression, 163, 165-166
Abdominal pain
  differential diagnosis of, 162
  left upper quadrant, 393-394
  negative examination in, 410
  right-sided, 409-410
Acetylcholinesterase, 369
Acid-base balance
  hypovolemic shock and, 396
  pregnancy and, 290
Acid-citrate-dextrose blood, 403-404
Activated coagulation time (ACT) test, 106-107
Acute respiratory failure, 31-50
Adenoidectomy, 431
Adrenal cortex, 237, 254-255, 255t
Adrenal gland, 236-237
Adrenal medulla, 237
Adrenalectomy, 256
Adrenergic antagonists, alpha and beta, 384
Adrenergic receptors
  alpha-1 and alpha-2, 383-384
  beta-1 and beta-2, 383, 384f
Adrenocortical tumor, 253-259
  intraoperative management of, 258-259
  postoperative complications in, 259
  preoperative evaluation and preparation in, 256-258
Adrenogenital syndrome, 255
Adult respiratory distress syndrome, 55
  manifestations and management of, 397-398
  oxygen therapy in, 35-37
Air embolism, 193-194, 211
Airway
  newborn, 183, 184t
  postoperative, cleft palate and, 433
Airway obstruction
  dyspnea and tachypnea in, 52
  thyrotoxicosis and, 231-232
  work of breathing and, 58-59
Allen test, 98
Amides, 216-217
Aminophylline, 16
Amniotic creatinine content, 293
Androgens, 255
Aneurysm, abdominal aortic, 148-158

Antibiotics
  prolonged neuromuscular blockade and, 283
  tracheoesophageal fistula and, 67
Anticoagulants, 106-107
Antithyroid resistant patient, "stealing" of, 230
Aortic aneurysm, abdominal, 148-158
Aortic clamping, 157
Aortic regurgitation, 131
Aortic valve measurement, 132
Apgar scoring system, 298t, 298-299
Apnea
  bronchoscopy and, 25
  postoperative, 372
    kidney transplant and, 282
  prolonged, 368-372, 371t
Arm, sympathetic nerve supply to, 215
Arrhythmias in hypothermia, 85
Arterial blood gases
  adult respiratory distress syndrome and, 35-37
  asthma and, 10
  cardiopulmonary bypass and, 115-116
  fetal, 323
  interpretation of, 9
  morbid obesity and, 446, 446t, 450
  surgical morbidity and mortality and, 22
Arterial circle of Willis, 202-203, 203f
Arterial CO_2 pressure ($PaCO_2$)
  hypothermia and, 389
  morbid obesity and, 444
Arterial O_2 pressure (PaO_2)
  morbid obesity and, 444
  normal, 9
Artery cannulation, 400
ASA physical status, 381
Aspiration, gastric
  bronchoscopy in, 327
  during intubation, 326-327
  intestinal obstruction and, 169
  mechanical ventilation in, 327-328
  signs and symptoms of, 54-55
Aspiration pneumonitis, 31-50
  bronchial irrigation in, 35
  continuous positive pressure ventilation in, 41-45
  management of, 33-35
  mechanical ventilation in, 37-41
  oxygen therapy in, 35-37
  prophylactic antibiotics in, 34
  steroid therapy in, 34-35
  weaning from ventilatory support in, 45-48
Aspirin and abnormal bleeding, 343

Asthma, 3-18
  cardiac, 5
  allergic vs idiosyncratic, 9-10
  arterial blood gases in, 10
  attacks of, 10
  differential diagnosis of, 5
  etiology of, 9-10
  inhalation vs intravenous anesthesia in, 14-15
  intraoperative management of, 13-17
  muscle relaxants in, 15
  postoperative management of, 18
  preoperative evaluation and preparation in, 11-12
  regional vs general anesthesia in, 15
  wheezing attack during surgery in, 15-17
Atelectasis
  pneumothorax vs, 53-54
  postoperative, 29-30, 452
Atropine
  asthma and, 12, 13
  bronchoscopy and, 23
  tracheoesophageal fistula and, 67-68
Autoregulation, 204
  cerebral blood flow, 435-436

Barbiturates and intracranial pressure, 197-198
Basedow's disease, 227
Bladder perforation, 270
Bleeding tonsil, 434-440
Blood
  normal values for, 447
  P 50 value of, 404
  stored, factors V and VIII in, 405
Blood coagulopathy, 339, 340t
Blood embolus, 53
Blood flow, obstructed, 201
Blood pH, 447
Blood pressure
  mean arterial, 382
  pediatric, 437
Blood sugar levels in cardiopulmonary bypass, 119
Blood transfusion
  acid-citrate-dextrose blood in, 403-404
  hemolytic reaction to, 405
  kidney transplant and, 275
  massive, alkalizing agent in, 404
  uncrossmatched blood in, 402
Blood volume, pediatric, 348, 436
Body temperature of burn patient, 387-389, 388t
Bohr equation (V_D/V_T), 8-9, 58, 444
Bowel distension, 163
Bradycardia
  ECG rhythm in, 138
  hypertension and, 236

Brain tumor, 189-199
  hypertonic solutions in, 195-196
  hyperventilation in, 194-195
  increasing room within head for surgery in, 194-197
  intracranial pressure and, 191
  intraoperative fluid restriction in, 196
  intraoperative management in, 193-198
  preoperative evaluation and preparation in, 192
  spinal fluid drainage in, 196
Breathing in airway obstruction, 58-59
Breech presentation, 319-328
  etiology of, 321
  incidence of, 320
  intraoperative management of, 324-328
  maternal morbidity and, 321
  perinatal morbidity and, 321-322
  postoperative management of, 328
  preoperative evaluation and preparation in, 322-324
  types of, 320-321
Bronchial irrigation, 35
Bronchodilation, 14
Bronchogenic carcinoma
  diagnosis of, 21
  metabolic manifestations of, 21
  types of, 20-21
Bronchoscopy, 19-30
  aspiration and, 327
  fiberoptic, 24-25
  intraoperative management of, 23-29
  preoperative evaluation and preparation in, 22-23
  types of, 24
BUN, 278
Burn, 373-391
  body temperature and, 387-389, 388t
  cholinesterase activity in, 390
  classification of, 374-375
  extent of, 375-376t
  intraoperative management of, 386-390
  major
    fluid formula in, 378-379
    pathophysiology of, 375-377
    resuscitation in, 378
    survival with, 377, 377f
  d-tubocurarine in, 390
  preoperative evaluation and preparation in, 381-386
  succinylcholine in, 389

Caffeine-contracture test, 362-363
Cannulation of arteries, 400
Carcinoma, bronchogenic, 20-21
Cardiac asthma, 5
Cardiac effects of thyrotoxicosis, 227-228

Cardiac index, 383
Cardioplegic solution, 117
Cardiopulmonary bypass, 106-120
  anesthesia in, 114
  anticoagulants in, 106-107
  arterial blood gases in, 115-116
  blood sugar levels in, 119
  defibrillation in, 119
  gas flow in, 115
  hypotension and hypertension in, 110-111
  hypothermia in, 113-114
  low heart rate in, 119
  low $PaCO_2$ in, 115
  monitoring in, 109-110
  muscle relaxants in, 114
  myocardium in, 117
  oxygenators for, 107-108
  perfusion in, 115
  platelet and coagulation factors in, 120
  priming solutions in, 108-109
  protamine in, 120-121
  pump flow during, 112-113
  pumps in, 109
  rewarming patient on, 118-119
  total vs partial, 107
  urine color after, 118
Cardiovascular system, 73-158
  end-stage renal disease and, 276-277
  hypovolemic shock and, 395
  lidocaine and, 220t
  morbid obesity and, 445
  toxic anesthetic reactions and, 315-316
Carotid endarterectomy, 200-207
  anesthesia in, 198
  intraoperative management of, 205-206
  postoperative management of, 206-207
  preoperative evaluation and preparation in, 203-205
Caudal epidural analgesia, 313
Causalgia, neuralgia vs, 214t
Central nervous system
  regional anesthesia and, 219-220
  toxic anesthetic reactions and, 315-316
Cerebral blood flow
  autoregulation of, 435-436
  cerebral artery clamping and, 206
  determinants of, 191, 204
  hypoxic vs normal, 435
  intracranial disease and, 192
  low, 203
  normal, 203
Cerebral steal syndrome, 192
Cesarean section
  emergency, 295
    anesthetic technique in, 324
    general anesthesia in, 297, 325-326
    intravenous agents in, 324-325
    premedication in, 324
  intravenous agents in, 296
  spinal vs epidural anesthesia in, 324

Cheiloplasty, 428-430
Chest wall compliance, 8
Child
  blood pressure in, 437
  blood volume in, 348, 436
  cerebral blood flow in, 435
  cleft palate in, 425
  endotracheal tubes for, 28, 184, 345
  fluid therapy in, 347
  larynx of, 345-346
  rule of nines and, 375
Cholinesterase, serum, 369-370, 371t
  burn patients and, 390
Chronic obstructive pulmonary disease (COPD), 3-18
  perioperative, 151-153, 152t
  preoperative preparations in, 11
  pulmonary function tests in, 155t
Chvostek's sign, 233
Cigarette smoking, 21
Circulation in pregnancy, 289-290
Cirrhosis, 172
Citrate intoxication, 406
Cleft lip, 423-433. *See also* Cleft palate
Cleft palate, 422-433
  definition of, 423
  etiology of, 424
  incidence of, 424
  intraoperative management of, 428-432
  pathophysiology of, 425
  postoperative airway protection in, 433
  postoperative management of, 432-433
  preoperative evaluation and preparation in, 427-428
  surgical procedures for, 426-427
Closed chest cardiac massage, newborn, 299
Closing capacity (CC), 7
Closing volume (CV), 7, 8
Coagulation factors in cardiopulmonary bypass, 120
Coagulation factor deficiency disorders, 340t
Colloid therapy, 402
Congenital heart disease, 75-87
Congestive atelectasis, 36
Conn's syndrome, 255
Continuous positive airway pressure (CPAP), 42
Continuous positive pressure ventilation (CPPV), 42-43
  aspiration pneumonitis and, 41-45
  complications with, 45
Convulsions, eclamptic, 307
Coronary arteries, 91, 92f
Coronary artery bypass graft, 88-124
  anesthesia induction in, 100-101
  anesthesia maintenance in, 101
  cardiopulmonary bypass in, 106-120
  digoxin and propranolol in, 94-95
  esophageal and rectal temperatures in, 98
  hypertension and hypotension in, 104

458 · Index

Coronary artery bypass graft (*continued*)
  indications for, 91-92
  inhalational vs intravenous agent in, 101-102
  intraoperative hypotension in, 94-95
  intraoperative management of, 97-122
  intraoperative propranolol in, 105
  monitoring before cardiopulmonary bypass in, 97
  muscle relaxant in, 103
  perioperative myocardial infarction in, 151
  postoperative management of, 122-124
  premedication in, 97
  preoperative evaluation and preparation in, 94-97
  preoperative tests in, 95-96
  respirator weaning in, 123-124
  ST segment depression in, 103-104
Corticosteroids, 255t
Craniotomy, 189-199
  hypotension in, 196-197
  postoperative management of, 198-199
Creatinine, serum, 278
Creatinine clearance, 154, 278
Creatinine-phosphokinase level, 362
Croup, postextubation, 186
Cry, hoarse, 440
Cryoprecipitate, 343
Cushing's syndrome, 254
Cyclopropane, 14

Da Nang lung, 36
Dead space ventilation to tidal volume (V_D/V_T) ratio, 8-9, 58, 444
Dextran, 399
Dehydration, newborn, 181t
Delirium, emergence, 349
Delivery, analgesia in, 317
Dexamethasone, 35
Dexamethasone suppression test, 257
Diabetes, 244-252
  classification of, 246
  complications of, 246
  etiology of, 245
  incidence of, 245
  insulin requirement in, 247
  intraoperative insulin in, 251
  intraoperative management of, 250-252
  monitoring control of, 247
  postoperative management of, 252
  preoperative evaluation and preparation in, 249-250
  treatment of, 246-247, 246f
Diabetic ketoacidosis, 248-249
Dibucaine number, 370
Diffusion hypoxia, 390-391
Digitalis, 266
Digoxin, 94

Diphenhydramine, 12
Diuretics, 407
Dopamine, 237-238
Droperidol, 12
Dyspnea, 52-53

Eclampsia
  etiology and incidence of, 304
  management of, 311
Edema
  laryngeal, 348-349
  postoperative, with spinal cord tumor, 212
Edrophonium, 420
Electrocardiogram monitoring, 100
Electrocautery
  muscle twitching during, 25-26
  pacemaker function and, 146-147
Electrolyte imbalance
  prolonged neuromuscular blockade and, 283-284
  renal disease and, 275-276
Embolism
  air, 193-194, 211
  blood, 53
  fat, 51-61
Embryology
  adrenal gland, 236-237
  of tracheoesophageal fistula, 65
  of transposition of great arteries, 77-78
Emergence delirium, 349
Endocrine system, 221-259
  pregnancy and, 291
Endotracheal intubation
  complications from, 40
  esophageal varices and, 174
  facial burns and, 387
  fat embolism and, 61
  morbid obesity and, 448
  thyrotoxicosis and, 231
  tracheoesophageal fistula and, 68-69
  transurethral resection of prostate and, 267-268
  vomiting and aspiration during, 326-327
Endotracheal tube size, pediatric, 28, 184, 345
Enflurane
  cardiovascular effects of, 102
  chemical structure of, 347f
  intracranial pressure and, 197
  metabolism of, 346-347
Epidural anesthesia, 312-314
  cesarean section and, 324
  toxic effects of, 315-316
Epidural blood patch, 318
Epinephrine
  biochemistry of, 237-238
  cleft palate surgery and, 428-429
  epidural anesthesia and, 313-314
  regional anesthetics and, 218

Erythrohepatic protoporphyria, 410-411
Erythropoietic porphyria, 410
Esophageal intubation, 167-168
Esophageal and rectal temperatures, 98
Esophageal varices, 171-175
Esters, 216-217
Eupnea, 52
Euthyroid patient, 229
Expiratory positive airway pressure (EPAP), 43
Expiratory reserve volume (ERV), 6
Extracorporeal membrane oxygenation (ECMO), 48-49
Extubation in morbid obesity, 451

Factor V, 405
Factor VIII
 blood storage and, 405
 units of, 342-343
Fat embolism, 51-61
 blood embolus vs, 53
 diagnosis of, 55-56
 treatment of, 56
Femur, fracture of, 51-61
Fentanyl
 cardiovascular effects of, 102
 intracranial pressure and, 198
Fetal blood gases, 323
Fetal heart rate
 baseline, 322
 beat-to-beat variability of, 322
 deceleration of, 322-323
Fetal nonstress test, 310-311
Fetus
 accurate assessment of, 292-293
 maturity of, 293
 muscle relaxants and, 297-298
 toxemia and, 306
Fick equation, 292
Fistula, tracheoesophageal, 62-72
Floppy valve syndrome, 127
Fluid replacement
 newborn, 180-181, 181t
 pediatric, 347
Fluoride, inorganic, 280-281
Forced expiratory volume, 10-11
Forced expiratory volume at 1 sec (FEV_1), 5-6
Forced vital capacity, 10-11
Fracture, femur, 51-61
Functional residual capacity (FRC), 6-8

Gallamine
 fetus and, 297-298
 renal failure and, 281

Gastrointestinal system, 159-186
 pregnancy and, 290
Gastrostomy, 67
General anesthesia
 asthma and, 15
 emergency cesarean and, 297, 325-326
 femur fracture and, 60
 malignant hyperthermia and, 364
 pacemaker insertion and, 144-145
 porphyria and, 415
Genitourinary system, 261-328
Glucocorticoids, 238, 254
Glucose metabolism, 250
Gram negative sepsis, 169-170
Graves' disease, 224, 226, 227

Halothane
 alveolar concentrations of, 416-418, 417f
 bronchodilation and, 14
 cardiovascular effects of, 102
 chemical structure of, 347f
 cleft palate surgery and, 428-429
 intracranial pressure and, 197
 metabolism of, 346-347
 uterine contractility and, 326
Heart block, 138-139, 140
Heart disease, ischemic, 88-124
Heart rate, fetal, 322-323
Heat intolerance, 228
Hematologic system, 329-349
Hemiblock, 140
Hemodialysis, chronic, 277
Hemodilution, 109
Hemoglobin levels in renal disease, 274
Hemolysis, intravascular, 405
Hemolytic transfusion reaction, 405
Hemophilia, 338-349
 aspirin and, 343
 differential diagnosis of, 342t
 induction techniques in, 346
 intraoperative management in, 344-348
 pediatric anesthetic equipment in, 344-345
 postoperative management in, 348-349
 preoperative evaluation and preparation in, 342-344
 types of, 340
Hemophilia A
 incidence and pathology of, 340-341
 preoperative preparation in, 342
Hemorrhage and replacement therapy, 437
Hemorrhagic diathesis, 344
Hemorrhagic shock. See Hypovolemic shock
Henderson-Hasselbalch equation, 447
Heparin
 cardiopulmonary bypass and, 106-107
 mechanism of action of, 205-206
 reversal of, 120
Hepatic porphyria, 410

Hespan, 399
Hetastarch, 399
Heterozygote, 332
High frequency positive pressure ventilation (HFPPV), 49
  bronchoscopy and, 25
  thoracotomy and, 28-29
Hoarse cry, 440
Horner's syndrome, 216
Hydrocortisone acetate, 12
Hydrocortisone phosphate, 12
Hyperaldosteronism, 255, 256
Hyperkalemia, 276
Hypertension
  bradycardia and, 236
  cardiopulmonary bypass and, 110-111
  causes of, 235-236
  coronary artery bypass graft and, 104
  definition of, 235
  maternal, 303-304
  perioperative, 151
  spinal cord tumor and, 211-212
  tachycardia in, 236
Hyperthermia, malignant, 358-367
Hyperthyroidism
  heat intolerance in, 228
  propranolol in, 229
  surgery in, 229-230
  treatment of, 228-229
Hypertonic solutions, 195-196
Hyperventilation
  brain tumor and, 194-195
  disadvantages of, 40
  maternal, 298
Hypoglycemic shock, 251-252
Hyponatremia
  dilutional, 269
  postoperative, 271
  treatment of, 269
Hypotension
  cardiogenic, 95
  cardiopulmonary bypass and, 110-111
  coronary artery bypass graft and, 104
  craniotomy and, 196-197
  maternal, 292
  PEEP and, 45
  protamine and, 121
  supine, pregnancy and, 294-295
  transurethral resection of prostate and, 270
Hypothermia
  arrhythmias in, 85
  cardiopulmonary bypass and, 113-114
  complications of, 86-87
  establishment of, 82
  metabolism and, 387-388
  oxygen dissociation curve and, 388
  $PaCO_2$ in, 389
  physiology of, 387, 388t
  physiology and pathology of, 84-85
  profound, 75-87, 83

prolonged neuromuscular blockade and, 284
  surface and core cooling in, 83-84
Hypoventilation, 17
Hypovolemic hypotension, 436
Hypovolemic shock
  blood loss volume in, 396
  colloid therapy in, 402
  pathophysiology of, 395-396
  resuscitative management of, 294
  signs and symptoms of, 395
  volume-expansion therapy in, 398-399
Hypoxemia, 9
Hypoxia, diffusion, 390-391
Hysteresis rate, 142

Infant
  breech, perinatal morbidity of, 321-322
  newborn
    airway of, 183, 184t
    Apgar score of 6 in, 328
    cleft palate in, 425
    closed chest cardiac massage in, 299
    dehydration in, 181t
    fluid replacement in, 180-181, 181t
    lungs of, 300
    maternal toxemia and, 317
    respiratory stimulation in, 300
    resuscitation of, 299
    thermoregulation in, 300
    thiopental sodium and, 296-297, 325
Inferior vena cava clamping, 175
Inhalation anesthesia
  asthma and, 14-15
  concentration effect of, 418
  coronary artery bypass graft and, 101-102
  halogenated, metabolism of, 280-281
  kidney transplant and, 280
  porphyria and, 416
  uterine contractility and, 326
Inspiratory capacity (IC), 6
Inspiratory positive airway pressure (IPAP), 43
Inspiratory reserve volume (IRV), 6
Insulin
  effect of anesthesia and surgery on, 250
  intraoperative, 251
  requirement of, 247
Intermittent assisted ventilation (IAV), 47
Intermittent demand ventilation (IDV), 47
Intermittent mandatory ventilation (IMV), 47
Intermittent positive pressure ventilation (IPPV), 43
  cardiovascular system and, 39-40
  lobectomy or pneumonectomy and, 29-30
Intestinal obstruction, 161-170

causes of, 162
diagnosis of, 162-163
esophageal intubation in, 167-168
fluid volume replacement in, 166
gastric aspiration and, 169
hemodynamic changes in, 164
intraoperative management of, 167-168
postoperative hypoventilation in, 168-169
postoperative management of, 168-170
premedication in, 166
preoperative evaluation and preparation in, 165-167
respiratory implications of, 165
small bowel, fluid shifts in, 164
small vs large bowel in, 162-163
Intraaortic balloon pump, 121-122, 134
Intracerebral steal, 202
Intracranial pressure
 anesthetic agents and, 197-198
 brain tumor and, 191
 determinants of, 190-191
Intraperitoneal injury, 394
Intravascular hemolysis, 405
Intravenous anesthesia
 asthma and, 14-15
 cesarean section and, 296, 324-325
 coronary artery bypass graft and, 101-102
 kidney transplant and, 280
Inverse steal, 202
Iodides, 228-229
Ischemic heart disease, 88-124
Isoflurane
 cardiovascular effects of, 102
 chemical structure of, 347f
 intracranial pressure and, 197
 metabolism of, 346-347
Isoproterenol, 16-17

Ketamine
 cesarean section and, 325
 cleft palate surgery and, 429
 intracranial pressure and, 198
Ketoacidosis, diabetic, 248-249
Kidney transplant, 272-285
 inhalation vs intravenous agents in, 280
 intraoperative management of, 279-284
 muscle relaxants in, 281
 neostigmine and, 282-283
 postoperative management of, 284-285
 postsurgical apnea in, 282
 preoperative evaluation and preparation in, 277-278
 preoperative transfusion in, 275
 regional anesthesia in, 281
 steroids in, 277
 succinylcholine in, 279

Labor
 analgesia in, 317
 caudal epidural analgesia in, 313
Laryngeal edema, 348-349
Laryngospasm, postoperative, 348
Larynx
 child's vs adult's, 345-346
 newborn, 184t
Lateral decubitus position, 26
Lecithin: sphingomyelin ratio, 293
Left ventricular stroke work index, 385
Lidocaine, 220t
Lip, cleft, 423-433
Lobectomy
 one-lung anesthesia in, 27
 patient evaluation in, 22-23
 postoperative management of, 29-30
Local anesthesia. See Regional anesthesia
Long-acting thyroid stimulator (LATS), 227
Lumbar epidural anesthesia, 312-313
Lung, newborn, 300
Lung compliance, 8
Luxury perfusion, 202

MAC (minimum alveolar concentration), 418-419
Magnesium
 antidote to, 310
 dosage and therapeutic levels of, 309
 effects of, 308
 muscle relaxants and, 310
 side effects and toxic effects of, 309
Malignant hyperthermia, 358-367
 clinical features of, 360
 clinical type and incidence of, 361
 crisis, 365-366
 etiopathology of, 362
 general anesthesia and, 364
 inheritance of, 361-362
 intraoperative management of, 364-366
 laboratory findings in, 361, 361t, 362
 postoperative management after, 366-367
 preoperative evaluation and preparation and, 363-364
 susceptibility to, 359, 360t
Mandibulofacial dysostosis, 426
Mannitol, 196
Maximal mid-expiratory flow rate (MMEFR), 5-6
Mechanical ventilation
 aspiration and, 327-328
 aspiration pneumonitis and, 37-41
 complications of, 40
 criteria for, 37-38
 intermittent mandatory, 47
 pressure-cycled vs volume-cycled, 38
 sigh volume on, 39

Mechanical ventilation (*continued*)
　T-piece adaptor for, 46-47
　valvular heart disease and, 135-136
　weaning from, 45-48, 123-124
Mendelson's syndrome, 33-34, 54, 328
Meningiomas, 194
Metabolic acidosis, 276
Metabolic alkalosis, 178, 181
Methimazole, 228
Methohexital, 13
Methoxyflurane, 14
Mineralocorticoids, 238, 255
Minimum alveolar concentration (MAC), 418-419
Mitral insufficiency, 127
Mitral regurgitation
　acute vs chronic, 129
　complications of, 127-128
　ECG findings in, 131
　myocardial oxygen consumption in, 131
　nitroprusside and nitroglycerine in, 133-134
Mitral valve, 132
Monro-Kellie hypothesis, 191
Morbid obesity, 441-452
　arterial blood gases in, 446, 446t, 450
　cardiovascular system in, 445
　extubation in, 451
　intraoperative management in, 448-450
　intubation in, 448
　metabolic problems in, 443
　muscle relaxants in, 449
　PaO_2 and $PaCO_2$ in, 444
　position and respiratory function in, 451
　postoperative atelectasis in, 452
　postoperative management of, 451-452
　preoperative evaluation and preparation in, 445-448
　Q_S/Q_T and V_D/V_T in, 444
　regional anesthesia and, 449-450
　respiratory function in, 443-444
　spirometry screening test in, 447
Morphine
　asthma and, 18
　cardiovascular effects of, 102
　intracranial pressure and, 198
Murmur, 128
Muscle contraction, 355-356
Muscle relaxants
　asthma and, 15
　cardiopulmonary bypass and, 114
　coronary artery bypass graft and, 103
　fetus and, 297-298
　kidney transplant and, 281
　magnesium and, 310
　morbid obesity and, 449
　nondepolarizing, 419-420
　porphyria and, 419
　recovery from, 421
　valvular heart disease and, 134
Muscle twitching, 25-26
Musculoskeletal disorders, 360t

Mustard procedure, 78-79
Myasthenia gravis, 353-357
　diagnosis of, 354
　intraoperative management of, 356
　muscle contraction in, 355-356
　neuromuscular transmission in, 355
　postoperative management of, 357
　premedication in, 356
Myocardial infarction
　abdominal aortic aneurysm and, 149-151, 150t
　intraoperative, 270-271
　perioperative, 149-150, 150t
　postoperative, 93-94, 271
Myocardial ischemia, 100
Myocardial oxygen consumption
　determinants of, 96
　mitral vs aortic regurgitation and, 131
Myocardial oxygen supply, 97
Myocardium in cardiopulmonary bypass, 117

Narcotics
　asthma and, 18
　intracranial pressure and, 198
　Oddi's sphincter and, 450
Neostigmine, 282-283, 420
Nephrotoxicity of inorganic fluoride, 280-281
Nervous system, 187-220
Neuralgia, 214t
Neuromuscular blockade, prolonged, 283-284
Neuromuscular transmission, 354-355
New York Heart Assoc Classification of heart disease, 128-129
Nifedipine, 95
Nitroglycerine
　IV infusion of, 111-112
　mitral regurgitation and, 133-134
Nitroprusside
　IV infusion of, 111-112
　mitral regurgitation and, 133-134
　pheochromocytoma and, 241-242
Nitrous oxide
　alveolar concentrations of, 416-418, 417f
　cardiovascular effects of, 102-103
　intracranial pressure and, 197
Nonrebreathing systems, 185
Norepinephrine, 237-238
Normothermia, 387

Obesity, morbid, 441-452
Obstructive lung disease, 5-6, 6t
Oddi's sphincter, 450
Oliguria
　prerenal, renal, and postrenal, 278
　recovery room, 406-407
One-lung anesthesia, 27-28

Overweight, 442
Oxygenation
　apneic, 284
　functional residual capacity and, 7-8
Oxygenators, cardiopulmonary, 107-108
Oxygen availability, 386
Oxygen consumption, 386
Oxygen content, 386
Oxygen dissociation curve, 388
Oxygen extraction ratio, 386
Oxygen therapy
　adult respiratory distress syndrome and, 35-37
　postoperative, asthma and, 18
Oxygen toxicity, 41-42
Oxytocin challenge test, 310

P 50, 388, 404
Pacemaker, 137-147
　atrial pacing in, 141-142
　AV sequential, 142
　electrocautery use with, 146-147
　environmental electromagnetic interference with, 146
　external, setting of, 142-143
　failure of, 146
　implanted demand, 144
　inhibition of, 147
　intraoperative management of, 144-145
　pacing threshold, sensing R-wave and resistance of, 142-143
　permanent
　　indications for, 139-140
　　specifications of, 142
　postoperative management of, 146-147
　preoperative evaluation in, 144
　types of, 141
Pacing threshold, 142-143
$PaCO_2$ (arterial CO_2 pressure)
　hypothermia and, 389
　morbid obesity and, 444
Palate, cleft, 422-433
Palatoplasty, 428-430
Pancuronium
　fetus and, 297
　renal failure and, 281
PaO_2 (arterial O_2 pressure)
　morbid obesity and, 444
　normal, 9
Parenchymal lung disease, 52
Parkland formula, 378-379
Pco_2, cerebral, 203-204
Pentobarbital, 23
Petechial hemorrhage, 53, 55
pH
　blood, 447
　regional anesthesia and, 218
　temperature correction factor for, 389

Pharyngeal flap operation, 431-432
Phentolamine
　IV infusion of, 111-112
　pheochromocytoma and, 241-242
Pheochromocytoma, 234-243
　intraoperative management of, 240-242
　phentolamine, propranolol, or nitroprusside in, 241-242
　postoperative hypotension in, 242-243
　postoperative management of, 242-243
　preoperative evaluation and preparation in, 239-240
　sites for, 238
　symptoms and diagnosis of, 238-239
Physical status, ASA, 381
Physiological dead space, 58
Physostigmine, 349
Pickwickian syndrome, 443
Pierre Robin syndrome, 425-426
Pituitary and thyroid function, 225-226
Placenta
　assessing function of, 293
　drug diffusion across, 292
Placenta praevia, 286-301
　definition, classification, incidence of, 288
　diagnosis of, 288-289
　emergency cesarean section in, 295
　etiology of, 289
　intraoperative management of, 296-301
　postoperative management of, 301
　preoperative evaluation and preparation in, 294-295
　shock in, 294
Placental barrier, 291
Platelets
　ACD stored blood and, 404
　cardiopulmonary bypass and, 120
　function of, 343
　renal disease and, 275
Pneumonectomy
　patient evaluation in, 22-23
　postoperative management of, 29-30
Pneumonia, atypical, 20
Pneumonitis, aspiration, 31-50
Pneumothorax
　atelectasis vs, 53-54
　tension, 401
Po_2, cerebral, 203-204
Porphyria, 408-421
　acute intermittent, 411-414
　　clinical manifestations of, 411-412
　　prognosis in, 414
　　treatment of, 413-414
　　triggering factors in, 412-413
　classification of, 410-411
　hereditary hepatic
　　laboratory findings in, 413
　　safe anesthetic agents in, 415-416
　inhalation agents in, 416
　intraoperative management in, 415-420
　metabolic defect in, 411

Porphyria (*continued*)
  muscle relaxants in, 419
  nervous system changes in, 411
  postoperative management of, 420-421
  preoperative evaluation and preparation in, 414
Portacaval anastomosis, 175
Portal pressure, 172
Positive end-expiratory pressure (PEEP), 42-45
  arterial oxygenation and, 43
  best or optimal, 44
  cardiovascular effects of, 44-45
  differential or selective, 48
  hypotension with, 45
  monitoring, 44
  ranges of, 43-44
Posterior cranial fossa pathology, 192
Posterior cranial fossa procedure, 199
Post-traumatic pulmonary insufficiency, 36
Preeclampsia
  etiology and incidence of, 304
  mild, management of, 307
  mild or severe, anesthesia in, 311-312
  severe, management of, 307-308
Pregnancy
  hypertension in, 303-304
  hypotension in, 292
  physiologic changes in, 289-291
  supine hypotension during, 294-295
Prerenal failure, 278t
Propranolol
  coronary artery bypass graft and, 94-95, 105
  hyperthyroidism and, 229
  pheochromocytoma and, 241-242
Propylthiouracil, 228
Prostate
  benign hyperplasia of, 264
  transurethral resection of, 263-271
    cardiac disease and, 264-265
    endotracheal intubation and, 267-268
    hypotension in, 270
    intraoperative fluids in, 268-269
    intraoperative management of, 267-271
    patient position for surgery in, 268
    postoperative management of, 271
    preoperative evaluation and preparation in, 266
    renal status of patient and, 266
Protamine, 120-121, 205-206
Pulmonary artery pressure
  coronary artery bypass graft and, 99
  surgical morbidity and mortality and, 22
Pulmonary capillary oxygen tension, 9
Pulmonary capillary wedge pressures, 105, 385
  increased, 105
  normal, 99
Pulmonary edema, 130-131
Pulmonary function tests, 154, 155t
Pulmonary infiltrate, 19-30

Pulmonary shunt, 57
Pulmonary system in hypovolemic shock, 395-396
Pulmonary vascular resistance, 385
Push back operation, 431-432
Pyloric stenosis, 176-186
  differential diagnosis of, 177
  intraoperative management of, 183-185
  metabolic findings in, 177-178, 178t
  postoperative management in, 185-186
  preoperative evaluation and preparation in, 182
  treatment of, 178-180
Pyridostigmine, 420-421

Q_S/Q_T (shunt equation), 57
  equation and normal values for, 8-9
  morbid obesity and, 444

Raskind balloon septostomy, 77
Rate pressure product, 96-97
Regional anesthesia
  asthma and, 15
  binding site of, 315
  epidural, 313-316
  epinephrine and, 218
  esters and amides for, 216-217
  femur fracture and, 60
  increased concentration of, 218
  kidney transplant and, 281
  malignant hyperthermia and, 365
  mechanism of action of, 314-315
  mixtures of, 218-219
  morbid obesity and, 449-450
  pacemaker insertion and, 144-145
  pH effects on, 218
  physicochemical properties of, 217, 217t
  porphyria and, 415
  systemic toxicity of, 219-220
Rectal and esophageal temperatures, 98
Reflex sympathetic dystrophy, 213-220
Reinfarction, perioperative, 92-93, 149-150, 150t
Renal blood flow, 407
Renal disease
  acute, diuretics in, 407
  chronic, etiology of, 273
  electrolyte imbalance in, 275-276
  end-stage, 274, 276-277
  hemoglobin level in, 274
  hyperkalemia in, 276
  metabolic acidosis correction in, 276
  platelet dysfunction and, 275
  prerenal vs, 278t

Renal function in pregnancy, 290-291
Renin-angiotensin-aldosterone system, 348
Residual volume (RV), 6
Respiratory failure, acute, 31-50
Respiratory function
  morbid obesity and, 443-444
  pregnancy and, 289
Respiratory system, 1-72
Restrictive lung disease, 5-6, 6t
Retroperitoneal injury, 394
Right-to-left shunt, 57
Right ventricular stroke work index, 385
Robin Hood syndrome, 202
Rule of nines, 375

Scopolamine, 349
Sellick's maneuver, 167-168
Sensing R-wave, 142-143
Sepsis, gram negative, 169-170
Septic shock, 379-381
  pathophysiology of, 380-381
  presurgical therapy in, 382-383
Shock
  classification of, 379, 394
  definition of, 379, 394
  hypoglycemia, 251-252
  hypovolemic hypotension vs, 436
  placenta praevia and, 294
Shock lung, 36
Shock syndrome, 379-380
Shunt equation, (Q_S/Q_T), 8-9, 57, 444
Sickle cell crisis, 333, 337
Sickle cell disease, 331-337
  clinical features of, 333
  intraoperative management of, 335-336
  postoperative management of, 336-337
  preoperative evaluation and preparation in, 333-334
  preoperative exchange transfusion in, 334
Sickle cell trait, 332
Sick sinus syndrome, 140
Sigh volume, 39
Smoke inhalation burn, 377-378
Spinal anesthesia for cesarean section, 324
Spinal cord tumor, 208-212
  hypertension and, 211-212
  postoperative edema and, 212
Spinal fluid drainage, brain tumor and, 196
Spinal puncture, inadvertent, 317-318
Spirometry screening test
  morbid obesity and, 447
  surgical morbidity and mortality and, 22
Stellate ganglion block, 215-216, 219
Stellate ganglion location, 215
Steroids
  aspiration pneumonitis and, 34-35
  asthma and, 11-12
  kidney transplant and, 277

Stridor, postoperative, 440
Stroke index, 385
ST segment depression, 103-104
Succinylcholine, 370
  burns and, 389
  fetus and, 297
  intracranial pressure and, 198
  kidney transplant and, 279
Swan-Ganz catheterization, 98, 99-100
Sympathetic nerve supply to arm, 215
Synchronized intermittent mandatory ventilation (SIMV), 47
Systemic vascular resistance, 385

Tachycardia
  blood loss and, 437
  hypertension and, 236
  sinus, differential diagnosis of, 406
Tachypnea
  blood loss and, 437
  definition and causes of, 52-53
Temperatures, esophageal and rectal, 98
Tension pneumothorax, 401
Tetany, 233
Thermoregulation, newborn, 300
Thiopental
  asthma and, 13
  intracranial pressure and, 197
  neonatal depression and, 296-297, 325
Thoracotomy, 19-30
  anesthesia in, 25
  HFPPV for, 28-29
  intraoperative management of, 23-29
  lateral decubitus position in, 26
  preoperative evaluation and preparation in, 22-23
  respiratory control in, 26-27
Thrombocytopenia, 342t
Thymectomy, 356-357
Thyroid
  hormones of, 224-225
  pituitary effects on, 225-226
Thyroid stimulating hormone (TSH), 225-226
Thyroid storm, 232
Thyrotoxic crisis, 232
Thyrotoxicosis, 223-233
  differential diagnosis of, 224
  endotracheal intubation in, 231
  heart and, 227-228
  intraoperative management of, 230-231
  postoperative management of, 231-233
  postsurgical airway obstruction in, 231-232
  preoperative evaluation and preparation in, 228-230
Thyroxine (T_4), 224-225
Tidal volume (V_T), 6

Tonsil, bleeding, 434-440
　cerebral hypoxia in, 435
　intraoperative management of, 438-439
　postoperative management of, 440
　preoperative evaluation and preparation in, 437-438
Tonsillectomy, 431
Total compliance, 8
Total lung capacity (TLC), 6
Toxemia, 302-318
　classification of, 304
　clinical courses in, 305-306
　fetus in, 306
　hematologic findings in, 306-307
　maternal death in, 306
　mechanism of, 305f
　pathophysiology of, 304-305
　postoperative management of, 317-318
　preoperative evaluation and preparation in, 307
Trachea, newborn, 184t
Tracheoesophageal atresia, 64-65
Tracheoesophageal fistula, 62-72
　antibiotics in, 67
　atresia vs, 64-65
　Calverley's classification of, 66
　diagnosis of, 63-64
　embryology of, 65
　fluid replacement in, 66-67
　gastrostomy in, 67
　intraoperative management in, 68-70
　intubation in, 68-69
　postoperative management of, 71-72
　premedication in, 67-68
　preoperative evaluation and preparation in, 65-68
　Waterston classification of, 66
Tracheostomy, 61
Transcapillary refill, 348
Transient ischemic attacks, 201
Transposition of great arteries
　corrected, 78
　embryology of, 77-78
　hypothermia for, 82-85
　intraoperative management of, 80-85
　most common form of, 78
　pathology in, 76-77
　postoperative management of, 85-87
　preoperative evaluation and preparation in, 79-80
　ventricular septal defect in, 79
Trauma, 392-407
　intraoperative management of, 400-406
　postoperative management of, 406-407
　preoperative evaluation and preparation in, 399-400
Treacher Collins syndrome, 426
Triiodothyronine (T_3), 224-225
Triple index, 96-97
Triple vessel coronary artery disease, 91
Trousseau's sign, 233

Tubal ligation, 333-334
d-Tubocurarine
　burns and, 390
　fetus and, 297
　renal failure and, 281
　reversal of, 420-421
　side effects of, 420
Tumor
　adrenocortical, 253-259
　brain, 189-199
　spinal cord, 208-212

Uterine blood flow, 316-317
Uterine contractility, 326
Uteroplacental circulation, 291

V_5 ECG lead, 100
Valvular heart disease, 125-136
　anesthetic management in, 133
　diagnosis in, 126-127
　intraoperative management of, 132-134
　muscle relaxant in, 134
　postoperative management of, 134-136
　postoperative ventilation in, 135-136
　premedication in, 132
　preoperative evaluation and preparation in, 129-132
　pulmonary edema in, 130-131
Varices, esophageal, 171-175
Vasopressors, 316-317
VATER, 65
V_D/V_T (dead space ventilation to tidal volume) ratio, 58
　equation and normal values for, 8-9
　morbid obesity and, 444
Velopharyngeal incompetence, 431
Venous admixture, 386
Venous oxygen content, 9
Ventilation/perfusion (V/Q) abnormality, 56
V/Q (ventilation/perfusion) abnormality, 56
Ventricular septal defect, 79
Vital capacity (V_C), 6
Volume expansion therapy, 398-399
Von Willebrand's disease, 341, 342t

Water intoxication, 268-269
Weight, normal, 442
Wheezing attack during surgery, 15-17

Zero end-expiratory pressure (ZEEP), 43